Optical Coherence Tomography of the Anterior Segment

Ludwig M. Heindl · Sebastian Siebelmann
Editors

Optical Coherence Tomography of the Anterior Segment

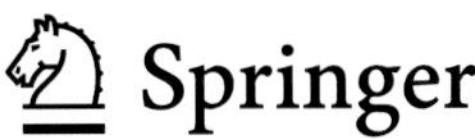 Springer

Editors
Ludwig M. Heindl
Department of Ophthalmology
University Hospital of Cologne
Cologne, Germany

Sebastian Siebelmann
Department of Ophthalmology
University Hospital of Cologne
Cologne, Germany

ISBN 978-3-031-07732-6   ISBN 978-3-031-07730-2   (eBook)
https://doi.org/10.1007/978-3-031-07730-2

This Springer imprint is published by the registered company Springer Nature Switzerland AG
The registered company address is: Gewerbestrasse 11, 6330 Cham, Switzerland

Preface

The introduction of Optical Coherence Tomography (OCT) in 1991 brought about enduring change in the field of ophthalmology. OCT technology uses light of invisible wavelengths and facilitates non-invasive and contact-free in vivo imaging of biological tissue and transparent non-biological materials of high, nearly histological, resolution. Especially the physiologically translucent structures of the eye, such as the cornea, anterior chamber, lens, and retina, are predisposed fields of use for the OCT. Nowadays at over 30 million annual clinical OCT examinations, ophthalmology is by far the largest specialty in which it is applied.

The OCT is the only procedure to date that enables separate visualization of the different layers of the retina. In combination with the introduction of antiangiogenic intravitreal treatments for exudative macular diseases, such as Age-Related Macular Degeneration (AMD), the OCT has revolutionized clinical diagnostics and therapeutic monitoring in retinology.

But shortly after the invention of the OCT, the first images of the anterior eye segment were published. This so-called Anterior Segment OCT (AS-OCT) has immense potential and provides important supplemental diagnostic information in diseases of the eyelid, conjunctiva, cornea, anterior chamber, iridocorneal angle, and the iris as well as the lens. The procedure is useful for early detection and treatment of diseases and monitoring therapeutic targets. However, AS-OCT is used in surgical preparation as well and recently also intraoperatively. In clinical practice, this patient-friendly procedure is already routinely utilized, as it currently has the highest resolution among the standard diagnostic tools in ophthalmology. The AS-OCT is therefore diagnostically an essential tool in any surgical eye clinic and its popularity is increasing among ophthalmologic practicians focusing on conservative treatment. Considering recent developments in automated image data analysis via artificial intelligence, the automatic evaluation of OCT image data might once again revolutionize ophthalmology entirely.

Currently available books on OCT focus solely or mainly on the posterior segment of the eye. In this book, however, we want to shed light on the utilization of OCT in the anterior chamber. It is the first book to clearly illustrate the most important conditions and applications of OCT in the anterior chamber with the help of several images. This guide intends to help with further education of ophthalmologists aiming to learn or improve in this highly relevant diagnostic procedure. It can also serve as a great reference guide for clinical findings of those already practicing AS-OCT. Furthermore, this book is intended to be of use to ophthalmologists in a preoperative, intraoperative, and postoperative setting.

Considering the optical coherence tomography to be applied ophthalmopathology, we hope this finds a broad readership and attains broad application for the benefit of all patients.

Cologne, Germany   Ludwig M. Heindl
January 2022   Sebastian Siebelmann

Contents

About the Editors

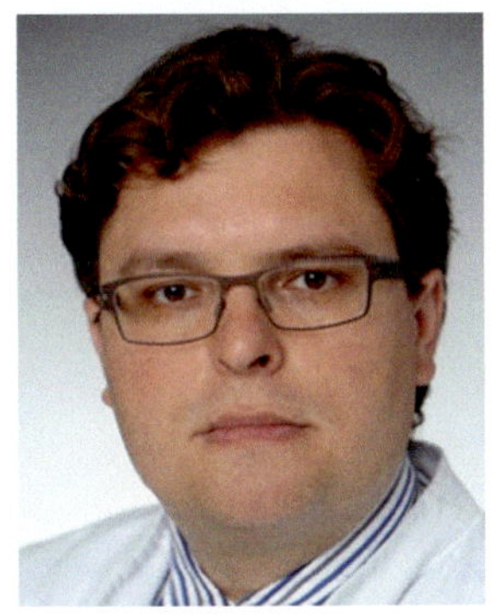

Ludwig M. Heindl Univ.-Prof. Dr. Dr. M.D., Ph.D., M.Sc. is a lifetime Professor at the Department of Ophthalmology at the University Hospital of Cologne, Germany. As the Director of the Clinic for ophthalmic oncology and ophthalmic plastic and reconstructive surgery, his clinical expertise is the diagnostics and treatment of diseases of the eyelid, lacrimal duct, orbit, and ocular surface as well as extraocular and intraocular tumors. He is the Director of the ophthalmic imaging and functional evaluation core and thus specialized in the most advanced high-resolution imaging of the eye. He is the author of more than 300 peer-reviewed publications in the most respected journals.

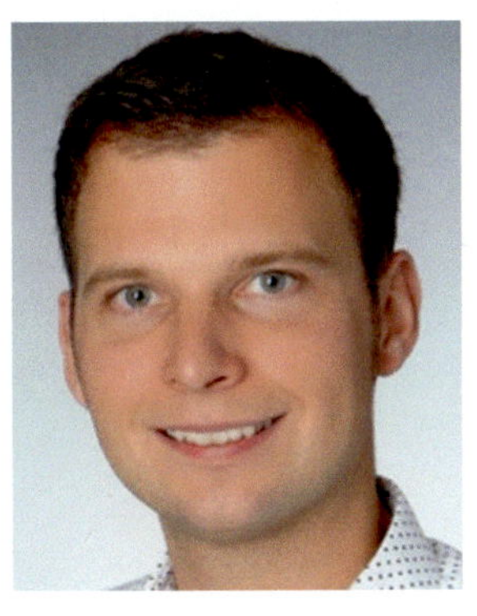

Sebastian Siebelmann, PD Dr. med. FEBO, MHBA is an Assistant Professor at the University Hospital of Cologne and Senior Physician in the field of corneal/refractive surgery at the Eye Center Erkelenz, Germany. His habilitation thesis was on the topic of intraoperative imaging via Optical Coherence Tomography (OCT) and his research now focuses on non-invasive OCT imaging for diagnostic purposes and the planning and postoperative evaluation of surgical procedures in the anterior segment. This research increasingly revolves around digital tools such as automated image recognition via artificial intelligence. Additionally, he is the Director of the research group "Digital Ophthalmology". He has meanwhile been given several national and international awards and in 2019 he was honored as Young Physician Leader, proposed by the Leopoldina National Academy of Sciences.

History and Future Prospects of Anterior Segment OCT

Jens Horstmann and Eva Lankenau

1 Introduction

Optical coherence tomography (OCT) is a non-invasive and non-contact method for imaging and measuring biological tissue and other partially transparent materials. In ophthalmology, OCT is mainly used in clinical diagnostics and therapy control, but also in research. In 1991, the method was published for the first time by the group around Prof. Fujimoto under the name OCT (optical coherence tomography) (Huang et al. 1991). Since then, hardly any other medical imaging technique has been established and disseminated more rapidly. To date, more than 10,000 patents have been granted for OCT and more than 45,000 publications have been written (https://worldwide.espacenet.com/patent/search?q=OpticalCoherenceTomography; https://pubmed.ncbi.nlm.nih.gov/?term=Optical+Coherence+Tomography).

The eye physiologically consists of light-transmitting optical elements such as the cornea, the lens, the aqueous humor and the retina. Therefore, since the development of OCT, it was obvious to look for application fields in the field of ophthalmology. To date, ophthalmology is by far the largest field of application of OCT worldwide, with currently 30 million clinical OCT examinations performed annually (Fujimoto and Swanson 2016).

OCT was the only technique capable of imaging the layers of the retina in vivo when it was first introduced and remains so today. It is possibly historically attributable to this particular novelty that a substantial part of the research, development and application was initially aimed at imaging the posterior segment of the eye. However, shortly after OCT was invented, the first images of the anterior segment

J. Horstmann (✉)
Departement of Ophthalmology, University Hospital of Cologne, Cologne, Germany
e-mail: jens.b.horstmann@gmail.com

E. Lankenau
University Modell-Augen-Manufaktur, Rondeshagen, Germany
e-mail: post@modell-augen-manufaktur.de

© The Author(s), under exclusive license to Springer Nature Switzerland AG 2022
L. M. Heindl and S. Siebelmann (eds.), *Optical Coherence Tomography of the Anterior Segment*, https://doi.org/10.1007/978-3-031-07730-2_1

(AS-OCT) were also published (Izatt et al. 1994) and the potential of OCT of the anterior segment was explored.

This chapter provides a descriptive overview of the most concise milestones of the historical development as well as the current status of AS-OCT and discusses current research and possible future prospects in the outlook. Underlying physical aspects and explanation of current technological concepts are presented in the second chapter "Physical principles of anterior segment OCT".

2   Profile and Nomenclature

As an optical imaging technique, OCT works with light - usually invisible infrared light. The light is targeted as a point on the surface of the tissue and penetrates several millimeters, depending on its nature. Different types of tissue can have different optical properties, so a part of the light is reflected or scattered at interfaces or in highly light-scattering tissue layers within. The part of the light that leaves the tissue against the direction of incidence is collected by the measuring apparatus and used for imaging. The detected light encodes the tissue depth from which it returns via its travel time - similar to the pulse-echo method in ultrasound imaging. Each partially reflecting layer of a specimen appears as a high peak in the OCT signal, while diffusely scattering layers appear in the OCT signal in varying strengths to very faint. Thus, the basic measurement in OCT is the one-dimensional measurement of the depth of all reflective layers and light-scattering structures below a point, such as on the tissue surface, to the maximum measurement depth. This one-dimensional measurement result is called an A-scan (amplitude-scan). For a depth sectional image, which is called a B-scan in OCT, the measurement results of laterally adjacent points are assembled one after the other column by column. For this purpose, the light beam is deflected laterally by a motorized mirror system within the OCT device. A volume scan can be assembled from several consecutive B-scans.

Time-domain OCT (TD-OCT) is the term used for the first generation of OCT systems, which plays a minor role today. Most clinical devices are currently based on the second generation, *spectral-domain OCT* (SD-OCT). Increasingly, *swept-source systems* (SS-OCT) are entering the market. The different technological concepts with their advantages and disadvantages are presented in the second chapter "Physical principles of anterior segment OCT".

3   The Origin of OCT

As described in the previous section, OCT is based on the measurement of the time of flight of light. Since light propagates much faster than (ultra-)sound, its direct time-of-flight measurement can only be achieved with a great technological effort.

In the 1970s, as part of developments for telecommunications, experiments were carried out at the *AT&T Bell Laboratories* in the USA to make the propagation time of light in a medium usable for measuring and imaging its interior. Using elaborate measurement techniques, it was possible for the first time to photographically detect light pulses in a specific propagation phase in the medium (Duguay 1971; Duguay and Mattick 1971). It was postulated that in this way it might also be possible to look inside tissue. A step in this direction was achieved in 1986 by Fujimoto and colleagues at the *Massachusetts Institute of Technology* in Cambridge, USA, by superimposing two light pulses, only one of which passes through the medium to be measured, while the other is reflected outside at a mirror (Fujimoto et al. 1986). After recombination of both pulses, the depth of reflective layers could be determined with a resolution of 15 µm (Fujimoto and Swanson 2016). However, the sensitivity of the method was not sufficient for measurements in highly light-scattering tissue and the equipment required for the method was considerable, so that alternative concepts were sought (Fujimoto and Swanson 2016).

Today, OCT can determine the time of flight of light indirectly by much simpler means. The next decisive step along the way was the implementation of white-light interferometry, the phenomena of which had already been described by Isaac Newton (1643–1727). White light interferometry is a non-contact optical measurement method that exploits the interference of broadband light (so-called white light), allowing 3D profile measurements of structures with resolutions down to a few micrometers. In the 1980s, again driven by developments in optical telecommunications, this method was rediscovered and exploited (Takada et al. 1987). By using white-light interferometry, the sensitivity of the time-of-flight measurement could be increased and the instrumental complexity significantly reduced, which turned out to be an important precursor for OCT.

In retrospect, technological developments in three unrelated areas outside the medical technology field have enabled the development of OCT.

1. Novel light sources

OCT requires light sources with an emission spectrum that is not too small and not too large. Developments in laser physics increasingly made this type of light source possible, even in the infrared range. One method of realizing an OCT light source could be, for example, a laser diode whose resonator was removed so that the light became spectrally more broadband. This so-called superluminescent diode (SLD) was developed by Gerard A. Alphonse at *Radio Corporation of America* (RCA Labs) in 1986 (IEEE 2020) and is a component of most *time-domain* and *spectral-domain devices*. More recent *swept-source OCT* has been made possible by the development of so-called tunable lasers, in which the emitted wavelength can be changed.

2. Computers

OCT requires computers for component control, sensor readout, signal processing, image display, image analysis, and data storage, among other tasks. The contemporary computing speed in the 1990s has been a limiting factor at the time of OCT development. Only with the development of more powerful computers was it possible to increase the measurement speed of OCT to such an extent that the first OCT medical products could be used around the turn of the millennium.

3. Fiber optic

The first OCT experiments took place on large optical tables on which the OCT light was guided in different directions via mirrors and beam splitters. These setups could not be integrated into a suitable medical device because they were extremely large and sensitive to adjustment. With the development of optical fiber technology for telecommunications, OCT systems could be made significantly smaller and less sensitive to adjustment (Fujimoto and Swanson 2016).

The following figure shows an early OCT setup from 1993 as well as a modern OCT system for outpatient diagnostics (Fig. 1).

The first published measurement of OCT was an A-scan representing the axial length of an eye (ex vivo) with a resolution of 10 μm (Fercher et al. 1988). The first B-scan of a retina (ex vivo) was published in 1991 (Huang et al. 1991), which is often considered the birth of OCT. The latter is shown in the following figure. In 1993, Swanson et al. published the first in vivo OCT image of a human retina (Swanson et al. 1993) (Fig. 2).

4 The Evolution of OCT Since Its Invention

The first OCT startup, *Advanced Optical Diagnostics* (AOD), was founded by Fujimoto, Puliafito, and Swanson in 1992 (Fujimoto and Swanson 2016). Two years later, AOD, along with working prototypes and basic patents, was purchased

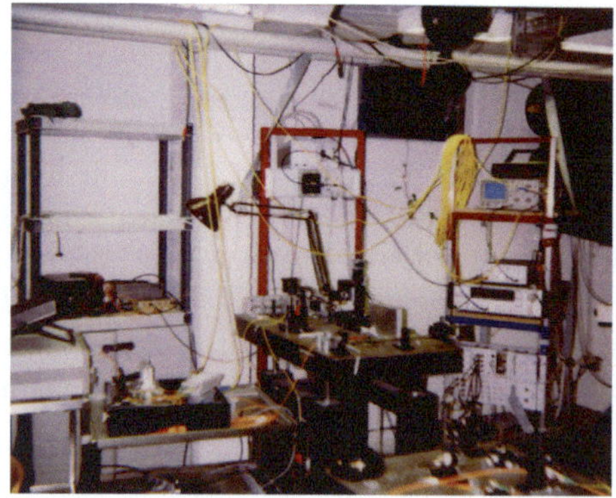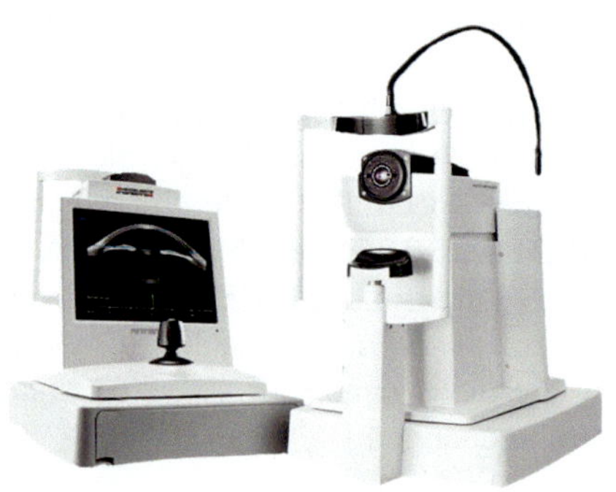

Fig. 1 OCT laboratory setup at the Lübeck Medical Laser Center from 1993 (left) and, for comparison, current OCT device *Anterion* from Heidelberg Engineering GmbH, Heidelberg, Germany (right)

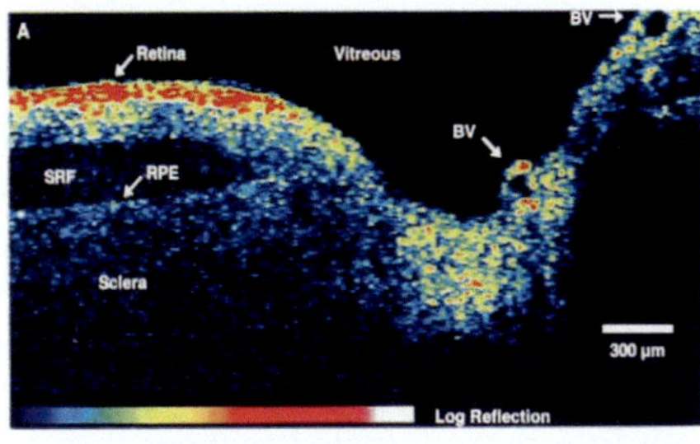

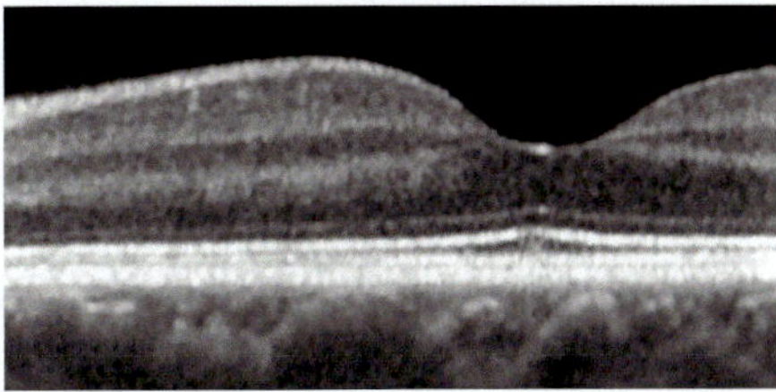

Fig. 2 First publication of an OCT image of the human retina (ex vivo) by Huang et al. from 1991 (Huang et al. 1991) and for comparison a contemporary image of a similar image section with a *Spectralis OCT* from Heidelberg Engineering GmbH (Heidelberg, Germany)

by *Humphrey Zeiss* (San Leandro, CA, USA). Another two years later, in 1996, *Zeiss* launched the first commercial OCT system (*OCT-1*). Since then, the main focus has been on acquisition speed, with the goal of keeping the overall duration of data collection as short as possible. Not only for convenience reasons: If the eye's own movements are "faster than the imaging" this can render images unusable. Especially elderly people and patients with eye diseases have problems to fixate a point for a longer time. The acquisition speed at the beginning was 100 A-scans per second, i.e. to acquire a cross-sectional image (B-scan) composed of 100 A-scans took one second.

In terms of the optical design, there is a significant difference between imaging the posterior or anterior segment of the eye. Due to the novelty of retinal imaging, a large part of the further development initially took place in the field of posterior segment OCT. Resolution is limited mainly by the imperfection of the crystalline lens and sensitivity is limited by the unwanted light absorption of the anterior segment and aqueous humor. Therefore, the anterior segment is basically easier accessible for OCT than the posterior segment (Hüttmann et al. 2009). However, for the anterior segment there were already methods available like ultrasound imaging, Scheimpflug imaging or confocal microscopy (Labbé et al. 2009; Swartz et al. 2007; Dada et al. 2007; Maldonado et al. 2006).

It took several years until the first OCT systems specifically designed for the anterior segment were commercialized (Izatt et al. 1994). The first *Anterior Segment OCT* device was launched by 4optics AG (Lübeck, Germany) in 2003 (Buchwald et al. 2003). Heidelberg Engineering GmbH (Heidelberg, Germany) acquired 4optics and commercialized the *Slitlamp OCT* for coupling to a *Haag-Streit* slit lamp in 2006. Meanwhile, the *Visante OCT* (Carl Zeiss Meditec, Dublin, CA, USA) appeared in 2005 as the first stand-alone device. The aforementioned devices were TD-OCT systems that were still relatively slow, with 2000 A-scans per second (*Visante*) and 200 A-scans per second (*SL-OCT*), respectively (Fujimoto and Swanson 2016). A quantum leap in speed with increases of up to three orders of magnitude was achieved with the realization of the second generation, so-called *spectral domain* (SD) OCT.

Since the first *SD-OCT* devices were developed for the posterior segment, an additional optical unit was necessary to make the anterior segment accessible for imaging. This initially limited the field of view considerably. One of the first commercialized devices of this type was the *RTView FD OCT* (Optovue, Fremont, CA, USA). The external anterior segment module provided a B-scan field of only 2 × 2 mm at full resolution. The first version of the *Cirrus HD-OCT* (Carl Zeiss Meditec, Dublin, USA) had an anterior segment-adapted field size of only 3 × 1 mm. Further developments of the *Cirrus OCT* have an internal switching optic, which can be adapted to the beam path in a more targeted manner than an external optic. The field of view of 15.5 × 5.8 mm is able to image the cornea completely ("angle-to-angle") including the underlying structures up to the part of the crystalline lens visible through the open iris. Similar performance is achieved by the current *Spectralis* (Heidelberg Engineering GmbH, Heidelberg, Germany) with a corresponding pre-switching module. Other current systems that can be converted to the anterior segment by means of a module are the *Copernicus HR* (Optopol, Technologies SA, Zawiercie, Poland) and the *Envisu* (Bioptigen Inc., USA, now part of Leica Microsystems, Wetzlar, Germany). The *Anterion* (Heidelberg Engineering GmbH, Heidelberg, Germany) is a system developed exclusively for the anterior segment. Due to the new technological concept of *swept-source OCT* (chapter "Physical Principles of Anterior Segment OCT"), this offers a very large imaging depth and even reaches beyond the complete crystalline lens to the surface of the retina for the purpose of axial length measurement. This makes it particularly suitable for cataract biometry, but also offers other quantitative measurements such as corneal topography and pachymetry.

5 The Evolution of the Clinical Acceptance of OCT

Around the turn of the millennium, the first approved OCT devices became available. In the same period first clinical studies on the efficacy of a new therapeutic approach for the treatment of age-related macular degeneration (AMD) in the exudative stage took place (E. S. 2002; Ng and Adamis 2005). It was shown that the efficacy of serial treatment with the so-called anti-vascular endothelial growth factor (VEGF) antibody was very good, but individually variable. Similarly, anti-VEGF antibody therapy is very costly, so individual monitoring of efficacy was essential. This monitoring was possible by observing the retinal structure using OCT and it played a crucial role in the clinical acceptance and dissemination of OCT (Fujimoto and Swanson 2016; Rosenfeld et al. 2005). With regular check-ups using OCT, it was possible in AMD treatment to check the efficacy of the therapy and thus to increase the success of the therapy on an individual basis (Cohen et al. 2007; Meyer et al. 2008; Pron 2014). At the same time, OCT saved costs in the health care system, since the expensive drug was only justified if the effect was good and the presence of retinal changes could be diagnosed much earlier, meaning a better outcome.

AMD monitoring certainly served as a kind of "door opener" for OCT in clinical routine, but other applications were quickly opened up. The novel possible in vivo imaging of the retina opened up the non-invasive diagnosis of highly relevant pathologies, such as macular edema or glaucoma by structural imaging and measurement (Puliafito et al. 1995; Schuman et al. 1995). Concerning the anterior segment, applications related to structural change were particularly considered (Kaluzny et al. 2006; Christopoulos et al. 2007; Ang et al. 2018). In 2010, the resolution of OCT images was sufficient to visualize and measure the individual layers of the cornea (Shousha et al. 2010; Sandali et al. 2013).

OCT has been used in the anterior segment of the eye, for example, for individual planning of corneal, cataract, and glaucoma surgery (Baikoff 2006; Haigis et al. 2000), for evaluation of tumor diseases (Buchwald et al. 2003; Failed 2016), pterygium (Nanji et al. 2015), corneal edema (Konstantopoulos et al. 2008), corneal injuries (Wylegala et al. 2009), and inflammatory diseases of the ocular surface such as dry eye disease (Yagci and Gurdal 2014). In differential diagnosis, OCT helped to distinguish corneal dystrophies according to the IC3D scheme (Siebelmann et al. 2018), as well as keratoconus (Fuentes et al. 2015). In the latter, OCT was shown to be at least equal to the well-established Scheimpflug imaging in monitoring progression and partly more sensitive in early detection by using epithelial thickness maps (Fujimoto et al. 2016). In research, it was discovered that the success of keratoconus treatment using corneal crosslinking was visible in the OCT image by a hyperreflective band representing the crosslinked stromal tissue (Doors et al. 2009). To date, combining treatment with monitoring by OCT is an important application and a standard clinical use of OCT. This includes photorefractive, photothermal, and photodynamic treatments (Ramos et al. 2009; Tarnawska and Wylegala 2010; Salinas-Alamán et al. 2005; Farhat et al. 2011; Lin et al. 2015; Gong et al. 2016; Koinzer et al. 2012; Wirbelauer and Pham 2004).

While OCT revolutionized diagnostic ophthalmology, ophthalmic surgery was based on the know-how of experienced surgeons who initially saw less benefit in OCT imaging during surgery. Parallel to the development of OCT for outpatient diagnostics, there were individual scientifically interested surgeons who modified OCT devices (Chavala et al. 2009; Dayani et al. 2009) or had special prototypes developed (Hüttmann et al. 2009) in such a way that they also allowed first OCT images in the operating room. For each image, however, the operation had to be interrupted and the surgical microscope had to be moved aside. For more acceptance in surgical ophthalmology, it was therefore required to integrate OCT into classic surgical microscopes in such a way that the intraoperative work flow was impaired as little as possible. In addition, intraoperative OCT, which was born in this way, could only be meaningfully realized with the newer and thus significantly faster OCT techniques. The first combinations of OCT with a surgical microscope were usefully implemented by Medizinisches Laserzentrum Lübeck GmbH (Lübeck, Germany) (Hüttmann et al. 2009; Geerling et al. 2005) and by Carl Zeiss Meditec AG (Jena, Germany) (Binder et al. 2010). In 2010, Optomedical Technologies GmbH, a company spin-off from the Medical Laser Center Lübeck, launched the first OCT fully integrated into a surgical microscope, the *Hi-R Neo*

900, from Haag-Streit Surgical (Wedel, Germany) as an approved medical device and coined the brand *iOCT* for intraoperative OCT (Lankenau et al. 2013; Mueller et al. 2010). In 2014, the company Carl Zeiss Meditec AG followed with the *Rescan 700* OCT integrated in its own *Lumera 700* surgical microscope, establishing intraoperative OCT in the market. Leica Microsystems followed in 2015, adapting the *EnFocus* OCT device developed by Bioptigen to the beam path of the Leica *Proveo 8* surgical microscope. Intraoperative OCT now allows surgeons to perform real-time, non-contact assessment of the different layers and structures in both the anterior and posterior segments of the eye at near histological resolution during surgery. In particular, OCT has benefited research in the development and monitoring of lamellar corneal transplantation techniques, and patients have been able to benefit from more targeted procedures (Steven et al. 2013; De Benito-Llopis et al. 2014; Siebelmann et al. 2015).

A clinically very useful mode of OCT imaging is in OCT angiography (OCT-A). As in many application areas, the posterior segment received initial attention. OCT-A provides vascular imaging of the retina, a clinically highly relevant feature that, unlike conventional angiography, does not rely on a contrast agent and is therefore non-invasive. During data collection for OCT-A, multiple B-scans are acquired sequentially at the same location and mathematically analyzed. This enables to visualize at which points in the image there have been changes over time, which also makes it possible to specifically depict blood flow in veins and arteries.

Usually, a volume of several hundred B-scans is visualized as a maximum intensity projection of the top view, which is similar in presentation to conventional angiography. However, it is also possible to isolate targeted vascular networks at specific depths (Spaide et al. 2015, Ishibazawa et al. 2015; Savastano et al. 2015). However, because OCT-A is a flow measurement, occluded vessels or leaks are not visible on OCT-A (Ang et al. 2016; Chua et al. 2019). Further disadvantageous is the susceptibility of OCT-A to motion artifacts, which is why a particularly high acquisition speed is mandatory. Among the established, commercialized, and approved OCT systems, the *swept-source* approach currently delivers the highest speeds. The *Plex Elite 9000* (Carl Zeiss Meditec, Dublin, CA, USA) measures at up to 200,000 A-scans per second, the *Spectralis* (Heidelberg Engineering GmbH, Heidelberg, Germany) at 85,000 A-scans per second, and the *Angiovue* (Optovue Inc., USA) at 70,000 A-scans per second. The *Plex Elite* and *Angiovue* offer OCT-A mode for the posterior and anterior segments of the eye; the *Angiovue* requires an additional optical lens. Clinically, AS-OCT-A is used primarily in the evaluation of iris and conjunctival vessels and pathologic corneal vessels (Ang et al. 2015; Roberts et al. 2017; Akagi et al. 2018).

6 Perspectives of Anterior Segment OCT

In the history and development of OCT, first the technology was invented and then application fields were sought, which made it difficult to establish in the beginning. A clinically highly relevant application had to be found first to really attract attention (Fujimoto and Swanson 2016). A better condition for development is often addressing "unmet needs" in the clinic, such as visualization of clinically invisible pathologic lymphatic vessels in the cornea (Horstmann et al. 2017) or the lack of depth resolution of conventional angiography (Spaide et al. 2015). However, the history of OCT impressively demonstrates that technological development has been mutually reinforcing with clinical and scientific testing and application (Fujimoto and Swanson 2016).

"Higher, faster, further"—this has been a credo in the development of OCT since its invention. The technologically most important parameters that can be optimized are, in addition to the image field size and the sensitivity, above all the acquisition speed and the resolution.

For in vivo measurements, the acquisition speed is significantly responsible for the image quality. This is especially true with respect to applications that go beyond purely structural imaging and require mathematical analyses of multiple consecutively acquired images, such as OCT angiography (Gorczynska et al. 2016). However, real-time imaging of image volumes (*4D-OCT*), which can be useful intraoperatively in microsurgery, for example, also relies on the highest acquisition rates (Zhang and Kang 2011).

Comparing the first clinically approved devices in the *time-domain* method with current devices in *spectral-domain* OCT, the speed of OCT has already increased approximately a thousandfold. Current systems in research, such as the *swept-source* method with particularly fast light sources (so-called FDML lasers, (Klein et al. 2013; Kolb et al. 2015)) or *full-field* OCT, which simultaneously acquires the entire image field instead of raster-scanning, are even faster by orders of magnitude (Hillmann et al. 2016). The methods are explained in more detail in the second chapter.

At speeds in the MHz range, the acquisition of two points occurs practically simultaneously, because within a few nanoseconds there is hardly any influential movement of the tissue itself. Due to the stable phase references, not only purely computational image enhancements are possible following data acquisition, as previously only possible with the aid of complex adaptive optics, but also special evaluations such as the visualization and measurement of pulse wave function in individual blood vessels or the physiological response of retinal nerve cell tissue to photostimulation (Hillmann et al. 2016; Spahr et al. 2015, 2018). The examples listed show that incremental technological progress can extend the structural imaging of OCT to include functional aspects and thus make it more specific.

OCT imaging is often criticized for being a purely morphological method that can depict structures but cannot methodically distinguish between specific structures. Especially with increasing resolution of the new OCT technologies, which allow a resolution down to the cellular level, it would be desirable to be able to specifically identify these cellular or even molecular structures (e.g. T-cells vs. B-cells). One approach to increase the specificity of the imaged structures by OCT is the use of nanoparticles, which are applied systemically or topically as contrast agents prior to imaging. Coupled to antibodies, they dock specifically to certain cell types and accumulate locally, for example in the case of inflammation or neovascularization. Since the particles with a size of a few 10 nm are invisible for OCT, external excitation of the particles in the tissue, e.g., by means of infrared radiation (photothermal OCT) or a magnetic field (magnetomotive OCT), is necessary for contrasting (Gordon et al. 2019; Oldenburg et al. 2005).

The general resolution of OCT imaging represents a further adjustment screw in order to be able to assign the structures thus depicted more specifically. Today's clinical devices achieve an axial resolution in the range of about 5 µm (Kiernan et al. 2010; Kanclerz 2019). This is not yet sufficient for imaging at the cellular level. However, microscopic OCT (mOCT) represents a particularly high-resolution approach, using a broadband light source for particularly high axial resolution and microscope optics for particularly high lateral resolution. Thus, resolutions below 1 µm are possible, with which, for example, flowing cells in a pathologic corneal blood vessel can be morphologically differentiated or clinically invisible pathologic corneal lymphatic vessels can be visualized (Horstmann et al. 2017). Corneal nerves can also be visualized (Shin et al. 2017).

Specificity in OCT imaging can identify biomarkers for diseases that enable early diagnosis. In this context, imaging performed on the basis of the eyes is not limited to the detection of ophthalmological diseases. Studies show that systemic diseases such as diabetes or Alzheimer's disease, diseases of the central nervous system and other neurodegenerative pathologies can also be detected by OCT imaging of the retina, in some cases even before the onset of clinical symptoms, and can thus be treated at an early stage (Knier et al. 2016; DeBuc and Somfai 2010; Sugimoto et al. 2005; Ascaso et al. 2014; He et al. 2012).

For diagnostics, reliable, objective and effective evaluation is just as important as optimal image quality. Disease-specific automatic measurements are already integrated in the system's operating software by many manufacturers (Garvin et al. 2008; Jahromi et al. 2014). In OCT angiography, the analysis and quantification of three-dimensional data play a crucial role for its use (Spaide et al. 2018; Jia et al. 2014).

Artificial intelligence is also finding its way into OCT (Hogarty et al. 2019; Lee et al. 2017; Treder et al. 2018). As in many other areas of life, methods such as *deep learning* will probably also play an important role in the data evaluation of OCT images in the future, e.g., in automated diagnostics and progress monitoring. In this context, hospital networks or secure cloud databases are already used to exchange image data between different practitioners or between the outpatient and surgical areas.

Further developments in OCT will continue to serve physicians, scientists and patients in the future and not only in ophthalmology. In the diagnostic field, in addition to the constant incremental progress, work is being done on telemedical concepts with the home use of simplified systems. Especially in the case of age-related eye diseases with necessary regular screenings, this can prospectively be relieving for patients as well as for practices and clinics, whereby diagnostics can even be improved by even closer monitoring (Koch et al. 2018; Miller and Fortun 2018). Classically interventional intraoperative OCT systems are being developed with regard to even better and faster imaging, automated real-time evaluation, and augmented reality overlays (Roodaki et al. 2015; Cahill and Mortensen 2010; Wieser et al. 2014). In special interventions such as microsurgery or laser surgery, OCT can make treatment more targeted, gentle, and safe, e.g., in robot-assisted interventions (Ourak et al. 2019; Garc-Vázquez et al. 2018; Borghesan et al. 2018), or enable individually better treatment outcomes through automated dosimetry and intervention monitoring (Katta et al. 2019; Wang et al. 2017; Kaufmann et al. 2018). OCT is even present in space: On the ISS there is a device for monitoring possible complications of astronauts' eyes caused by weightlessness (SPECTRALIS 2020).

The clinical development and use of the full potential is currently hindered by the fact that innovative approaches with physically feasible performance have not yet been commercialized, since their clinical translation is inhibited by high equipment requirements and costs as well as regulatory hurdles in the approval process.

In summary, OCT has revolutionized ophthalmology within a quarter of a century. With the help of OCT, eye diseases could be better visualized and understood and thus new therapies could be developed. In the future, combinations of OCT with other diagnostic and therapeutic procedures will continue to protect patients' vision.

References

Akagi T, et al. Conjunctival and intrascleral vasculatures assessed using anterior segment optical coherence tomography angiography in normal eyes. Am J Ophthalmol. 2018;196:1–9.

Ang M, et al. Optical coherence tomography angiography for anterior segment vasculature imaging. Ophthalmology. 2015;122(9):1740–7.

Ang M, et al. Optical coherence tomography angiography and indocyanine green angiography for corneal vascularization. Br J Ophthalmol. 2016;100(11):1557–63.

Ang M, et al. Anterior segment optical coherence tomography. Prog Retin Eye Res. 2018;66:132–56.

Ascaso FJ, et al. Retinal alterations in mild cognitive impairment and Alzheimer's disease: an optical coherence tomography study. J Neurol. 2014;261(8):1522–30.

Baikoff G. Anterior segment OCT and phakic intraocular lenses: a perspective. J Cataract Refract Surg. 2006;32(11):1827–35.

Binder S, Falkner-Radler CI, Hauger C, Matz H, Glittenberg CG. Clinical applications of intrasurgical SD-optical coherence tomography. Invest Ophthalmol Vis Sci. 2010;51(13):268.

Borghesan G, et al. Single scan oct-based retina detection for robot-assisted retinal vein cannulation. J Med Robot Res. 2018;3(02):1840005.

Buchwald H-J, Müller A, Kampmeier J, Lang GK. Optical coherence tomography versus ultrasound biomicroscopy of conjunctival and eyelid lesions. Clin Monbl Ophthalmolog. 2003;220(12):822–9.

Cahill RA, Mortensen NJ. Intraoperative augmented reality for laparoscopic colorectal surgery by intraoperative near-infrared fluorescence imaging and optical coherence tomography. Minerva Chir. 2010;65(4):451–62.

Chavala SH, Farsiu S, Maldonado R, Wallace DK, Freedman SF, Toth CA. Insights into advanced retinopathy of prematurity using handheld spectral domain optical coherence tomography imaging. Ophthalmology. 2009;116(12):2448–56.

Christopoulos V, et al. In vivo corneal high-speed, ultra-high-resolution optical coherence tomography. Arch Ophthalmol. 2007;125(8):1027–35.

Chua J, et al. Future clinical applicability of optical coherence tomography angiography. Clin Exp Optom. 2019;102(3):260–9.

Cohen SY, et al. Monitoring anti-VEGF drugs for treatment of exudative AMD. J Fr Ophtalmol. 2007;30(4):330–4.

Dada T, Sihota R, Gadia R, Aggarwal A, Mandal S, Gupta V. Comparison of anterior segment optical coherence tomography and ultrasound biomicroscopy for assessment of the anterior segment. J Cataract Refract Surg. 2007;33(5):837–40.

Dayani PN, Maldonado R, Farsiu S, Toth CA. Intraoperative use of handheld spectral domain optical coherence tomography imaging in macular surgery. Retina. 2009;29(10):1457.

De Benito-Llopis L, Mehta JS, Angunawela RI, Ang M, Tan DTH. Intraoperative anterior segment optical coherence tomography: a novel assessment tool during deep anterior lamellar keratoplasty. Am J Ophthalmol. 2014;157(2):334–41.

DeBuc DC, Somfai GM. Early detection of retinal thickness changes in diabetes using optical coherence tomography. Med Sci Monit. 2010;16(3):MT15–MT21.

Doors M, Tahzib NG, Eggink FA, Berendschot TTJM, Webers CAB, Nuijts RMMA. Use of anterior segment optical coherence tomography to study corneal changes after collagen cross-linking. Am J Ophthalmol. 2009;148(6):844–51.

Duguay MA. Light photographed in flight: ultrahigh-speed photographic techniques now give us a portrait of light in flight as it passes through a scattering medium. Am Sci. 1971;59(5):550–6.

Duguay MA, Mattick AT. Ultrahigh speed photography of picosecond light pulses and echoes. Appl Opt. 1971;10(9):2162–70.

European Patent Office. https://worldwide.espacenet.com/patent/search?q=OpticalCoherenceTomography. Accessed 19 May 2020.

E.S. Group and others. Preclinical and phase 1A clinical evaluation of an anti-VEGF pegylated aptamer (EYE001) for the treatment of exudative age-related macular degeneration. Retina. 2002;22(2):143–152.

Farhat G, Czarnota GJ, Kolios MC, Yang VXD. Detecting cell death with optical coherence tomography and envelope statistics. J Biomed Opt. 2011;16(2):26017.

Fercher AF, Mengedoht K, Werner W. Eye-length measurement by interferometry with partially coherent light. Opt Lett. 1988;13(3):186–8.

Fuentes E, et al. Anatomic predictive factors of acute corneal hydrops in keratoconus: an optical coherence tomography study. Ophthalmology. 2015;122(8):1653–9.

Fujimoto JG, De Silvestri S, Ippen EP, Puliafito CA, Margolis R, Oseroff A. Femtosecond optical ranging in biological systems. Opt Lett. 1986;11(3):150–2.

Fujimoto J, Swanson E. The development, commercialization, and impact of optical coherence tomography history of optical coherence tomography. Invest Ophthalmol Vis Sci. 2016;57(9):OCT1–OCT13.

Fujimoto H, et al. Quantitative evaluation of the natural progression of keratoconus using three-dimensional optical coherence tomography. Invest Ophthalmol Vis Sci. 2016;57(9):OCT169–OCT175.

Garc-Vázquez V, et al. Navigation and visualization with HoloLens in endovascular aortic repair. Innov Surg Sci. 2018;3(3):167–77.

Garvin MK, Abràmoff MD, Kardon R, Russell SR, Wu X, Sonka M. Intraretinal layer segmentation of macular optical coherence tomography images using optimal 3-D graph search. IEEE Trans Med Imaging. 2008;27(10):1495–505.

Geerling G, et al. Intraoperative 2-dimensional optical coherence tomography as a new tool for anterior segment surgery. Arch Ophthalmol. 2005;123(2):253–7.

Gong P, et al. Optical coherence tomography for longitudinal monitoring of vasculature in scars treated with laser fractionation. J Biophotonics. 2016;9(6):626–36.

Gorczynska L, Migacz JV, Jonnal RS, Zawadzki RJ, Werner JS. Influence of speed and resolution on OCT angiography and Doppler OCT imaging in human retinal and choroidal capillary systems. In: IEEE photonics conference (IPC). 2016;2016:140–1.

Gordon AY, Lapierre-Landry M, Skala MC, Penn JS. Photothermal optical coherence tomography of anti-angiogenic treatment in the mouse retina using gold nanorods as contrast agents. Transl vis Sci Technol. 2019;8(3):18.

Haigis W, Lege B, Miller N, Schneider B. Comparison of immersion ultrasound biometry and partial coherence interferometry for intraocular lens calculation according to Haigis. Graefe's Arch Clin Exp Ophthalmol. 2000;238(9):765–73.

He X-F, Liu Y-T, Peng C, Zhang F, Zhuang S, Zhang J-S. Optical coherence tomography assessed retinal nerve fiber layer thickness in patients with Alzheimer's disease: a meta-analysis. Int J Ophthalmol. 2012;5(3):401.

Hillmann D, Spahr H, Pfäffle C, Sudkamp H, Franke G, Hüttmann G. In vivo optical imaging of physiological responses to photostimulation in human photoreceptors. Proc Natl Acad Sci. 2016;113(46):13138–43.

Hogarty DT, Mackey DA, Hewitt AW. Current state and future prospects of artificial intelligence in ophthalmology: a review. Clin Experiment Ophthalmol. 2019;47(1):128–39.

Horstmann J, et al. Label-free in vivo imaging of corneal lymphatic vessels using microscopic optical coherence tomography. Invest Ophthalmol vis Sci. 2017;58(13):5880–6.

Huang D et al. Optical coherence tomography. Science. 1991;254(5035):1178–1181.

Hüttmann G, Lankenau E, Schulz-Wackerbarth C, Müller M, Steven P, Birngruber R. Overview of apparative developments in optical coherence tomography: from imaging the retina to supporting therapeutic interventions. Klin Monbl Ophthalmolog. 2009;226(12):958–64.

IEEE. https://web.archive.org/web/20131213191449/http://www.ieeeusa.org/volunteers/presidents/alphonse.asp. Accessed 27 May 2020.

Ishibazawa A, et al. Optical coherence tomography angiography in diabetic retinopathy: a prospective pilot study. Am J Ophthalmol. 2015;160(1):35–44.

Izatt JA, et al. Micrometer-scale resolution imaging of the anterior eye in vivo with optical coherence tomography. Arch Ophthalmol. 1994;112(12):1584–9.

Jahromi MK, et al. An automatic algorithm for segmentation of the boundaries of corneal layers in optical coherence tomography images using gaussian mixture model. J Med Signals Sens. 2014;4(3):171.

Jia Y, et al. Quantitative optical coherence tomography angiography of choroidal neovascularization in age-related macular degeneration. Ophthalmology. 2014;121(7):1435–44.

Kaluzny BJ, et al. Spectral optical coherence tomography: a novel technique for cornea imaging. Cornea. 2006;25(8):960–5.

Kanclerz P. Optical biometry in a commercially available anterior and posterior segment optical coherence tomography device. Clin Exp Optom. 2019.

Katta N, et al. Laser brain cancer surgery in a xenograft model guided by optical coherence tomography. Theranostics. 2019;9(12):3555.

Kaufmann D, et al. Selective retina therapy enhanced with optical coherence tomography for dosimetry control and monitoring: a proof of concept study. Biomed Opt Express. 2018;9(7):3320–34.

Kiernan DF, Mieler WF, Hariprasad SM. Spectral-domain optical coherence tomography: a comparison of modern high-resolution retinal imaging systems. Am J Ophthalmol. 2010;149(1):18–31.

Klein T, Wieser W, Reznicek L, Neubauer A, Kampik A, Huber R. Multi-MHz retinal OCT. Biomed Opt Express. 2013;4(10):1890–908.

Knier B, et al. Optical coherence tomography indicates disease activity prior to clinical onset of central nervous system demyelination. Mult Scler J. 2016;22(7):893–900.

Koch P, et al. A compact off-axis full-field time-domain OCT device for home-care applications. Invest Ophthalmol vis Sci. 2018;59(9):1440.

Koinzer S, et al. Correlation of temperature rise and optical coherence tomography characteristics in patient retinal photocoagulation. J Biophotonics. 2012;5(11–12):889–902.

Kolb JP, Klein T, Kufner CL, Wieser W, Neubauer AS, Huber R. Ultra-widefield retinal MHz-OCT imaging with up to 100 degrees viewing angle. Biomed Opt Express. 2015;6 (5):1534–52.

Konstantopoulos A, Kuo J, Anderson D, Hossain P. Assessment of the use of anterior segment optical coherence tomography in microbial keratitis. Am J Ophthalmol. 2008;146(4):534–42.

Labbé A, Niaudet P, Loirat C, Charbit M, Guest G, Baudouin C. In vivo confocal microscopy and anterior segment optical coherence tomography analysis of the cornea in nephropathic cystinosis. Ophthalmology. 2009;116(5):870–6.

Lankenau EM, Krug M, Oelckers S, Schrage N, Just T, Hüttmann G. iOCT with surgical microscopes: a new imaging during microsurgery. Adv Opt Technol. 2013;2(3):233–9.

Lee CS, Tyring AJ, Deruyter NP, Wu Y, Rokem A, Lee AY. Deep-learning based, automated segmentation of macular edema in optical coherence tomography. Biomed Opt Express. 2017;8 (7):3440–8.

Lin T, Gong L, Liu X, Ma X. Fourier-domain optical coherence tomography for monitoring the lower tear meniscus in dry eye after acupuncture treatment. Evidence-Based Complement Altern Med. 2015;2015.

Maldonado MJ, Nieto JC, D\\iez-Cuenca M, Piñero DP. Repeatability and reproducibility of posterior corneal curvature measurements by combined scanning-slit and placido-disc topography after LASIK. Ophthalmology. 2006;113(11):1918–1926.

Meyer CH, Helb HM, Eter N. Monitoring of AMD patients on anti-vascular endothelial growth factor (VEGF) treatment. Practical notes on functional and anatomical examination parameters from drug approval studies, specialist information and case series. Der Ophthalmol J Dtsch Ophthalmol Gesellschaft. 2008;105(2):125–138.

Miller KP, Fortun JA. Home monitoring for age-related macular degeneration. Curr Ophthalmol Rep. 2018;6(1):53–7.

Mueller M, et al. Intraoperative OCT (iOCT) for Anterior and Posterior Segment Surgery. Invest Ophthalmol Vis Sci. 2010;51(13):5817.

Nanji AA, Sayyad FE, Galor A, Dubovy S, Karp CL. High-resolution optical coherence tomography as an adjunctive tool in the diagnosis of corneal and conjunctival pathology. Ocul Surf. 2015;13(3):226–35.

Ng EWM, Adamis AP. Targeting angiogenesis, the underlying disorder in neovascular age-related macular degeneration. Can J Ophthalmol. 2005;40(3):352–68.

Oldenburg A, Toublan F, Suslick K, Wei A, Boppart S. Magnetomotive contrast for in vivo optical coherence tomography. Opt Express. 2005;13(17):6597–614.

Ong SS, Vora GK, Gupta PK. Anterior segment imaging in ocular surface squamous neoplasia. J Ophthalmol. 2016;2016.

Ourak M, et al. Combined oct distance and fbg force sensing cannulation needle for retinal vein cannulation: in vivo animal validation. Int J Comput Assist Radiol Surg. 2019;14(2):301–9.

Pron G. Optical coherence tomography monitoring strategies for A-VEGF-treated age-related macular degeneration: an evidence-based analysis. Ont Health Technol Assess Ser. 2014;14 (10):1.

Puliafito CA, et al. Imaging of macular diseases with optical coherence tomography. Ophthalmology. 1995;102(2):217–29.

Pubmed. https://pubmed.ncbi.nlm.nih.gov/?term=Optical+Coherence+Tomography Accessed 19 May 2020.

Ramos JLB, Li Y, Huang D. Clinical and research applications of anterior segment optical coherence tomography–a review. Clin Experiment Ophthalmol. 2009;37(1):81–9.

Roberts PK, Goldstein DA, Fawzi AA. Anterior segment optical coherence tomography angiography for identification of iris vasculature and staging of iris neovascularization: a pilot study. Curr Eye Res. 2017;42(8):1136–42.

Roodaki H, Filippatos K, Eslami A, Navab N. Introducing augmented reality to optical coherence tomography in ophthalmic microsurgery. In: IEEE international symposium on mixed and augmented reality, vol 2015. 2015. p 1–6.

Rosenfeld PJ, Moshfeghi AA, Puliafito CA. Optical coherence tomography findings after an intravitreal injection of bevacizumab (Avastin®) for neovascular age-related macular degeneration. Ophthalmic Surgery Lasers Imaging Retin. 2005;36(4):331–5.

Salinas-Alamán A, Garc\\ia-Layana A, Maldonado MJ, Sainz-Gómez C, Alvárez-Vidal A. Using optical coherence tomography to monitor photodynamic therapy in age-related macular degeneration. Am J Ophthalmol. 2005;140(1):23–e1.

Sandali O, et al. Fourier-domain optical coherence tomography imaging in keratoconus: a corneal structural classification. Ophthalmology. 2013;120(12):2403–12.

Savastano MC, Lumbroso B, Rispoli M. In vivo characterization of retinal vascularization morphology using optical coherence tomography angiography. Retina. 2015;35(11):2196–203.

Schuman JS, et al. Optical coherence tomography: a new tool for glaucoma diagnosis. Curr Opin Ophthalmol. 1995;6(2):89–95.

Shin JG, Hwang HS, Eom TJ, Lee BH. In vivo three-dimensional imaging of human corneal nerves using Fourier-domain optical coherence tomography. J Biomed Opt. 2017;22(1):10501.

Shousha MA, et al. Use of ultra-high-resolution optical coherence tomography to detect in vivo characteristics of Descemet's membrane in Fuchs' dystrophy. Ophthalmology. 2010;117 (6):1220–7.

Siebelmann S, Steven P, Cursiefen C. Intraoperative optical coherence tomography: ocular surgery on a higher level or just nice pictures? JAMA Ophthalmol. 2015;133(10):1133–4.

Siebelmann S, et al. Anterior segment optical coherence tomography for the diagnosis of corneal dystrophies according to the IC3D classification. Surv Ophthalmol. 2018;63(3):365–80.

Spahr H, Pfäffle C, Koch P, Sudkamp H, Hüttmann G, Hillmann D. Interferometric detection of 3D motion using computational subapertures in optical coherence tomography. Opt Express. 2018;26(15):18803–16.

Spahr H, Hillman D, Hain C, Sudkamp HM, Franke GL, Huttmann G. Numerical aberration correction in optical coherence tomography and holoscopy by optimization of image quality. Proc SPIE. 2015;9312:93123B.

Spaide RF, Klancnik JM, Cooney MJ. Retinal vascular layers imaged by fluorescein angiography and optical coherence tomography angiography. JAMA Ophthalmol. 2015;133(1):45–50.

Spaide RF, Fujimoto JG, Waheed NK, Sadda SR, Staurenghi G. Optical coherence tomography angiography. Prog Retin Eye Res. 2018;64:1–55.

SPECTRALIS OCT2 module from Heidelberg Engineering on its way to the International Space Station. https://www.heidelbergengineering.com/de/pressemitteilungen/spectralis-oct2-modul-von-heidelberg-engineering-auf-dem-weg-zur-internationalen-raumstation/. Accessed 29 Nov 2020.

Steven P, et al. Optimizing descemet membrane endothelial keratoplasty using intraoperative optical coherence tomography. JAMA Ophthalmol. 2013;131(9):1135–42.

Sugimoto M, Sasoh M, Ido M, Wakitani Y, Takahashi C, Uji Y. Detection of early diabetic change with optical coherence tomography in type 2 diabetes mellitus patients without retinopathy. Ophthalmologica. 2005;219(6):379–85.

Swanson EA, et al. In vivo retinal imaging by optical coherence tomography. Opt Lett. 1993;18 (21):1864–6.

Swartz T, Marten L, Wang M. Measuring the cornea: the latest developments in corneal topography. Curr Opin Ophthalmol. 2007;18(4):325–33.

Takada K, Yokohama I, Chida K, Noda J. New measurement system for fault location in optical waveguide devices based on an interferometric technique. Appl Opt. 1987;26(9):1603–6.

Tarnawska D, Wylegala E. Monitoring cornea and graft morphometric dynamics after descemet stripping and endothelial keratoplasty with anterior segment optical coherence tomography. Cornea. 2010;29(3):272–7.

Treder M, Lauermann JL, Eter N. Automated detection of exudative age-related macular degeneration in spectral domain optical coherence tomography using deep learning. Graefe's Arch Clin Exp Ophthalmol. 2018;256(2):259–65.

Wang L, Jiang L, Hallahan K, Al-Mohtaseb ZN, Koch DD. Evaluation of femtosecond laser intrastromal incision location using optical coherence tomography. Ophthalmology. 2017;124 (8):1120–5.

Wieser W, Draxinger W, Klein T, Karpf S, Pfeiffer T, Huber R. High definition live 3D-OCT in vivo: design and evaluation of a 4D OCT engine with 1 GVoxel/s. Biomed Opt Express. 2014;5(9):2963–77.

Wirbelauer C, Pham DT. Continuous monitoring of corneal thickness changes during LASIK with online optical coherence pachymetry. J Cataract Refract Surg. 2004;30(12):2559–68.

Wylegala E, Dobrowolski D, Nowińska A, Tarnawska D. Anterior segment optical coherence tomography in eye injuries. Graefe's Arch Clin Exp Ophthalmol. 2009;247(4):451–5.

Yagci A, Gurdal C. The role and treatment of inflammation in dry eye disease. Int Ophthalmol. 2014;34(6):1291–301.

Zhang K, Kang JU. Real-time intraoperative 4D full-range FD-OCT based on the dual graphics processing units architecture for microsurgery guidance. Biomed Opt Express. 2011;2(4):764–70.

Physical Principles of Anterior Segment OCT

Jens Horstmann and Eva Lankenau

1 Introduction

In this chapter, the underlying physical and technological concepts for optical coherence tomography (OCT) are highlighted. The goal is to clearly convey the key ideas and their fundamentals, which should contribute to a better understanding of OCT images.

As an optical imaging technique, OCT works with light. Various models are used in the physical description of optical phenomena, including the wave and particle models. The most important aspects of optical metrology for OCT are best described in wave-optical terms. Beyond metrology, it is advantageous to also understand fundamental processes of light-tissue interaction, as these shape the appearance of OCT images and the possibilities and limitations of OCT imaging are also determined by tissue-optical aspects. The underlying phenomena are often described in terms of particle optics.

The original version of this chapter was revised: Figures 1, 3, 4, 5, 6, 8, 9, 10, 11, 12, 13, 14, 15, 16 have been replaced, then section 6.2 and figure 16 have been deleted. The correction to the chapter is available at https://doi.org/10.1007/978-3-031-07730-2_14

J. Horstmann (✉)
Zentrum für Augenheilkunde, Uniklinik Köln, Köln, Germany
e-mail: jens.b.horstmann@gmail.com

E. Lankenau
Modell-Augen-Manufaktur, Rondeshagen, Germany
e-mail: post@modell-augen-manufaktur.de

L. M. Heindl and S. Siebelmann (eds.), *Optical Coherence Tomography of the Anterior Segment*, https://doi.org/10.1007/978-3-031-07730-2_2

2 Particle Optical Aspects: Light Propagation in Tissue

The basic assumption of particle optics is that light consists of tiny, massless particles called photons or quanta (Pfeiler 2016). Each photon has a discrete energy; therefore, a given intensity of light causes a given number of photons. The propagation of photons in biological tissue is subject to various influences. For example, a disturbance in propagation can be the collision of a photon with microscopic matter such as cell nuclei and cell membranes. The consequences of this vary and depend in detail on the exact nature of the photon and its obstacle, as well as the collision geometry. The most important particle-optical phenomenon for OCT is light scattering, which affects the propagation direction of a photon. Furthermore, however, it can also be absorbed by the obstacle, making it unavailable for OCT imaging. With regard to absorption, it should be noted that photon energy is transferred to the absorber (e.g., the tissue cell) and converted into thermal energy (Wang and Wu 2012). To ensure that the tissue is not thermally damaged in the process, there are strict guidelines on the maximum permissible irradiation (MPE), without compliance with which a device cannot be approved under the *Medical Device Regulation* (MDR), the EU regulation on medical devices.

Only photons that leave the tissue exactly against the direction of incidence can be used for OCT. The reason for this is that OCT uses the same optics for irradiation and detection. Figure 1 shows various scenarios relevant to OCT that can arise after a photon enters matter. Path A represents the direct absorption of a photon by a molecule inside. In path B, the photon is first scattered several times before being absorbed. In both cases, it can no longer contribute to imaging by OCT. The paths of detectable photons are shown in paths C to E. Path C depicts direct reflection (i.e., *backscattering*) at the surface. Path D also shows direct backscattering, only deeper in the matter. Paths C and D describe the significant portion of photons contributing to the OCT image. In strongly light-scattering tissue, a photon can also change its direction very frequently before randomly leaving the matter again against the direction of propagation (path E). These multiple-scattered photons can interfere with the OCT image, but this plays only a minor role in ophthalmic OCT imaging. A photon can also leave matter in a different direction after multiple random scattering, after which it is no longer usable by OCT (path F). Since only those few photons that are directly backscattered (paths C and D) are useful for OCT, most of the incident light is lost. Therefore, OCT devices require very high sensitivity and dynamic range in terms of measurement.

The penetration depth of light into tissue is limited by light absorption and light scattering. In the wavelength range of the so-called optical window from 700 to 1400 nm, the penetration depth is particularly high, since the light absorption of water is relatively low here (Shi and Alfano 2017). For shorter wavelengths in the diagnostic window, light absorption is somewhat lower than for longer wavelengths (Kodach et al. 2010). Therefore, central wavelengths around 840 nm are more commonly used for posterior segment OCT applications. For applications in the anterior segment of the eye, less aqueous humor needs to be penetrated.

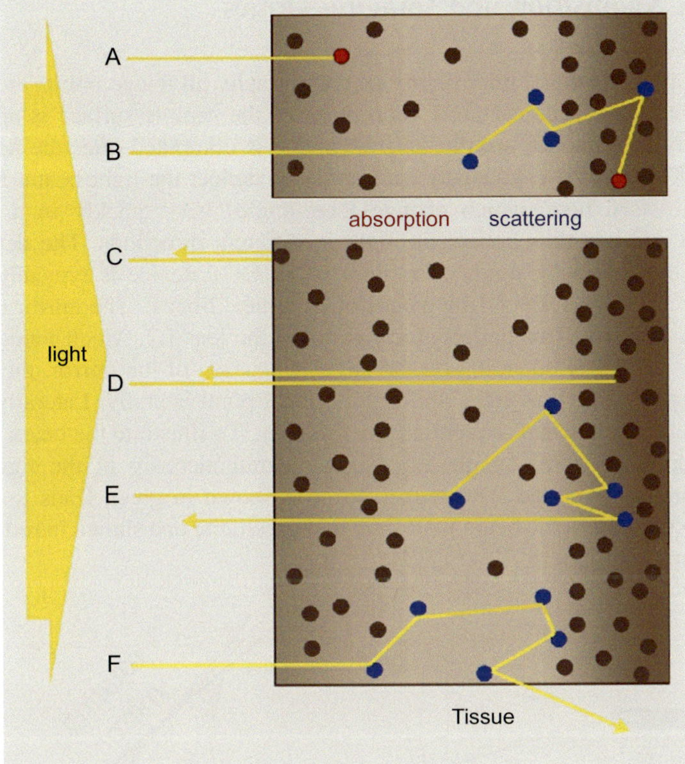

Fig. 1 Different photon paths are shown in yellow, light-absorbing structures in red, light-scattering ones in blue. Since tissue structures are inhomogeneous, the density varies in the figure of the points. Photon paths: **A** Absorption, **B** Absorption after multiple scattering, **C** Reflection at the surface, **D** backscattering at a tissue structure, **E** diffuse multiple scattering with final Backscatter into the detection optics, **F** Diffuse multiple scattering finally in another direction (Horstmann et al. 2017; © Georg Thieme Verlag KG Stuttgart New York, DOI: 10.1055/s-0042-119126)

Accordingly, the absorption of water has less influence here. Central wavelengths around 1300 nm are also used here. The chamber angle behind the sclera can also be visualized using OCT.

Light scattering varies with tissue properties. The cornea as a window to the eye normally hardly scatters at all. Its special anatomical structure allows most photons to pass through it unhindered. The iris, which serves as an aperture, scatters light very strongly. Consequently, for anterior segment OCT, this means that the iris appears much brighter in the OCT image than the cornea. However, the wide dynamic range of OCT also allows analysis of the cornea. The different layers of the cornea also stand out well in appropriately high-resolution systems due to their slightly different optical properties.

3 Data Acquisition and Imaging Optics

Whereas in conventional microscopy or photography all image points are acquired simultaneously, in classical OCT each point of the sample surface is approached individually in sequence and the overall image is computed after the acquisition. Most OCT systems use so-called scan optics to deflect the light beam. Motorized mirrors are used here, which change their angles very quickly in a rotational movement and can thus deflect the light in different directions. The deflection is shown in the following figure. The light of an OCT device is typically fed to a scanning mirror via a lens L1 by means of an optical fiber F. The mirror directs the light to the lens L1. This deflects the light onto the lens L2, which focuses it onto the sample surface. Depending on the angular position of the mirror, the light hits L2 at a slightly different angle, shifting the focal point laterally. Laterally adjacent points can be approached sequentially in this way. To illustrate the beam guidance, three different deflection angles are shown simultaneously in the figure as an example and color-coded. The mirror position shown in green leads to the focus point P1 according to the beam path shown in green, the one shown in red to P2 and the one shown in blue to P3 (Fig. 2).

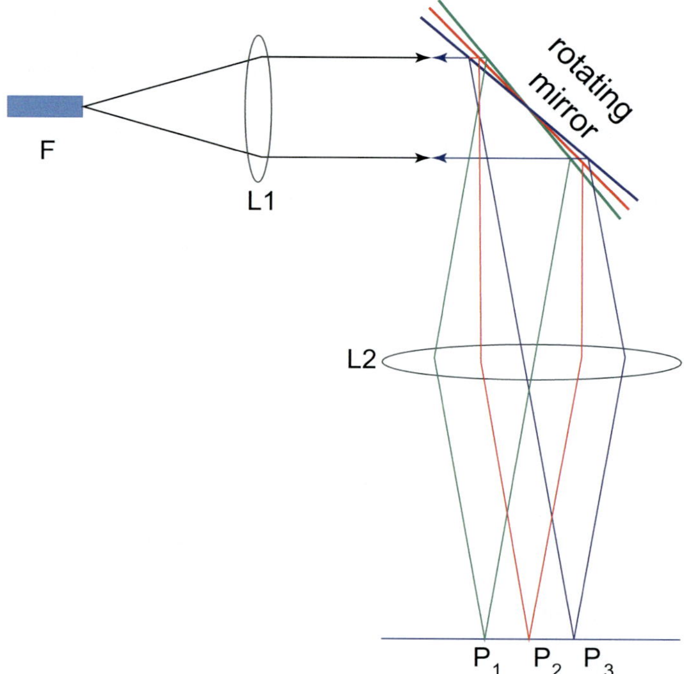

Fig. 2 In order to successively approach different points on the object surface with the OCT measuring beam, the angle of the scan mirror is changed slightly. The mirror position shown in green corresponds to the green beam path leading to P1, the red and blue positions analogously to points P2 and P3 (F = optical fiber, L1 = collimating lens, L2 = focusing lens, P = points on the object surface)

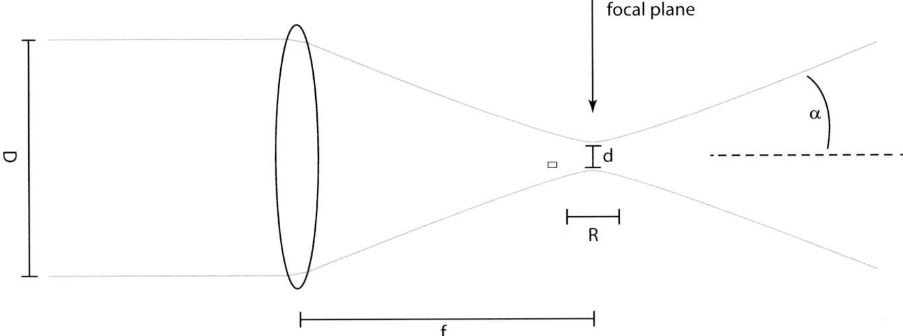

Fig. 3 Focusing by means of a lens results in a beam waist with the lateral extent d and the axial extent R, the so-called Rayleigh length, which is determined by definition by a certain intensity ratio in front of and behind the focal plane. The waist diameter d is smallest at the focal distance f to the lens; furthermore, d depends significantly on the beam diameter D

In reality, a focal point always has some extension both laterally and axially, which has great practical importance for the resolution and sharpness of OCT images. Figure 3 shows schematically the theoretical focus geometry.

The lens L deflects the incident light in the direction of the optical axis so that it is collected near the axis in the focal plane. In addition to the wavelength under consideration, the exact beam geometry determines how large the diameter d of this collection point actually is. If the beam can continue to propagate unhindered behind the focal plane, it subsequently diverges again. The localized tapering of the beam in the area around the focal plane is called the beam waist. The axial extension of the beam waist in front of and behind the focal plane up to a specified ratio is called Rayleigh length R. Rayleigh length also has great practical significance for OCT imaging. As indicated earlier, OCT uses the same optics to irradiate the tissue and detect the backscattered light. This gives OCT confocal properties, meaning that light from the focal area—that is, the axial and lateral extent of the beam waist within the Rayleigh length—is detected. Outside this range, backscattered light can no longer return to the measuring apparatus. Colloquially, this is known as "depth of field." For typical OCT parameters, the Rayleigh length is, for example, 2 mm in biological tissue. For retinal imaging, the exemplary 2 mm is largely sufficient. However, especially in anterior segment imaging, there is a desire to make the measurement window depth particularly large, for example, to represent the entire anterior chamber of the eye (front of the cornea to back of the lens) in one OCT image. As in photography, an aperture that reduces the diameter of the input beam D can increase the depth of field (see Fig. 4). However, this is done at the expense of lateral resolution because the waist diameter d increases at the same time. Thus, in practice, the balance between depth of focus and measurement depth is usually a compromise. Sophisticated OCT systems work with multifocal optics at large measurement window depths or adjust the focus within an A-scan in order to largely preserve the lateral resolution even at large measurement

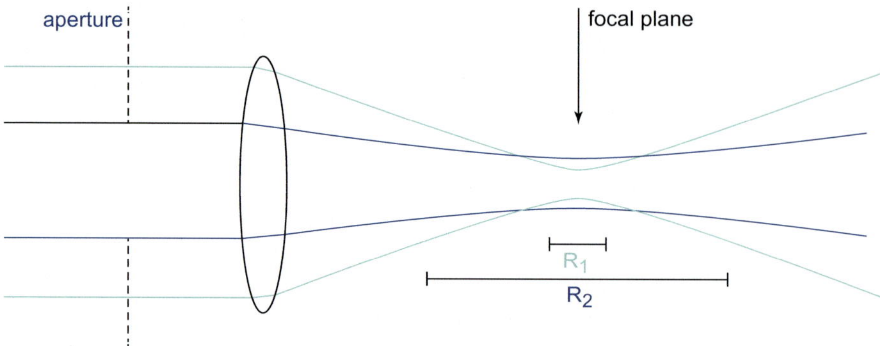

Fig. 4 For high resolution, the waist diameter should be small, which requires a large diameter of the input beam. However, this results in a small Rayleigh length (R1 compared to R2) and thus a shallow depth of field. If the depth of field is to be large, the diameter of the input beam is reduced with an aperture. This in turn affects the resolution due to a larger waist diameter

window depths. Quality differences in this respect can be clearly seen in devices from different manufacturers.

Basically, it should be noted that the best lateral resolution can only be achieved in the exact depth position of the focal plane. The lateral OCT image resolution specified by device manufacturers usually refers to the beam waist diameter d in exactly the focal position and thus represents an optimum. Outside the focal plane, the lateral resolution usually deteriorates.

4   Wave Optical Aspects: Interference

As already mentioned, OCT works with indirect time-of-flight measurement of light to determine the depth of light-scattering structures. Indirect here means that it is not actually the time taken for the light to travel from emission to re-detection that is determined, but the distance it has traveled in the process. For this purpose, OCT uses interferometry, which takes advantage of the wave character of light.

Light waves can interact with each other under certain circumstances. If they are observed together at one point, they can reinforce each other (*constructive inter-ference*) or weaken each other to the point of extinction (*destructive interference*). The decisive factor is the path difference *between the* two waves under consideration, which is illustrated in the figure (Fig. 5).

A fundamental approach to the metrological use of interferometry is the Michelson interferometer (see following figure). Here, a partially transparent mirror (also known as a beam splitter) is used in both directions, which serves to both split and recombine the light. After the first beam splitter pass, the partial waves are each reflected at a mirror and recombined again in the second beam splitter pass. A path

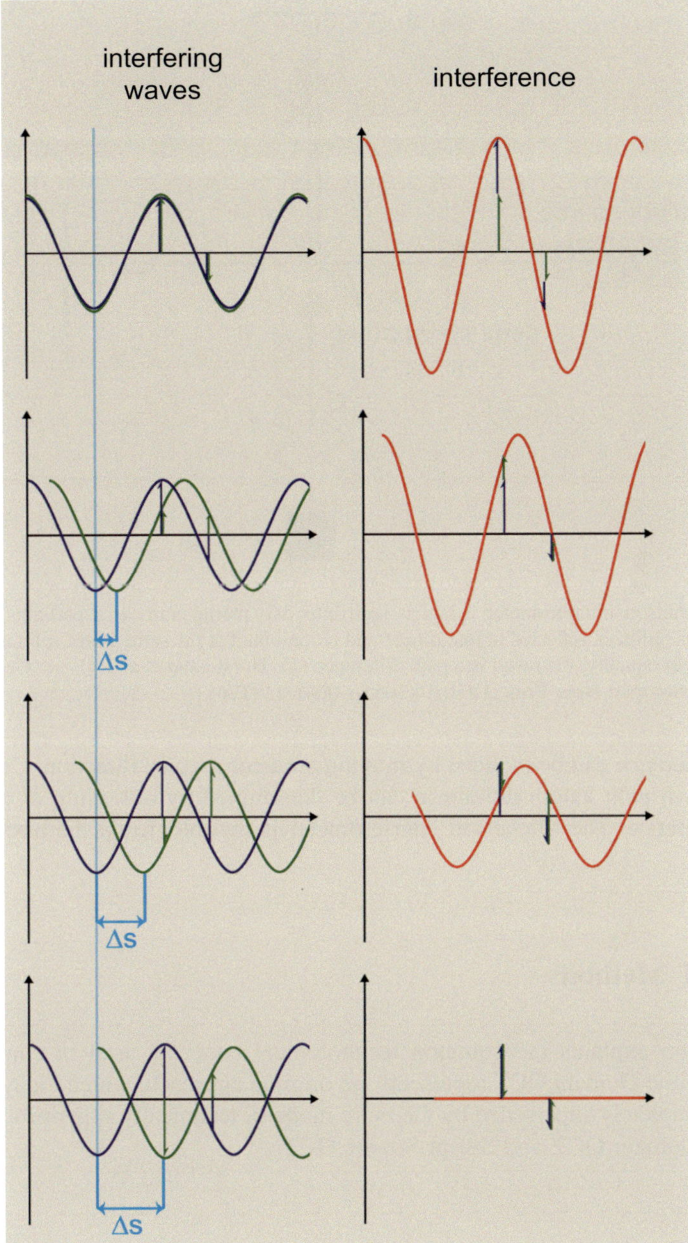

Fig. 5 Left column: The path difference of two waves increases from top to bottom. Right column: Resulting interference of the two waves. The amplitudes of the waves in the respective oscillation state add up, which is exemplarily shown by arrows in some places (Horstmann et al. 2017; © Georg Thieme Verlag KG Stuttgart New York, DOI: 10.1055/s-0042-119126)

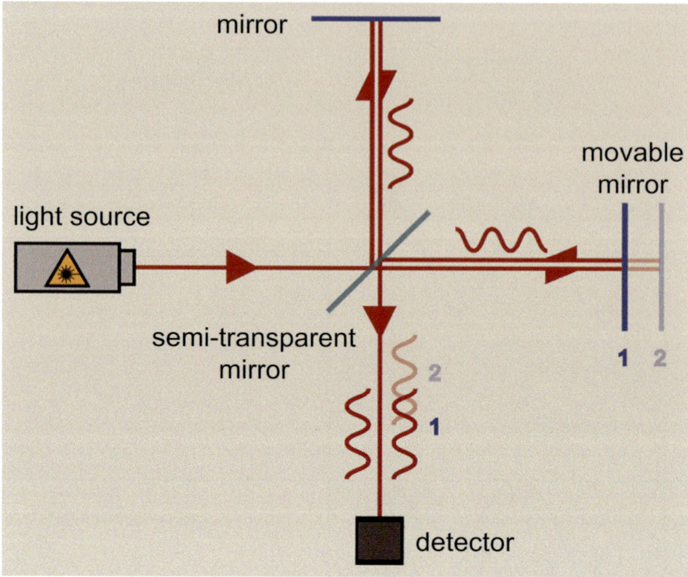

Fig. 6 Michelson interferometer. Light is split into two partial arms at a partially transparent mirror (beam splitter), reflected at one mirror and recombined at the same beam splitter. If there is no path length equality, the result is a path difference (2) (Horstmann et al. 2017; © Georg Thieme Verlag KG Stuttgart New York, DOI: 10.1055/s-0042-119126)

length difference can be induced by moving a mirror in axial direction. Conversely, an unknown path length difference can be determined by observing or measuring the interference. The Michelson interferometer is metrologically the basis of OCT (Fig. 6).

5   OCT Methods

This section explains the common technological concepts used in clinical OCT devices. Time Domain OCT represents the original approach, which today has been almost completely superseded by the more modern, technically superior methods of Spectral Domain OCT and Swept Source OCT.

5.1   *Time Domain OCT*

For time domain OCT, a broadband light source in the near-infrared spectral range is used in a Michelson interferometer. Interference then only occurs in a very small spatial range of e.g. 10 μm around a path length delay of 0. By selective axial adjustment of a reference mirror, the interference-capable spatial range of the light can be shifted axially, causing the sensitive measurement range to be shifted in front of or behind a reference plane. The first generation of OCT devices is referred to as time domain OCT because it scans the different depths of the object to be measured in time sequence. An A-scan represents the one-dimensional depth measurement of the light scattering structures below the irradiated point on the surface. To acquire an A-scan, the mechanical displacement of the reference mirror is necessary in time domain OCT. In this way, it is possible to measure successively at different depths how strongly the light is reflected or scattered at the respective object depth. In the next figure, three reference mirror positions and the corresponding measurement depth positions in the object are shown for illustration. If the reference mirror is at position 1, only the light from sample position 1 is picked up by the OCT detector, and the same applies to the other positions. In real time domain OCT instruments, about 1000 depth positions are acquired for one A-scan. For targeted, fast and reproducible displacement of the reference mirror, it is motorized in the axial direction (Fig. 7).

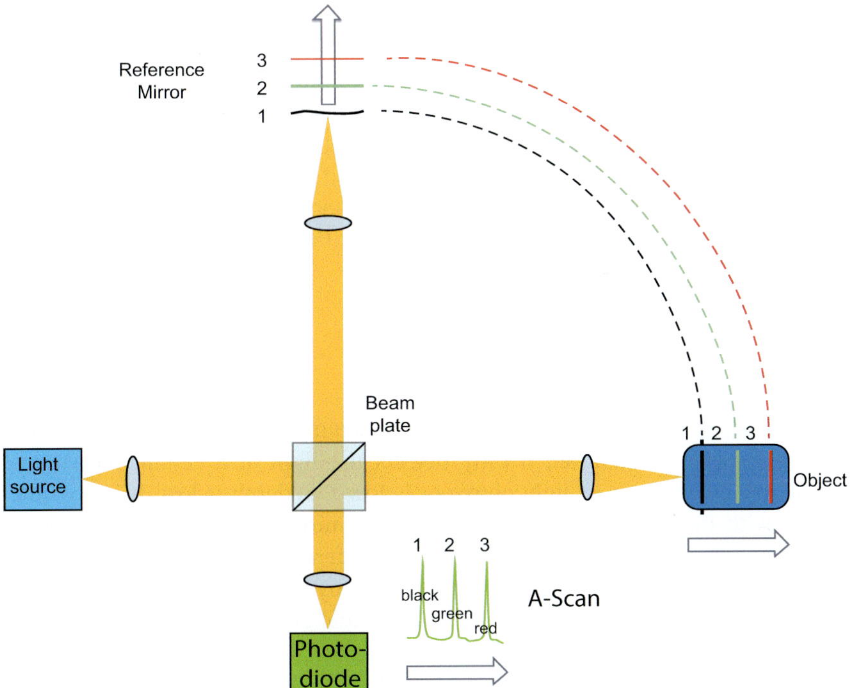

Fig. 7 The core of time domain OCT is based on the Michelson interferometer (see previous figure). Due to the broadband nature of the light source, the OCT light can only interfere when the reference and object arms have equal path lengths. Due to the delay of the reference wave, the sensitive measurement plane is also located further back, for example below the surface of an object

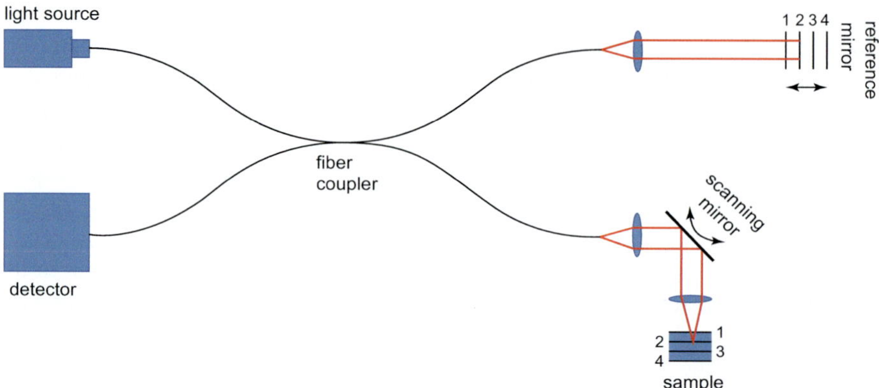

Fig. 8 Fiber-based realization of time domain OCT. The beam splitter is integrated into the fiber as a so-called fiber coupler, which makes the beam guidance much more robust. The reference mirror is shown in four different positions with the corresponding depths in the object. The scanning mirror can be used to move to the next point on the object surface after a simultaneous depth measurement

A rigid setup with a beam splitter takes up a lot of space and is very susceptible to adjustment. Therefore, the Michelson interferometer is usually realized with optical fibers and fiber couplers (fiber-based beam splitters). In addition to the resulting improved stability, this also allows the light source and detector unit to be flexibly separated from the rest of the instrument. This is illustrated in the next figure, which also shows the scanning optics and various corresponding positions of reference mirrors and depth planes in the object (Fig. 8).

5.2   Spectral Domain OCT

Due to the necessary motorization of the reference mirror, time domain OCT works relatively slowly. In addition, it only detects the light at a certain measurement depth at any given time; all light above or below this depth is lost. It is possible to dispense with the motorization of the reference mirror if, instead of detecting the interference intensity at one point, the entire interference light is detected spectrally split with one sensor line. Practically, this is done by using a refractive element such as a prism or a diffractive element such as an optical grating to split the wavelengths and a line-scan camera for detection, which together is called a spectrometer. This approach represents the second generation of OCT and is called spectral domain OCT (Fig. 9).

To illustrate how the information from which depth the photons originate can be derived from the detected spectrum of light from all object depths, individual wavelengths (W1 to W4) at different transit time differences relative to the fixed reference mirror are considered as examples in the next figure (Fig. 10).

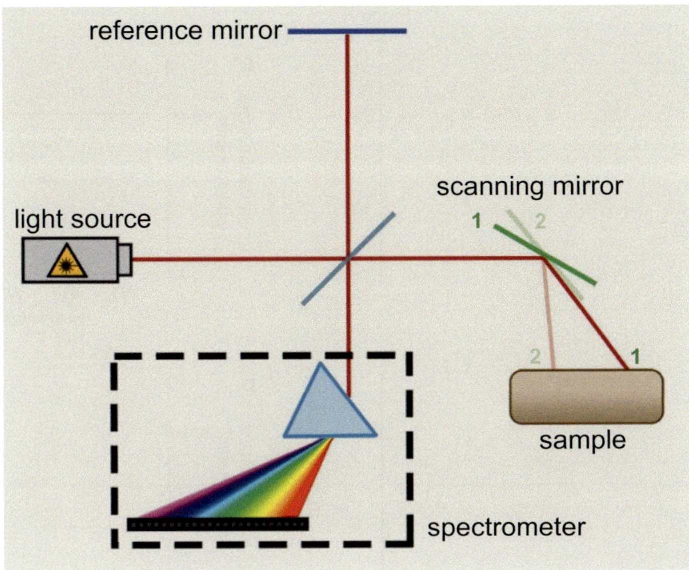

Fig. 9 In spectral domain OCT, the interference light is detected wavelength-dependently with a spectrometer. Here, too, a scanner mirror is used to move to different points on the object surface (Horstmann et al. 2017; © Georg Thieme Verlag KG Stuttgart New York, DOI: 10.1055/s-0042-119126)

If the transit times of reference light R and sample light P are exactly the same, there is constructive interference at all wavelengths. The spectrometer outputs a maximum signal for all wavelengths. If the transit time of the sample light P is slightly longer than that of the reference light R, because the waves have been backscattered slightly deeper in the object, the waves W1 of reference light and sample light are in destructive interference , so that at this position an intensity of 0 is displayed at the line sensor of the spectrometer. For W4, constructive interference is almost present again. For the waves W2 and W3 intermediate values are reached.

For all wavelengths and sample depths, the interference behavior of the different wavelengths remains qualitatively the same, i.e. constructive interference is present for certain wavelengths and destructive interference for certain wavelengths. This modulates the spectrum. The modulation increases with increasing path length difference (see the following figure). Since the modulation frequency increases with increasing depth, the maximum measurement depth depends on the resolution of the spectrally resolved detection.

By simultaneous detection of the entire spectrum, the totality of all reflecting or light-scattering structures below a surface point can be detected up to the maximum measurement depth without moving the reference mirror. The detected spectrum has finally undergone a characteristic modulation for a certain depth structure (Fig. 11).

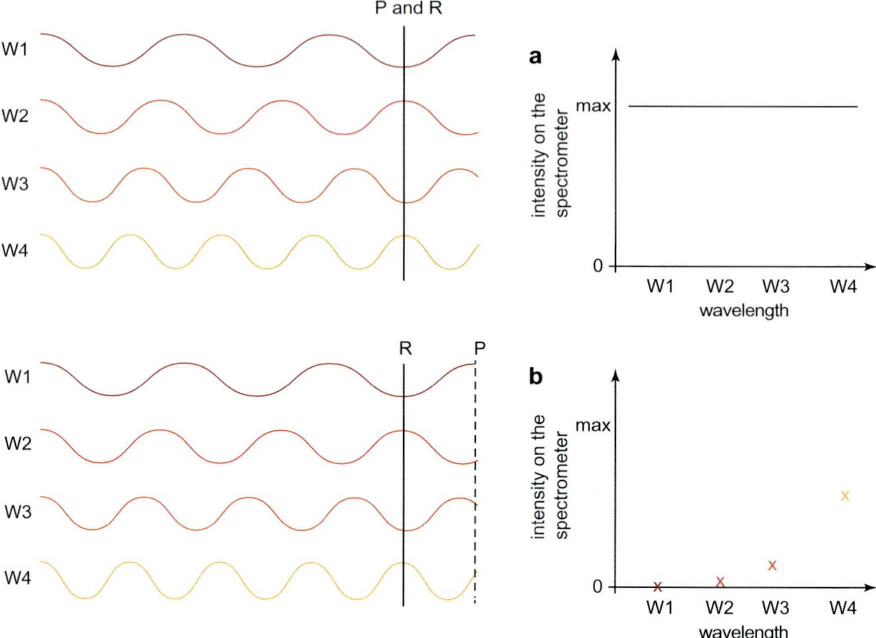

Fig. 10 Time-of-flight-dependent interference. Four wavelengths W1-4 are considered. At the top, the light is reflected at the reference mirror (R) and at the sample depth P at the same distance. Therefore, there is no difference in travel time and the considered wavelengths interfere constructively. The result is a maximum signal of all wavelengths at the spectrometer (**a**). Bottom: If there is a difference in travel time due to deviating depths of P and R, the spectrometer signal is wavelength dependent (**b**).

The mathematical operation for decoding the depth information from the measured spectra is called Fourier transform. The core of the signal processing is schematically shown in the next figure (Fig. 13).

The spectral domain version of OCT has significant advantages over time domain OCT. On the one hand, it is significantly faster, since the reference mirror procedure is not required. On the other hand, it is metrologically much more sensitive, since it utilizes the light of all depths, whereas time domain OCT discards all light outside the approached detection depth (Hüttmann et al. 2009).

5.3 Swept Source OCT

Instead of a broadband light source, tunable lasers ("swept sources") can also be used. Instead of a spectrometer, a point detector is then used, as in time domain OCT, which records the different wavelengths one after the other in time. Such detectors are available from optical telecommunication technology up to the GHz

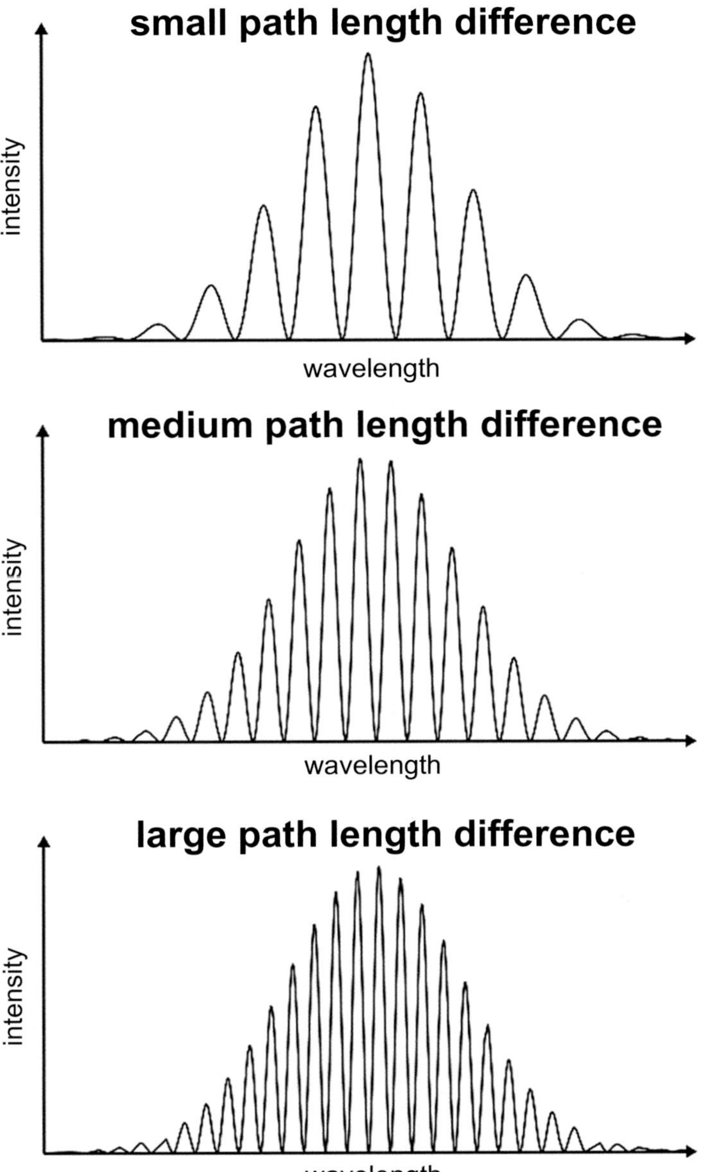

Fig. 11 The modulation frequency, i.e. the position and number of maxima and minima in the interference spectrum, depends on the path length difference (schematic representation). A mirror is used here as a sample to represent the discrete sample depths (Horstmann et al. 2017; © Georg Thieme Verlag KG Stuttgart New York, DOI: 10.1055/s-0042-119126)

Fig. 12 The superposition of the depth-dependent modulation for all measurable depths results in a characteristic spectrum, which contains information about the presence of light-scattering structures at certain depths (schematic representation) (Horstmann et al. 2017; © Georg Thieme Verlag KG Stuttgart New York, DOI: 10.1055/s-0042-119126)

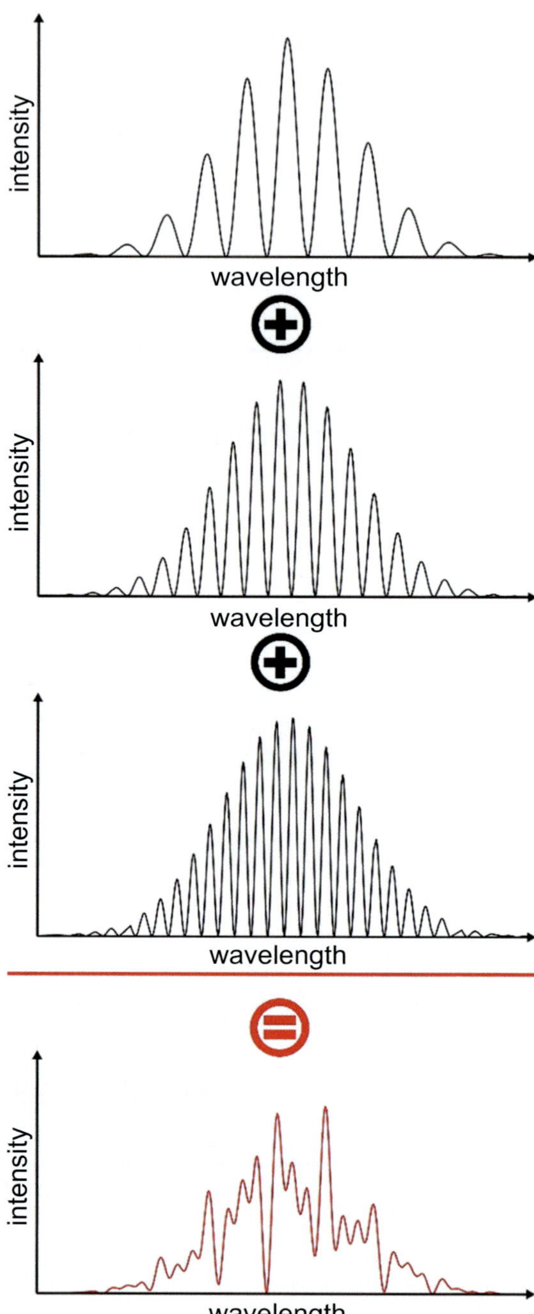

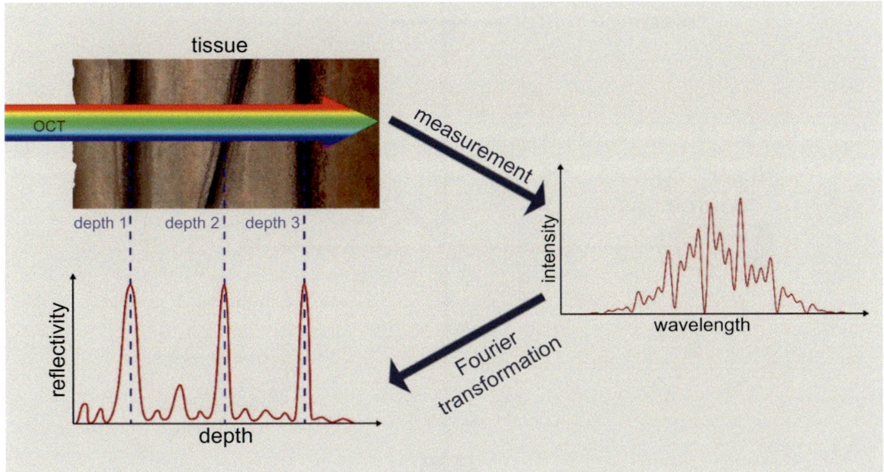

Fig. 13 Backscattering of light at certain tissue depths causes a characteristic modulation of the interference spectrum. Mathematically, the position and intensity of the backscattering can be decoded by the Fourier transform (schematic representation) (Horstmann et al. 2017; © Georg Thieme Verlag KG Stuttgart New York, DOI: 10.1055/s-0042-119126)

range. Furthermore, modern tunable swept source light sources offer a very high modulation rate, making swept source OCTs currently the fastest clinical systems (Aumann et al. 2019). Furthermore, swept source light sources with medium wavelengths in the range between 1000 and 1300 nm are available. The higher penetration depth (cf. section on tissue optics) is particularly interesting for imaging deep and subretinal structures, for axial length measurements or for imaging the lens up to its posterior interface (Grulkowski et al. 2012; Huang et al. 2015). The principle setup of an SS-OCT is shown in the figure (Fig. 14).

6 OCT Imaging of the Anterior Segment of the Eye-Practical Examples

6.1 *Example from Research: Influence of Focus Geometry*

As explained in Section 3, the optical imaging system of an OCT device has a great influence on the appearance of the images. In the anterior segment, this applies in particular to the Rayleigh length of the focusing optics. When designing an OCT optic, a trade-off must be made between lateral resolution and Rayleigh length, colloquially depth of field. In OCT, this is not just a question of imaging sharpness at a given depth. Rather, because of the confocal properties of OCT, the focal geometry is also critical in determining how many photons can be detected from a

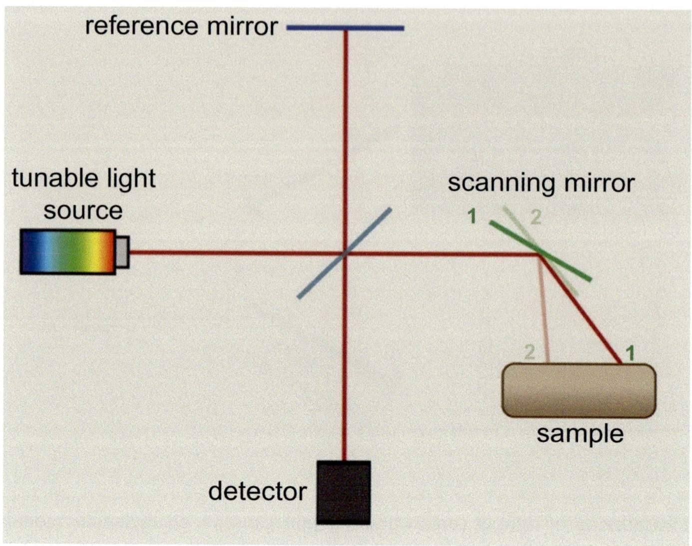

Fig. 14 In swept-source OCT, a tunable light source is used. The interference light of the different wavelengths is detected in time sequence by a single detector (Horstmann et al. 2017; © Georg Thieme Verlag KG Stuttgart New York, DOI: 10.1055/s-0042-119126)

given depth. An extreme case from research is shown in the following figure (Fig. 15).

Since the cornea of mice (BALB/c) is examined, the measurement window depth shown here is very small at about 200 μm. The thickness of the normal murine cornea is centrally 100 to 150 μm. In this approach, a sharply focusing objective with a numerical aperture of 0.5 was used for microscopic imaging (Horstmann et al. 2017). Outside the focus (dashed focal plane), the loss of sharpness and intensity is clearly visible. Thus, in the example for the best possible image of the epithelium in Figure A, the focus has been shifted to its height, the stromal fibrils approximately centered in the cornea (B), and the very thin epithelium just before its depth (C). Comparing A and C, it is noticeable that the structure at the other end of the cornea is almost invisible. The benefit of sharp focusing is evident in Figure D. At the focal position, the resolution is very high at about 1 μm, allowing visualization of individual flowing blood cells in a pathological murine corneal blood vessel.

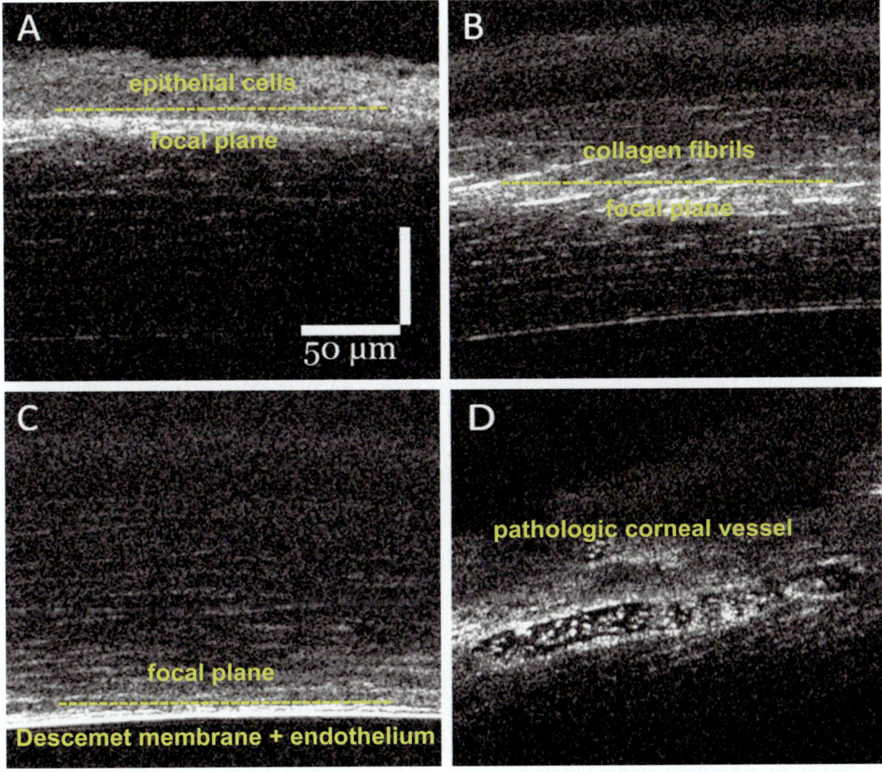

Fig. 15 OCT images A to C are acquired with the same optical coherence microscope directly one after the other and show the same location of a murine cornea in depth section (corneal thickness approx. 100 µm). Between the images, only the focal position was shifted posteriorly. The dependence of image sharpness and brightness on the focal position is clearly visible. Figure D shows a pathological blood vessel. Since this is in focus, individual flowing blood cells can be seen here (Horstmann J et al (2017) OCT verstehen – Teil 1: Physikalische Grundlagen. Klin Monbl Augenheilkunde 234(01):131–143. https://doi.org/10.1055/s-0042-119126. Georg Thieme KG, Stuttgart/New York)

6.2 Application Example: Intraoperative OCT

The requirements for OCT devices that can be used in the operating room differ greatly from the requirements for OCT devices used in outpatient settings. Table 1 lists the most important differences in the respective requirements.

Figure 16 schematically shows a possible realization concept of OCT integration in a stereo operating microscope (A) and a modern microscope with fully integrated OCT. For example, OCT can be integrated at the so-called camera port (Lankenau

Table 1 The most important differences regarding the requirements for OCT devices

	Outpatient OCT devices for eye diagnostics	OCT devices for imaging during surgical procedures
Device location	• Usually as an independent (*stand-alone*) device	• Usually integrated into a surgical microscope for reasons of space
Sterility	• Basic hygiene conditions • Patient may come into contact with the device	• Operating room hygiene conditions • Patient and surgeon should not come into contact with the device • Touchable parts sterilely covered
Measuring speed	• Data acquisition and evaluation can be done sequentially • Diagnostics in principle also possible with slower devices (at least fast enough to compensate for eye movements)	• Real-time display essential • Strong movements on the patient's eye during the procedure • High measuring speed absolutely necessary
Lateral scan width	• Fixed for the respective diagnostics	• Ideally synchronized with the zoom of the surgical microscope • Scan ranges between about 5 mm and 30 mm reasonable
Working distance	• Less than 50 mm	• As large as possible for handling surgical instruments • Greater than or equal to 160 mm useful
Software requirements	• User-friendly user interface • Many setting options useful • Data processing and evaluation following the exposure	• Imaging runs parallel to surgery and should require as little additional time as possible • Real-time data processing and display useful • Clear software useful • Automatic adjustment in real time if possible

et al. 2013). These are beam splitters (ST) that couple or decouple part of the light of the main beam path. Other ways of coupling the OCT light are possible, for example coupling in or out between the zoom optics and the objective or integrating a separate optics channel for the OCT into the surgical microscope. The OCT sample light is guided by optical fibers so that all other components such as light source, spectrometer, reference unit and computer) are positioned in the stand system of the microscope. The enumerated realizations ensure that no additional space in the operating room needs to be set up for OCT.

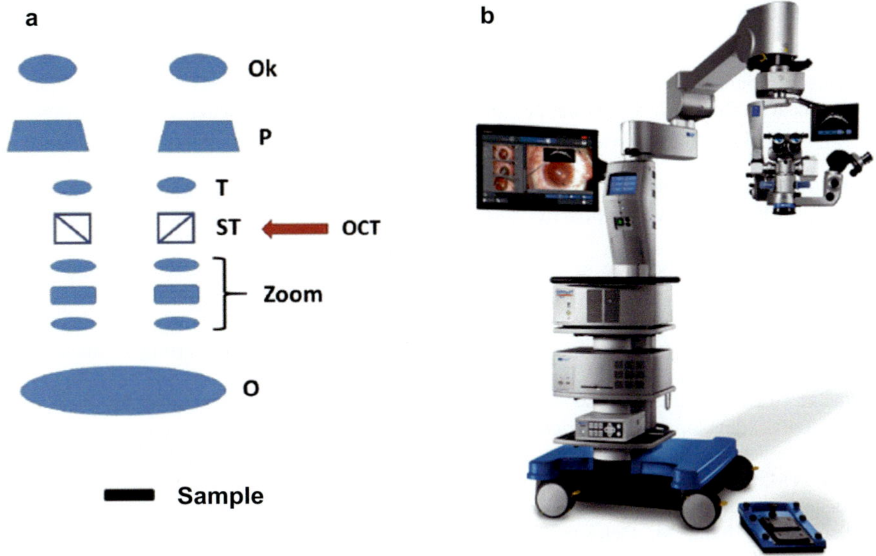

Fig. 16   **a** Schematic representation of the beam path of a surgical microscope with eyepieces (Ok), prisms (P), tube lenses (T), beam splitters (ST), zoom optics (Zoom) and objective lens (O). **b** Modern Hi-R 900 surgical microscope (Haag-Streit Surgical, Wedel, Germany) with integrated OCT system from Optomedical Technologies GmbH (Lübeck, Germany). The OCT image can optionally be transparently mirrored into the field of view of the eyepieces (small image on the right)

7   Summary

In this chapter, the basic principles of OCT and differences between various technological concepts with their advantages and disadvantages were discussed. The influence of the optical imaging system on OCT images was clarified. When designing an OCT system, physical limitations ultimately often require compromises between different imaging parameters. For example, a large field of view with fine spatial sampling stands in the way of a short acquisition time and vice versa. A trade-off must also be made between high spatial resolution and large depth of field.

Furthermore, some physical principles and its practical relevance for OCT imaging of the anterior eye segment regarding image sharpness and brightness as well as measurement window depth were described. In the following chapters, OCT images of the anterior segment of the eye are discussed, which were acquired with different stand-alone OCT devices of outpatient diagnostics as well as intraoperative OCT.

References

Aumann S, Donner S, Fischer J, Müller F. Optical Coherence Tomography (OCT): principle and technical realization. In: Bille JF, editor. High resolution imaging in microscopy and ophthalmology: new frontiers in biomedical optics. Cham: Springer International Publishing; 2019. p. 59–85.

Grulkowski I, et al. Retinal, anterior segment and full eye imaging using ultrahigh speed swept source OCT with vertical-cavity surface emitting lasers. Biomed Opt Express. 2012;3 (11):2733–51.

Horstmann J, et al. Label-free in vivo imaging of corneal lymphatic vessels using microscopic optical coherence tomography. Invest Ophthalmol Vis Sci. 2017;58(13):5880–6.

Huang D, Li Y, Tang M. Anterior eye imaging with optical coherence tomography. In: Optical coherence tomography: technology and applications. 2nd edn. Springer International Publishing; 2015. p 1649–1683.

Hüttmann G, Lankenau E, Schulz-Wackerbarth C, Müller M, Steven P, Birngruber R. Overview of apparative developments in optical coherence tomography: from imaging the retina to supporting therapeutic interventions. Klin Monbl Ophthalmolog. 2009;226(12):958–64.

Kodach VM, Kalkman J, Faber DJ, van Leeuwen TG. Quantitative comparison of the OCT imaging depth at 1300 nm and 1600 nm. Biomed Opt Express. 2010;1(1):176–85.

Lankenau EM, Krug M, Oelckers S, Schrage N, Just T, Hüttmann G. iOCT with surgical microscopes: a new imaging during microsurgery. Adv Opt Technol. 2013;2(3):233–9.

Pfeiler W. Quanta, atoms, nuclei, particles. Walter de Gruyter GmbH & Co KG; 2016.

Shi L, Alfano RR. Deep imaging in tissue and biomedical materials: using linear and nonlinear optical methods. CRC Press; 2017.

Wang LV, Wu H. Biomedical optics: principles and imaging. John Wiley & Sons; 2012.

Anatomy and Traumatology of the Anterior Segment of the Eye with Optic Coherence Tomography

Sebastian Siebelmann, Stefan J. Lang, Takahiko Hayashi,
Atsuyuki Ishida, Alexander Händel, and Alexandra Lappas

Anatomy

Optical Coherence Tomography (OCT) allows high-resolution, real-time imaging of the ocular tissue at the anterior and posterior segment of the eye. In this process, cross-sectional images with near histologic resolution of transparent structures are generated in a very short time. Depending on the type of OCT, even ocular structures that are not optically transparent can be visualized. However, the penetration depth may sometimes be significantly reduced. The limiting factor is the optical density of the tissue to be examined. Thus, transparent structures such as the conjunctiva or the cornea can be better visualized than opaque, very dense or pigmented structures like the deeper lid skin, the sclera or the pigment epithelium of the iris. Significant differences in terms of penetration, depth and resolution can be observed between Time-domain (TD-OCT) and Spectral-domain OCT (SD-OCT) (Siebelmann et al. 2016) (Fig. 1). Swept-source OCT also provides a much better overview of the anterior segment of the eye, which makes it ideal for planning surgical interventions.

While SD-OCT achieves very high resolution at low penetration depth, TD-OCT provides a very good overview of almost the entire anterior chamber of the eye. However, the resolution achieved by TD-OCT is inferior to that of SD-OCT.

S. Siebelmann (✉) · A. Händel · A. Lappas
Department of Ophthalmology, University Hospital of Cologne, Cologne, Germany
e-mail: siebelmann@augenarzt-solingen.de

S. J. Lang
Klinik für Augenheilkunde, Uniklinik Freiburg, Freiburg im Breisgau, Germany

T. Hayashi
Division of Ophthalmology, Department of Visual Sciences, Nihon University School of Medicine, Itabashi, Tokyo, Japan

A. Ishida
Department of Ophthalmology, Kikuna Yuda Eye Clinic, Yokohama, Japan

© The Author(s), under exclusive license to Springer Nature Switzerland AG 2022
L. M. Heindl and S. Siebelmann (eds.), *Optical Coherence Tomography of the Anterior Segment*, https://doi.org/10.1007/978-3-031-07730-2_3

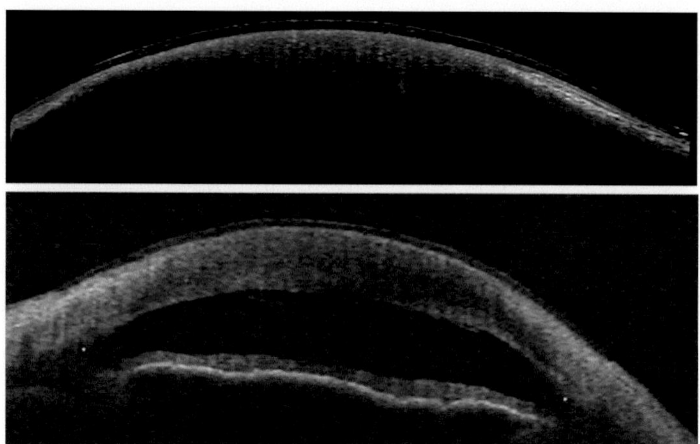

Fig. 1 Comparison of Spectral-domain and Time-domain OCT. Visualization of a peripheral graft detachment after DMEK in SD-OCT (top) and in TD-OCT (bottom). While SD-OCT is significantly higher in resolution, TD-OCT provides much greater depth of penetration

Swept-source OCT offers a very good combination of high penetration depth and good tissue resolution. This is made possible by the fact that the wavelengths of the radiation source are adjusted, i.e. changed. Therefore, it operates without a spectrometer and enables very fast imaging.

Since swept source technology is currently still very cost-intensive, the examiner usually has to decide which structures are to be imaged with which OCT modality. A large number of ocular structures can be imaged quickly and without contact in almost histological resolution. Both the resolution and the penetration depth of the OCT are usually limited by particularly dense or opaque ocular structures, such as the sclera or the pigment epithelium of the iris. The following is an overview of the possibilities and limitations of OCT in imaging the physiological anatomy of the anterior segment of the eye.

Optical coherence tomography is also increasingly used in the dermatological field for differential diagnosis of dermal processes. The dermatological OCT uses a different wavelength to allow an adequate penetration depth into the optical denser epidermis Fig. 2. It is, however, possible to visualize the epidermal layers. In some cases, glands such as sweat glands can be distinguished from one another. Epidermal imaging is limited by very dense structures like nevi or hemorrhages. In some cases, tattoos may reduce the penetration of the laser light of the OCT into the deeper tissue due to the iron-containing ink used (Figs. 2, 3, 4, 5 and 6).

Limitations

Limitations are mainly the penetration depth and the blockage of the OCT-image by dense tissue, blood or pigmented structures. Swept-source OCT devices, however, are capable of partially penetrating scleral tissue, as shown above. Further limitations may occur due to dislocated or damaged ocular tissue in ocular trauma.

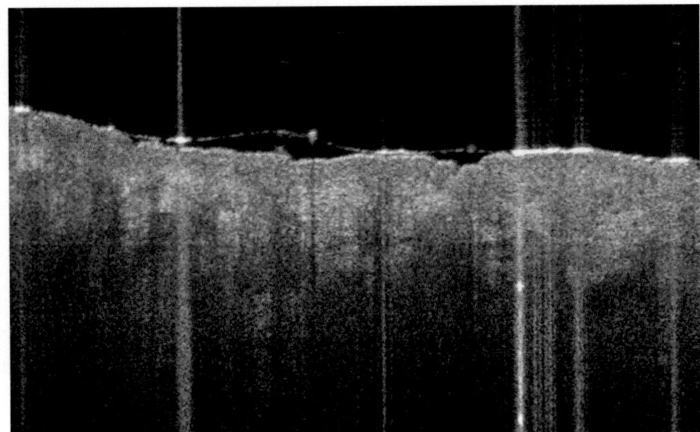

Fig. 2 OCT of the healthy eyelid skin. The image is courtesy of Vivosight®, Michelson Diagnostics, UK

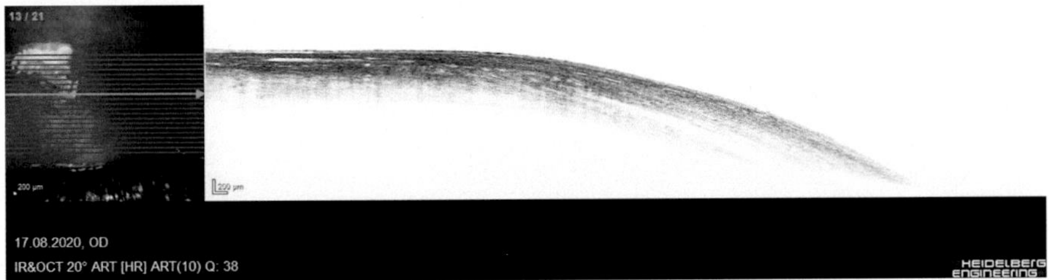

Fig. 3 Illustration of the physiological conjunctiva in OCT. The conjunctival epithelium, the underlying conjunctival stroma with conjunctival vessels can be seen. The underlying sclera can also be delineated. Due to the optical density of the sclera, the penetration depth of OCT into deeper scleral tissue is limited

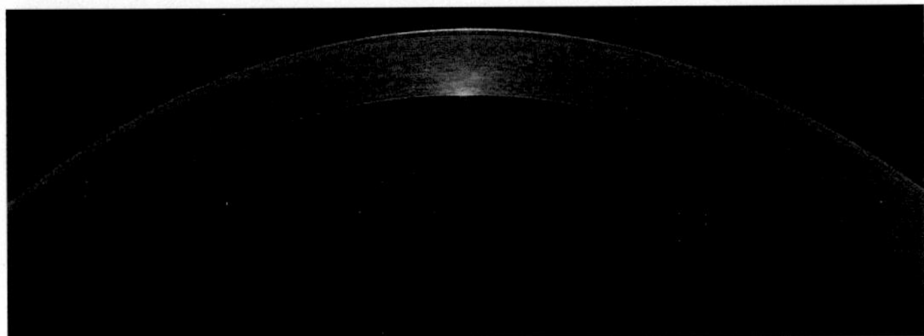

Fig. 4 Physiologic cornea in OCT. Almost complete visualization of all corneal layers in near histologic resolution can be seen. The epithelium with underlying Bowman's lamella is clearly delineated, and the underlying corneal stroma shows heterogeneous reflectivity, presumably caused by the arrangement of corneal collagen fibrils. Descemet's membrane with indicated endothelium is also recognizable. However, the posterior corneal complex is poorly delineated in respect to the Dua's layer

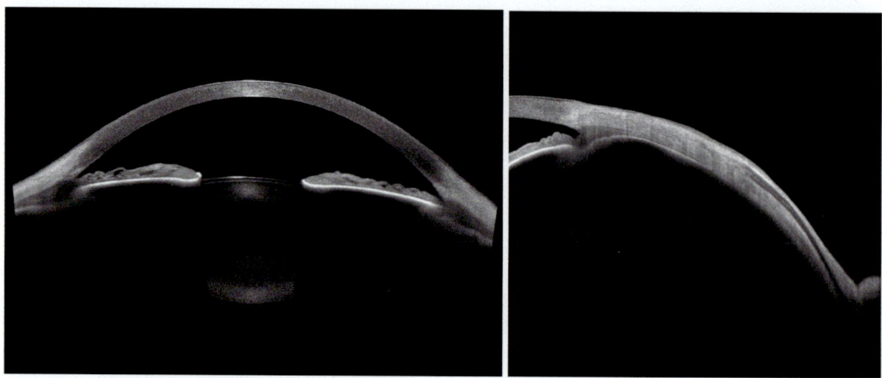

Fig. 5 Imaging of the complete anterior segment of the eye by swept-source OCT (ACE, Bausch and Lomb, Rochester, New York, USA). Courtesy of Bausch and Lomb

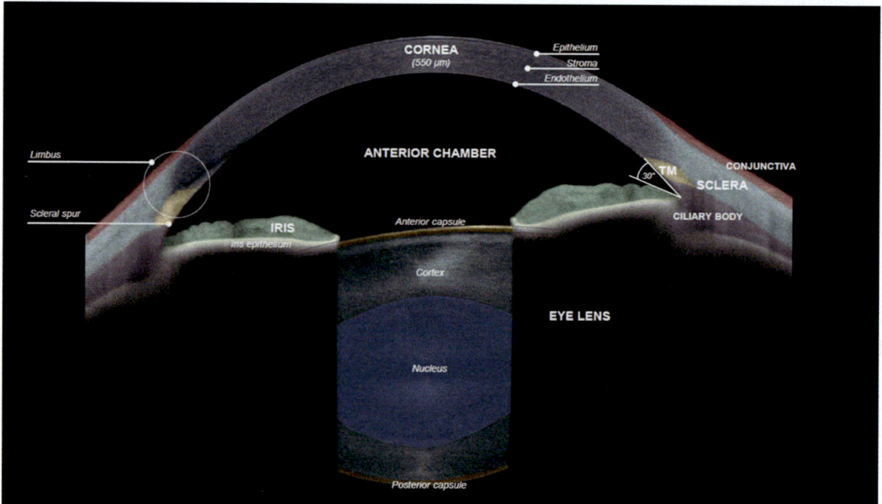

Fig. 6 Illustration of the anatomy of the anterior segment of the eye, shown by swept-source OCT (ACE, Bausch und Lomb, Rochester, New York, USA). Courtesy of Bausch and Lomb

Examples may include corneal edema, iris prolapse, or intraocular foreign bodies. In the following, we will further specify the capabilities of OCT to evaluate the anterior segment of the eye in ocular trauma.

Traumatology

As shown in the previous section, using different OCT devices with wavelengths and optics adapted to the respective tissues provides a very good representation of almost all structures of the anterior segment of the eye. This is only limited by pigmented or opaque structures such as the pigment sheet of the iris.

A particularly interesting area of application in this context is the imaging of non-physiological conditions of ocular structures, e.g. after ocular trauma. In trauma the view into the anterior chamber of the eye may be reduced because of corneal edema, iris prolapse or anterior chamber hemorrhage.

In addition to traditional ultrasound biomicroscopy (UBM), OCT can provide important diagnostic information to assess further diagnostic or therapeutic procedures. Of particular note is that OCT is a non-contact imaging technique compared to UBM. In surgical treatment of, e.g. penetrating corneal and scleral injuries, it is usually essential not to compress and thus further destabilize the eye by contact with an ultrasound probe.

Although OCT is appropriate for imaging the traumatized eye and the use of the OCT specifically in the posterior segment of the eye is well-established, there is very little literature on its use in trauma to the anterior segment of the eye (Cauduro et al. 2012; Pham et al. 2007).

Ophthalmic trauma is characterized by a localized force acting on the ocular globe. Ocular distinction is made between non-penetrating and penetrating ocular trauma, with or without intraocular foreign bodies. Especially in penetrating trauma, there is usually ocular hypotony involved, which makes accurate diagnosis difficult.

In addition, it is not only the direct trauma site that is affected, but also—depending on the intensity of the applied force—its neighboring structures. This overarching characteristic of trauma requires thorough diagnostics to identify all traumatized structures involved. Only then can a strategy for adequate therapy be made.

Traditional preoperative imaging diagnostics are based primarily on slit lamp examination, gonioscopy, and ultrasound biomicroscopy. These can be used to diagnose injuries to the cornea, iris, lens, and chamber angle. Unfortunately, after trauma, the transparency of the ocular structures is often impaired by corneal edema or anterior chamber hemorrhage. Therefore, the classical examination methods can only be used in a limited way. If hypotony is also present, then contact-based examinations such as gonioscopy and ultrasound biomicroscopy are too invasive and thus not applicable. Structures such as the iris, the chamber angle and the ciliary body are particularly difficult to access in such cases.

Here, OCT can significantly expand the diagnostic possibilities and thus increase the safety of preoperative diagnostics, therapy planning and postoperative follow-up. It is not contact-bound and provides fast imaging speeds, which can be very helpful in the case of structural damage to the globe in acute ocular trauma.

Akil et al. were able to show in a small case series that in acute trauma diagnostics the use of an anterior segment OCT allowed 360° visualization of the anterior chamber angle within a few seconds. This allowed preoperative assessment of cyclodialysis or iridodialysis and thus improved the quality of surgical care (Akil et al. 2016).

Of note, OCT was also able to generate images in the presence of corneal edema, which may impede diagnosis by slit lamp (Ryan et al. 2013). In another study descemetolysis that was not detectable by slit lamp could well be diagnosed by OCT (Wylegala et al. 2009). Moreover, children that are often insufficiently examinable by slit lamp microscopy after ocular trauma, could be examined by OCT to assess any traumatic change in the eye (Cauduro et al. 2012).

OCT may also be used to examine traumata with intraocular foreign bodies. In a case series with 104 patients, foreign body injuries of the cornea, the anterior chamber, the chamber angle, and the lens were examined by OCT. The foreign bodies could be characterized by OCT in terms of material, size, localization, and penetration depth (Ryan et al. 2013). The depth of penetration of an ocular foreign body is particularly crucial for further surgical planning in this context. Mahendradas et al. were able to localize a foreign body intralentally by OCT, which was not possible by slit lamp due to traumatic lens opacification, and thus could choose an anterior approach for surgical therapy (Mahendradas et al. 2010). Various foreign body materials of metal, glass, wood, and graphite could be visualized by OCT (Armarnik et al. 2019). Glass, in particular, is often difficult to detect with most traditional imaging techniques: Arora et al. were able to visualize glass foreign bodies in the cornea using OCT and found otherwise undetectable endothelial involvement, which influenced further treatment planning (Arora et al. 2015).

A limitation to foreign body visualization, however, even with OCT, is, that potential hyperreflectivity of foreign bodies may obscure underlying structures due to posterior blockage phenomena.

OCT also has some advantages in postoperative follow-up. It was shown, for example that the measurement of the central corneal thickness was very well possible by OCT, so that a postoperative quantitative evaluation of the cornea allowed an estimation of the endothelial cell function after trauma (Kim et al. 2008).

In a pilot study, Wyegala et al. demonstrated in 38 eyes of 34 patients after ocular trauma that optical coherence tomography is suitable for initial diagnosis after trauma as well as for follow-up examinations after surgical treatment (Wylegala et al. 2009). The corneal healing process could even be followed beneath a transplanted amniotic membran. Specifically, in the case of concomitant corneal edema, OCT was clearly superior to the slit-lamp microscope alone, as visualization of the anterior chamber structures was possible despite reduced visibility. Surprisingly, even in the case of a patient with hematocornea, visualization of the anterior chamber was possible by OCT, although blood significantly reduced the penetrance of the laser light. Again, wound healing of the corneal epithelium after corneal cauterization and subsequent amniotic membrane grafting could be followed even through the amniotic membrane.

In addition to the cornea, the anterior chamber angle could also be better documented postoperatively using OCT: anterior synechiae formation was detected earlier and could be quantified (Ryan et al. 2013). Angle closure glaucoma could be better diagnosed, even in the presence of hemorrhage (Wylegala et al. 2009). In addition, despite a reduced view into the anterior chamber of the eye, lens subluxation could also be visualized.

Beyond the studies mentioned here, however, only single case reports regarding the use of anterior segment OCT in anterior segment injuries, such as perforating corneal injuries, scleral perforations, and lens dislocations, are available to date (Madhusudhana et al. 2007; Prakash et al. 2009).

Nevertheless, OCT is also limited in these cases by transparency reduction, especially due to pigment and severe hemorrhage.

Overall, the advantages of OCT can be summarized as follows:

As a noncontact technique, it allows for less invasive and rapidly performable diagnostics in the acute event of bulbar trauma. Thus, it may demonstrate superiority in the examination of the anterior segment compared to the more invasive ultrasound biomicroscopy and gonioscopy. OCT can prove superior to traditional slit-lamp examination because it allows visualization through a traumatically opacified cornea. OCT itself requires some transparency for image generation, but the long wavelength of low-coherence light allows for an expansion of the diagnostic spectrum compared to conventional light sources used in slit lamp microscopy. This can expand the range of examinations through structures that are actually transparent, as the cornea, the anterior chamber, the anterior chamber angle, and the lens, even in the presence of mild opacities.(Wylegala et al. 2009).

OCT can confirm the results of classical diagnostics, but also go beyond them and provide valuable insights for further treatment planning in an acute trauma setting.

Intraoperative OCT is another feature worth mentioning. It allows for additional diagnostic information even during surgery, but is tied to separate equipment.

Another possible use of OCT is observation of postoperative wound healing and of possible posttraumatic pathologies. In particular, angle-closure glaucoma, which is difficult to visualize by slit lamp, can still threaten late visual rehabilitation—even with otherwise successful trauma management.

> **Infobox OCT Findings**
>
> OCT of the anterior segment of the eye has distinct advantages over the slit lamp, especially in traumatologic cases. Since the cornea or the view into the anterior chamber is often reduced, injuries of all structures of the anterior eye segment can be detected. This can be e.g. perforations and erosions of the cornea, but also iris carcerations and lens luxations. Especially in the presence of a foreign body, its depth and position can be determined in many cases. Also, the configuration of the chamber angle can be assessed despite a reduced view. Post-traumatic pathologies, such as scars, synechiae and vitreous bodies, can also be seen on OCT, making it an excellent tool for surgical planning.

In the following, different examples of ocular trauma are presented and explained on the basis of OCT images (Figs. 7, 8, 9, 10, 11, 12, 13, 14, 15, 16, 17, 18, 19 and 20).

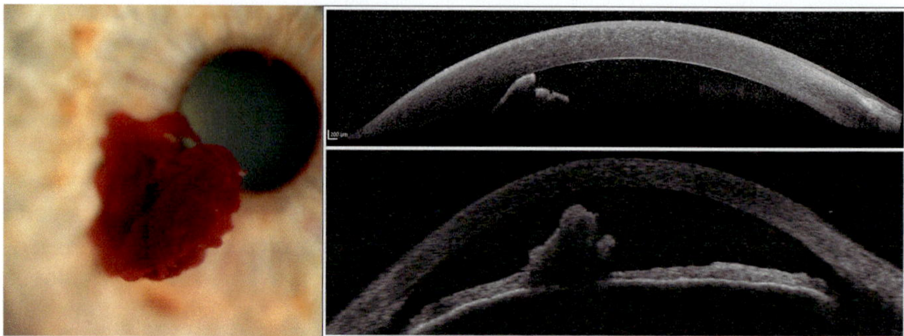

Fig. 7 Isolated iris hemorrhage. Comparing SD- and TD-OCT, the significantly deeper penetration depth of TD-OCT is evident. By means of OCT it can be confirmed that there is a hemorrhage originating from the iris

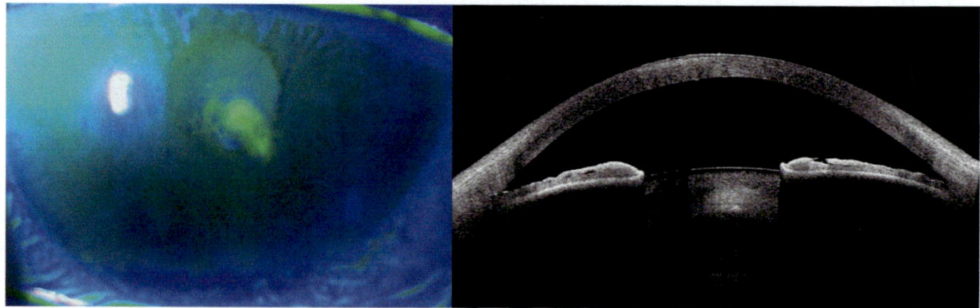

Fig. 8 Small, superficial erosion of the cornea. Slit lamp shows fluorescein staining of the cornea. OCT displays a superficial abrasion of the epithelium. The corneal stroma is also slightly swollen in this area

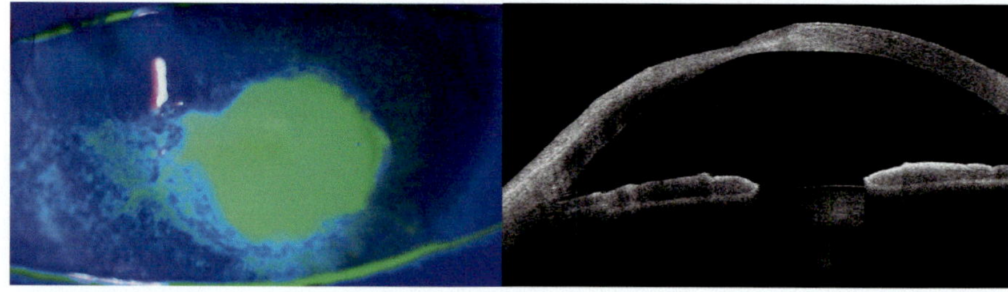

Fig. 9 Traumatic corneal erosion with a stromal defect. While slit lamp imaging using fluorescein shows only an epithelial defect, OCT imaging allows a detailed visualization of the corneal defect. It reveals that there is not only an epithelial defect, but also a large ablation of the anterior corneal stroma

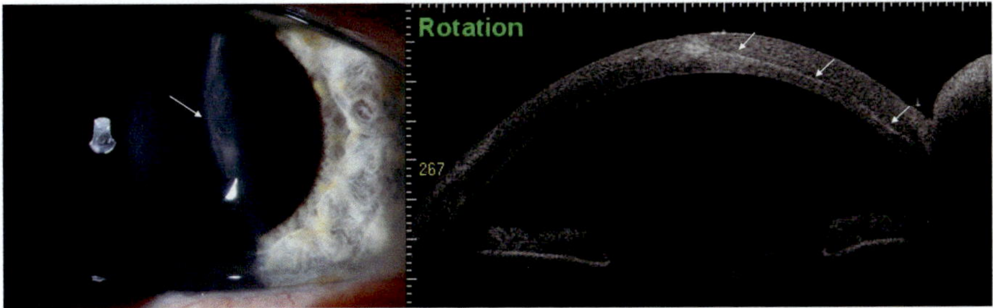

Fig. 10 Lamellar corneal injury. The clinical picture shows an injury with unclear depth extension. OCT reveals a lamellar injury extending into the posterior stroma (arrows)

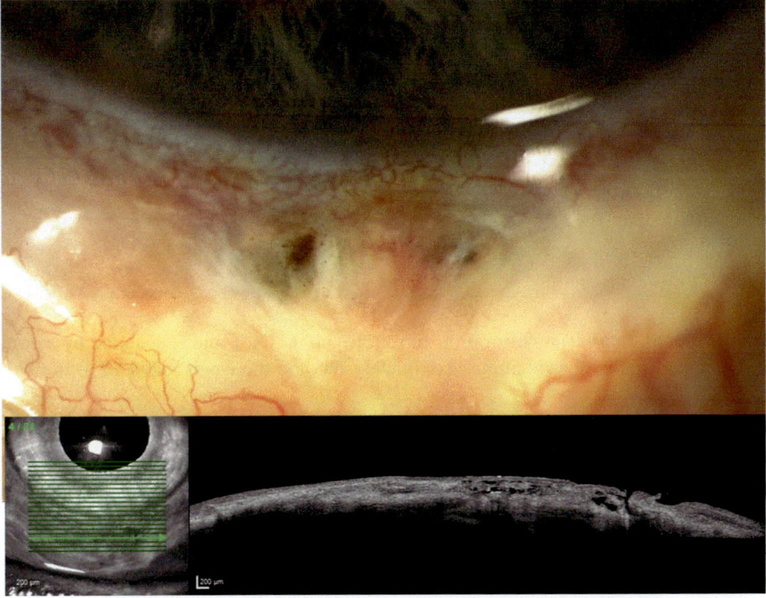

Fig. 11 Perforating eye injury at 6 o'clock. Two perforation sites are clearly visible by slit lamp. OCT confirms the presence of a fistula

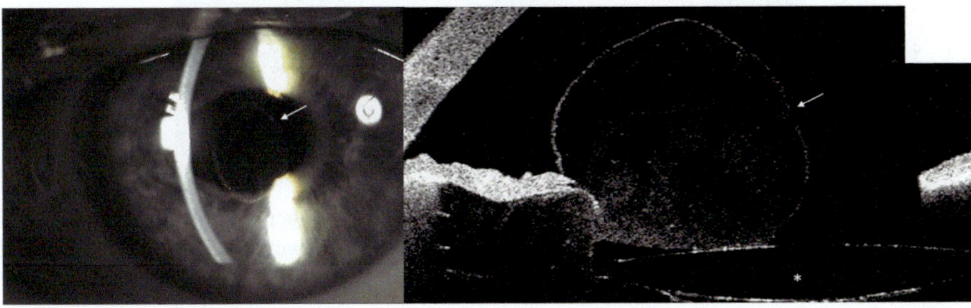

Fig. 12 Vitreous prolapse (arrows) into the anterior chamber after blunt bulbar trauma. OCT shows pseudophakia (*)

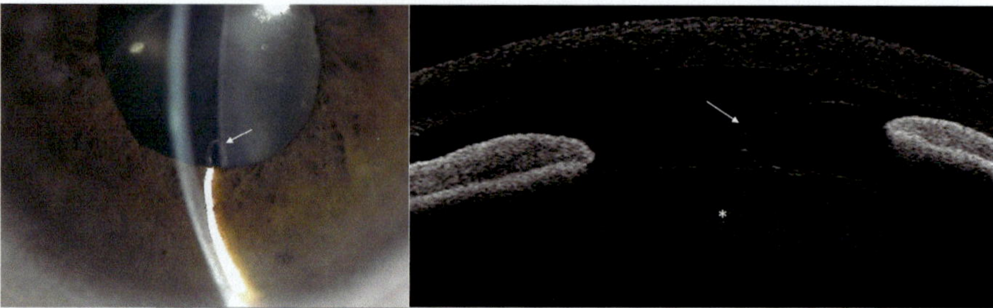

Fig. 13 Vitreous prolapse (arrows) into the anterior chamber after blunt bulbar trauma. The eye is phakic (*)

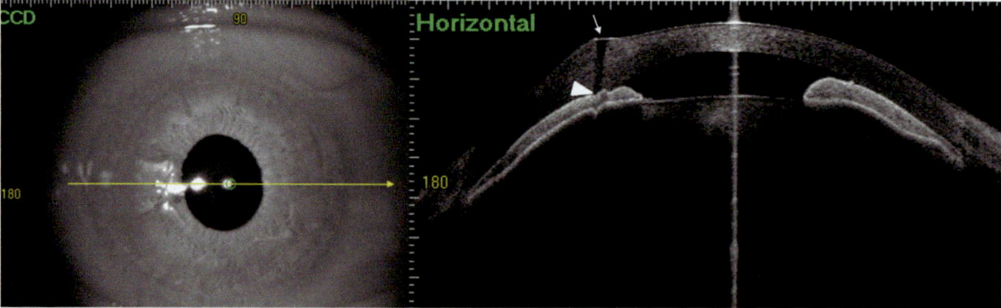

Fig. 14 Perforating injury.The perforation site shows up on OCT and is spanned by a contact lens (arrow). The anterior chamber is almost completely flat and the iris is adjacent to the wound gap

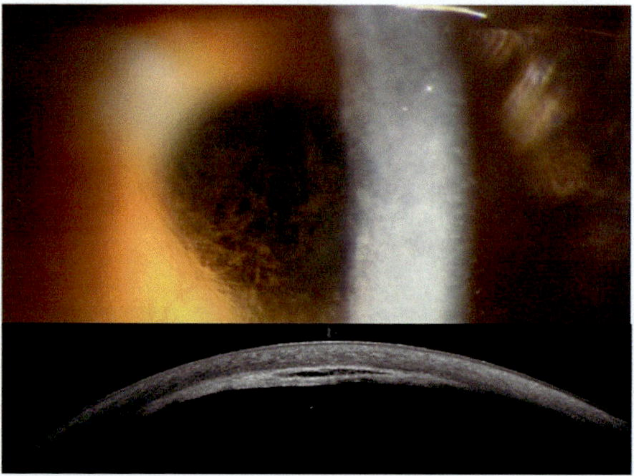

Fig. 15 Corneal scars after cataract surgery. Slit lamp findings show multiple endothelial corneal lesions. These can be precisely localized by OCT. Circumscribed swelling of the posterior part of the cornea and cystic spaces are visible

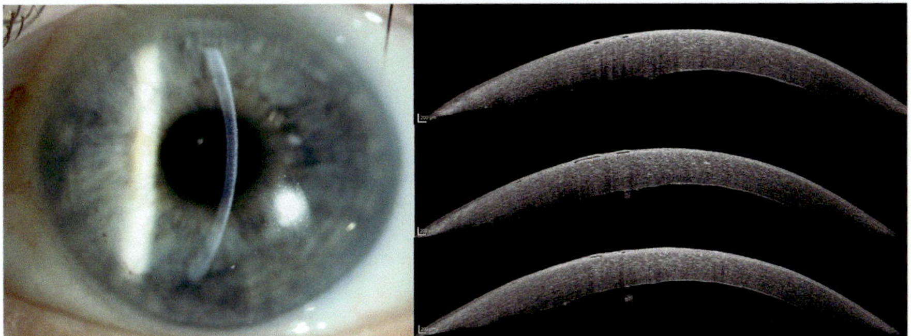

Fig. 16 Postoperative sequelae, e.g. after traumatic rupture of the posterior capsule during cataract surgery, with vitreous strands to the cornea, can also be followed by OCT. Here, OCT shows exactly the adhesion site of the vitreous strand. Its course within the anterior chamber can also be followed well by OCT. In the future, intraoperative OCT could help to exclude vitreous adhesions after posterior capsule rupture during cataract surgery

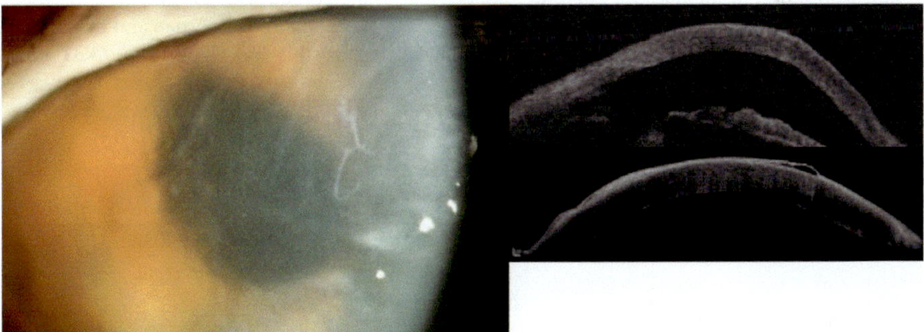

Fig. 17 Finding after blunt bulbar ocular trauma. The slit lamp image shows corneal edema and an only partially round pupil. The view into the anterior chamber is reduced. TD-OCT imaging shows an iris defect in the periphery. SD-OCT shows marked bullous corneal edema

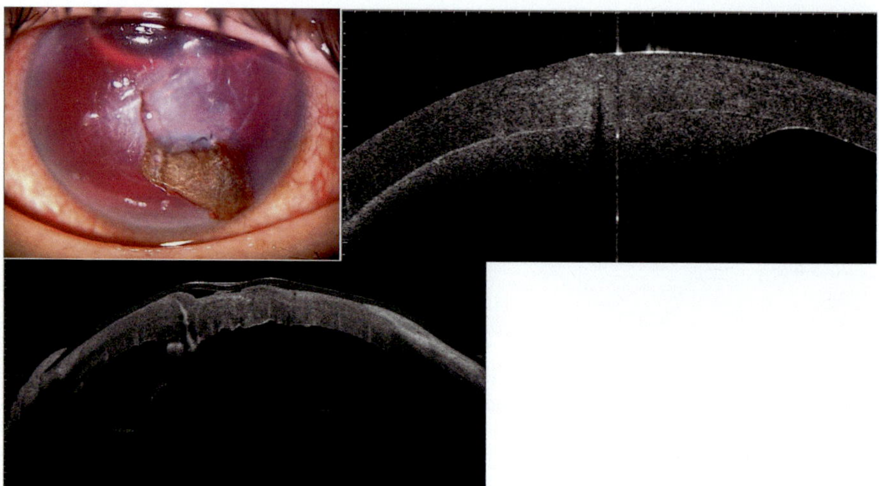

Fig. 18 Rupture of the globe as visualized by OCT. Top left: Clinical photograph showing ocular rupture with blood in the anterior chamber, a large tear in the cornea with incarcerated iris tissue. Top right: OCT imaging at presentation. OCT imaging shows a tear in the cornea and blood in the anterior chamber. The anterior chamber appears to be deep in this image. Bottom: OCT image using Swept-source OCT after initial wound closure. The anterior chamber is deep; however, incarcerated iris tissue is still evident. The cornea is covered with a therapeutic contact lens

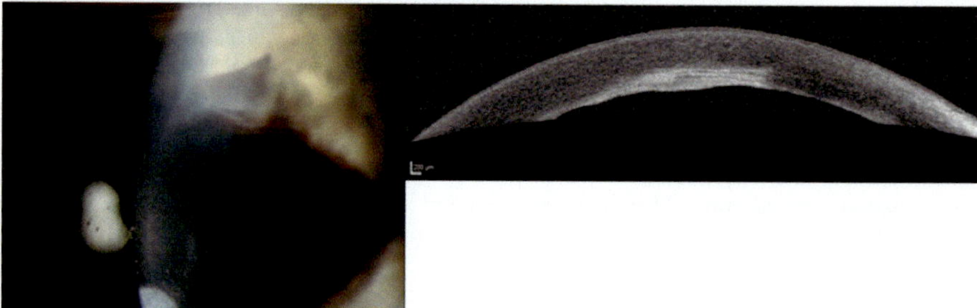

Fig. 19 Long-term follow up after perforating traumatic injuries to the anterior segment of the eye can also be assessed using OCT. Slit lamp microscopy shows an old penetrating corneal scar, as well as an old iris defect in the background. OCT can be used to accurately assess the depth and extent of the remaining corneal scar

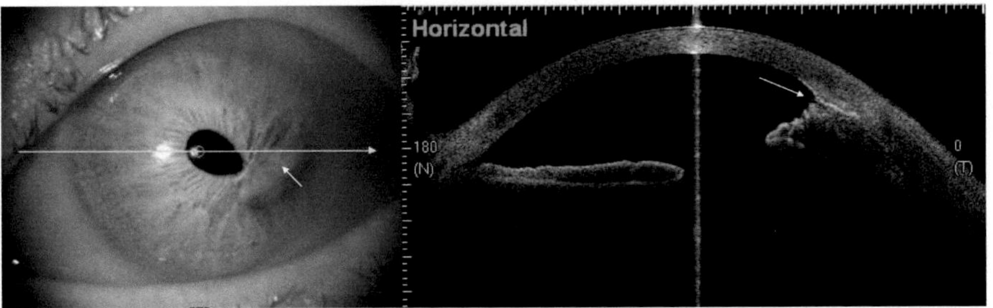

Fig. 20 Anterior synechiae after an old trauma. The synechiae are adjacent to the cornea in the area of the perforation site (arrows). This is accompanied by a distorted pupil

References

Akil H, Minasyan L, Francis BA, Chopra V. Utility of anterior segment swept-source optical coherence tomography for imaging eyes with antecedent ocular trauma. Am J Ophthalmol Case Rep. 2016;3:18–21.

Armarnik S, Mimouni M, Goldenberg D, et al. Characterization of deeply embedded corneal foreign bodies with anterior segment optical coherence tomography. Graefes Arch Clin Exp Ophthalmol. 2019;257(6):1247–52.

Arora T, Arora S, Sinha R. Management of intrastromal glass foreign body based on anterior segment optical coherence tomography and Pentacam analysis. Int Ophthalmol. 2015;35(1):1–1.

Cauduro RS, Ferraz CdA, Morales MSA, et al. Application of anterior segment optical coherence tomography in pediatric ophthalmology. J Ophthalmol. 2012;2012

Kim HY, Budenz DL, Lee PS, Feuer WJ, Barton K. Comparison of central corneal thickness using anterior segment optical coherence tomography vs ultrasound pachymetry. Am J Ophthal. 2008;145(2):228–32. e1.

Madhusudhana K, Hossain P, Thiagarajan M, Newsom R. Use of anterior segment optical coherence tomography in a penetrating eye injury. Br J Ophthalmol. 2007;91(7):982–3.

Mahendradas P, Vijayan PB, Avadhani K, Garudadri S, Shetty BK. Usefulness of anterior segment optical coherence tomography in the demonstration of intralenticular foreign body in traumatic cataract. Can J Ophthal/J Canadien D'ophtalmologie. 2010;4(45):413–4.

Pham TQ, Chua B, Gorbatov M, Mitchell P. Optical coherence tomography findings of acute traumatic maculopathy following motor vehicle accident. Am J Ophthalmol. 2007;143(2):348–50.

Prakash G, Ashokumar D, Jacob S, Kumar KS, Agarwal A, Agarwal A. Anterior segment optical coherence tomography–aided diagnosis and primary posterior chamber intraocular lens implantation with fibrin glue in traumatic phacocele with scleral perforation. J Cataract Refract Surg. 2009;35(4):782–4.

Ryan DS, Sia RK, Colyer M, et al. Anterior segment imaging in combat ocular trauma. J Ophthalmol. 2013;2013.

Siebelmann S, Gehlsen U, Le Blanc C, Stanzel TP, Cursiefen C, Steven P. Detection of graft detachments immediately following Descemet membrane endothelial keratoplasty (DMEK) comparing time domain and spectral domain OCT. Graefes Arch Clin Exp Ophthalmol. 2016;254(12):2431–7.

Wylegala E, Dobrowolski D, Nowińska A, Tarnawska D. Anterior segment optical coherence tomography in eye injuries. Graefes Arch Clin Exp Ophthalmol. 2009;247(4):451–5.

Optical Coherence Tomography in Conjunctival and Eyelid Lesions

Alexander C. Rokohl, Sebastian Siebelmann, and Ludwig M. Heindl

Optical coherence tomography (OCT) has been established in ophthalmology for several years and is currently of great importance, especially in the diagnosis and therapy monitoring of retinal, optic nerve, and corneal diseases (Berufsverband der Augenarzte Deutschlands e V, Deutsche Ophthalmologische G, Retinologische Gesellschaft e V. 2017). Although the acquisition of an OCT image can be integrated very well into a clinical routine due to its rapid feasibility and low patient burden, this technique does not currently play a major role in routine clinical diagnostics for lesions of the eyelids and conjunctiva. However, OCT technology is undergoing continuous and rapid development and is becoming increasingly important in the field of imaging of eyelid and conjunctival lesions. In particular, OCT can be helpful in the diagnosis of conjunctival diseases such as lymphoma and amyloidosis (Venkateswaran et al. 2019). OCT technology is also opening up new areas of application in the imaging of periocular skin and skin tumors in the periocular region including basal cell carcinoma or squamous cell carcinoma of the eyelid. With special dermal OCT devices with a longer wavelength of 1305 nm, which are already established in this field, the extent of basal cell carcinomas of the skin can be determined up to a penetration depth of approx. 1 cm, as well as peripheral palisading, can be visualized (Coleman et al. 2013). In addition, dermal OCT helps to differentiate basal cell carcinomas from other disease entities such as actinic keratoses (Olsen et al. 2016). Also, dermal OCT shows a good correlation between preoperative OCT images and histopathology, especially in basal cell carcinomas (Pelosini et al. 2013). While these dermal OCT devices are already used in routine dermatologic diagnosis, these devices are not yet established in clinical practice in the field of ophthalmology (Pelosini et al. 2015). However, in the future, these dermal OCT devices could not only contribute to finding the correct diagnosis already preoperatively but could also be of great importance in preoperative inci-

A. C. Rokohl (✉) · S. Siebelmann · L. M. Heindl
Department of Ophthalmology, University hospital of Cologne, Cologne, Germany
e-mail: alexander.rokohl@uk-koeln.de

L. M. Heindl and S. Siebelmann (eds.), *Optical Coherence Tomography of the Anterior Segment*, https://doi.org/10.1007/978-3-031-07730-2_4

sion margin planning in periocular tumors. Thus, the routine establishment might even reduce the number of resections and at the same time reduce the loss of healthy tissue being essential for ophthalmoplastic reconstruction (Kakkassery et al. 2020; Kakkassery and Heindl 2020; Rokohl et al. 2020a). Also, preoperative dermal OCT could potentially prevent complications and further improve the safety profile of surgery. In particular, the ability to image all layers of the skin using dermal optical coherence tomography and, for example, to detect invasive pathology at an early stage would be of great benefit. The increasing resolution in the field of dermal OCT in recent years, the development of new diagnostic modules, such as the imaging of vascularization of the skin or tumors, as well as the possibility of volume calculation and three-dimensional imaging of specific structures, will most likely lead to the establishment of dermal OCT in clinical routine in the coming years.

The following chapter will give a short overview of OCT findings in different diseases of the conjunctiva and eyelids.

1 Eyelid Diseases

Basal cell carcinoma of the eyelid

Basal cell carcinoma is the most common malignant tumor in ophthalmology, but also one of the most common malignant tumors overall (Rokohl et al. 2020a). In most cases, periocular basal cell carcinomas are localized to the lower eyelid and present clinically as waxy, shiny, indurated lesions with a pearly cord-like marginal rim, surrounding telangiectasia and/or central ulceration, as well as madarosis (Rokohl et al. 2020a, b). Clinico-histopathologically, three main forms can be distinguished: nodular, nodular-ulcerative, and morphea basal cell carcinoma (Hou et al. 2020). In contrast, pigmented, superficial, or metatypical basal cell carcinoma are rather rare. Histopathologically, there are usually undermining infiltrates of a basaloid tumor with balled trabecular growth, sometimes with peripheral palisading of the cells. The cells were predominantly monomorphic with isolated pleomorphic nuclei and partly enclosed mitoses (Figs. 1 and 2).

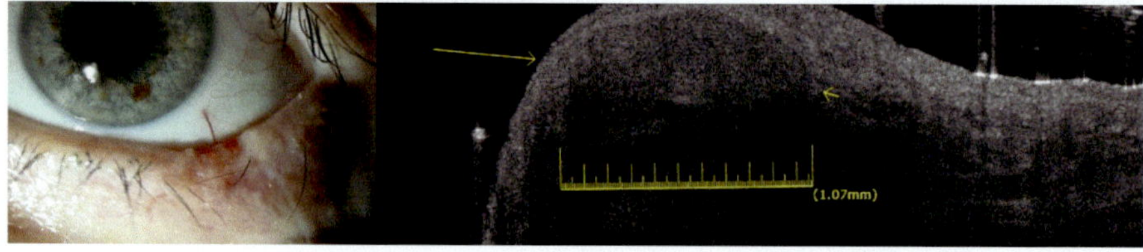

Fig. 1 Nodular basal cell carcinoma of the lower eyelid. Clinically, telangiectasia and ulceration with madarosis are present. Dermal OCT shows a 1.07 mm wide, low-reflective nodular tumor directly at the lid margin, sharply demarcated from the lighter surrounding stroma

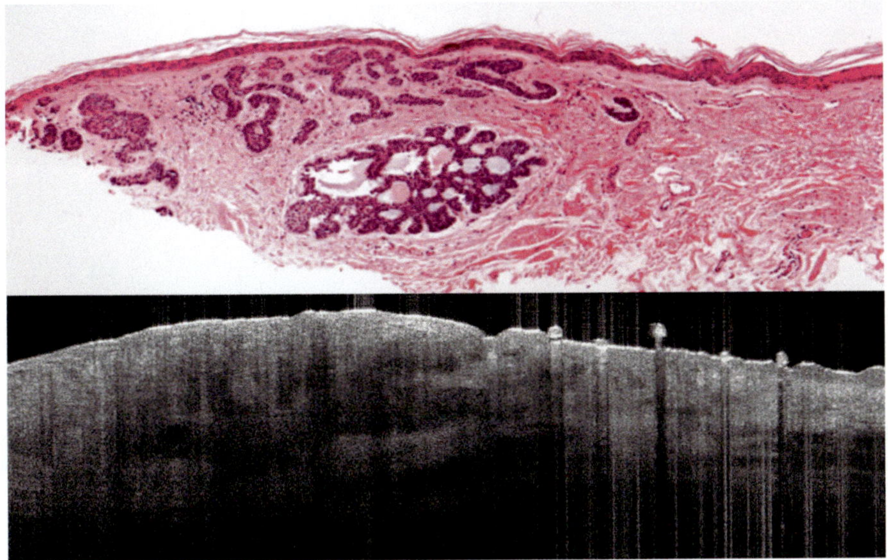

Fig. 2 Basal cell carcinoma with invasive growth in histologic HE cut and matching dermal OCT. Starting from the basal cells of the epidermis, the basal cells have formed nests in the dermis. These consist of variable cells with large nuclei and mitosis. OCT shows multiple hyporeflective tumor nests in the dermis. Image courtesy of Vivosight®, Michelson Diagnostics, UK

Capillary hemangioma of the eyelid

Capillary hemangiomas are often congenital and usually grow rapidly during the first months of life. Clinically, they appear as a reddish mass. Periocular capillary hemangiomas are mostly localized on the upper eyelid. Histologically, capillary hemangiomas show small capillaries with clots (Fig. 3).

Squamous cell carcinoma of the eyelid

Squamous cell carcinoma is the most common skin tumor besides basal cell carcinoma. The most important etiological factor is chronic UV exposure. Therefore, it occurs predominantly on chronically light-exposed skin sites, including the eyelids. The clinical picture of squamous cell carcinoma is very variable and depends mainly on the duration of the tumor. Squamous cell carcinomas can appear skin-colored to dirty-gray or brownish yellow to reddish. The growth can be nodular-tumorous, exophytic, ulcerative, or plaque-like. Histologically, there is usually the proliferation of eosinophilic cells originating from the surface epithelium. These contain variously differentiated keratinocytes that infiltrate the different layers of the dermis or the subcutis in a finger-like pattern or broad cell bonds. Frequently, the tumor contains a pronounced cell polymorphism with partly extensively differentiated keratinocytes and also small epithelial bulbs. In these, concentrically arranged keratinocytes are grouped around a horny bead. Increasing de-differentiation of the cells in the deeper layers is often observed (Fig. 4).

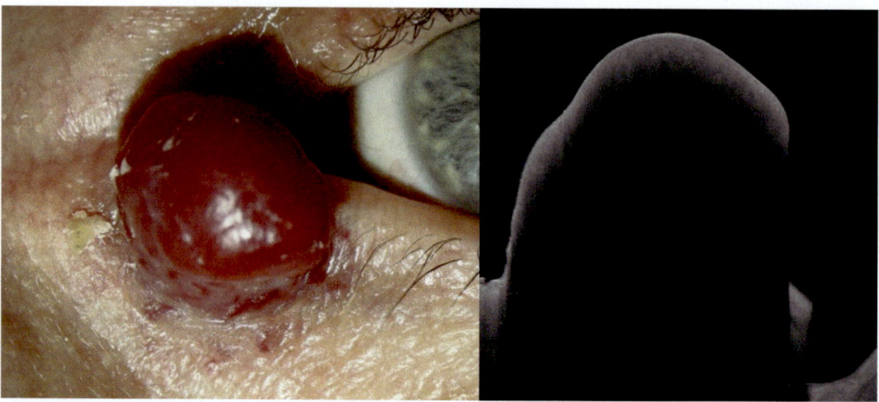

Fig. 3 Capillary hemangioma of the lower eyelid. Clinically, there is a deep red nodular mass with surrounding telangiectasia. OCT shows a hyperreflective outer layer followed by a hyporeflective tumor interior due to the high tumor density

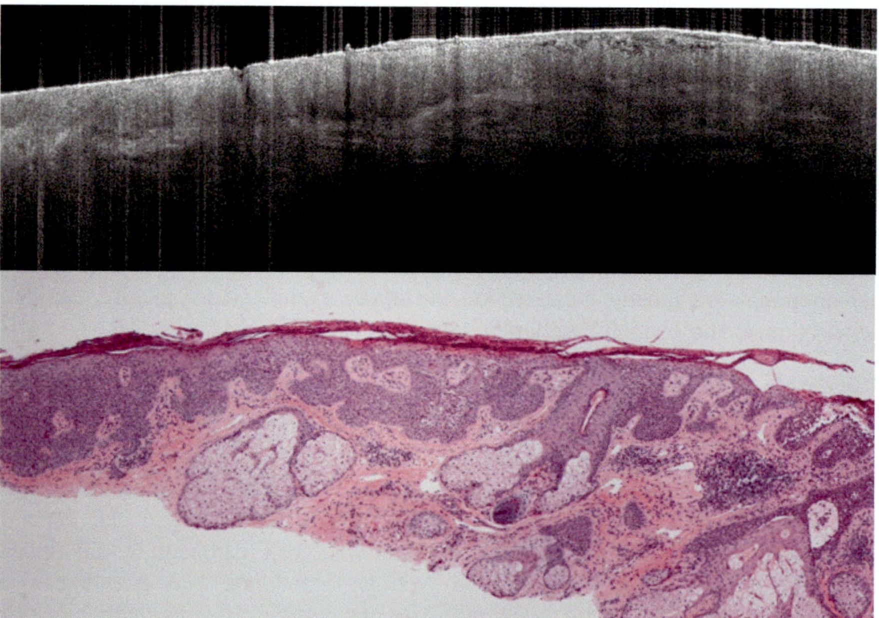

Fig. 4 Squamous cell carcinoma in situ. Dermal OCT shows a widened epidermis, a partially irregular dermo-epidermal junctional zone, and irregular hyperreflective structures in the dermis. Histologically, there is a proliferation of eosinophilic cells originating from the surface epithelium with variously differentiated keratinocytes infiltrating the different layers of the dermis in finger-like or broad cell bonds. Figure provided courtesy of Vivosight®, Michelson Diagnostics, UK

2 Diseases of the Conjunctiva

Primary acquired melanosis of the conjunctiva

In primary acquired melanosis (PAM) of the conjunctiva, blurred and irregularly circumscribed conjunctival hyperpigmentation usually occurs after the age of 40. These are usually located bulbar and/or near the limbus. These hyperpigmentations can spread in the further course and also form a prominence. In addition, inflammatory reactions appear regularly. The clinical picture is pathognomonic for acquired melanosis of the conjunctiva and helps to differentiate it from stationary conjunctival nevus. Both degeneration tendencies and disappearance of lesions without therapy may occur. Histologically, pigment proliferation is found in the conjunctival epithelial layers, particularly in the basal cell layer (Naumann 1980). However, pigment proliferation can in principle occur in any cell layer (Fig. 5).

Conjunctival nevus

Nevi of the conjunctiva are considered hamartomas and account for a large proportion of all excised conjunctival tumors (Naumann 1980). Conjunctival nevi can be congenital or acquired and usually manifest unilaterally. Clinically, they typically present as solitary, slightly raised to nodular, circumscribed thickenings of the conjunctiva with highly variable pigmentation and pseudocysts. The presence of pseudocysts is an important criterion to differentiate nevi from conjunctival melanosis. Pigmentation may not appear until puberty and may then mimic growth. Conjunctival nevi are usually localized to the limbus, lid margins, or caruncle (Fig. 6).

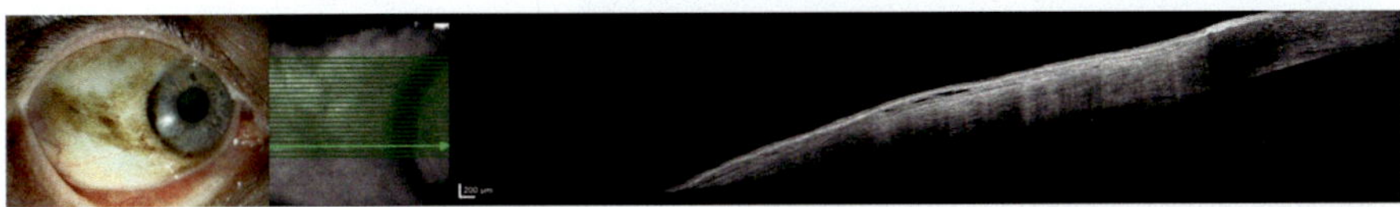

Fig. 5 Unilateral primary acquired melanosis. OCT imaging shows hyperreflectivity of the basal epithelial cell layer of the conjunctiva. In addition, a small cleavage of the conjunctiva, most likely due to an inflammatory reaction, is present

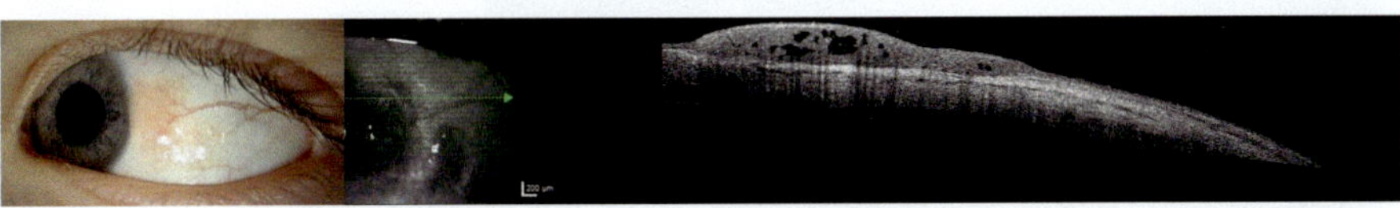

Fig. 6 Amelanotic conjunctival nevus. OCT imaging shows marked thickening of the conjunctiva near the limbus with pseudocysts

Conjunctival papillae

Papillae of the conjunctiva usually occur in the context of chronic conjunctivitis vernalis, but also more often in contact lens wearers. Clinically, there are bulges of the conjunctiva with a very variable size expression. The papillae appear hyperemic due to the central vessel. Histologically, the increased epithelium overlaps the hyperplastic stroma (Naumann 1980) (Fig. 7).

Conjunctival follicles

Conjunctival follicles can occur in the setting of both acute and chronic conjunctivitis. Common causes are infections with adenoviruses, herpesviruses, or chlamydia. Allergic reactions and various topical medications such as iodine and atropine may also be causative. Clinically, follicles appear as whitish to gray, oval to round conjunctival elevations. Vessels are seen only at the margin but, unlike the conjunctival papillae, do not reach the center. Histologically, there is a thinned epithelium with underlying lymphoid hyperplasia with secondary vascularization (Naumann 1980) (Fig. 8).

Pinguecula

A Pinguecula appears as a yellowish prominence of the conjunctiva in the palpebral fissure area and usually occurs in middle adulthood. The pinguecula itself is of no clinical significance but may cause discomfort due to secondary changes in the tear

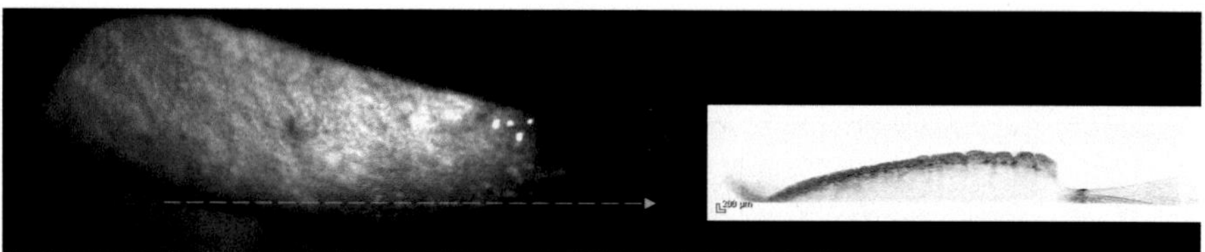

Fig. 7 OCT of the upper tarsus (the upper lid was ectropinated for this purpose) shows small protrusions of the conjunctiva. This papillary hypertrophy is reminiscent of so-called cobblestones

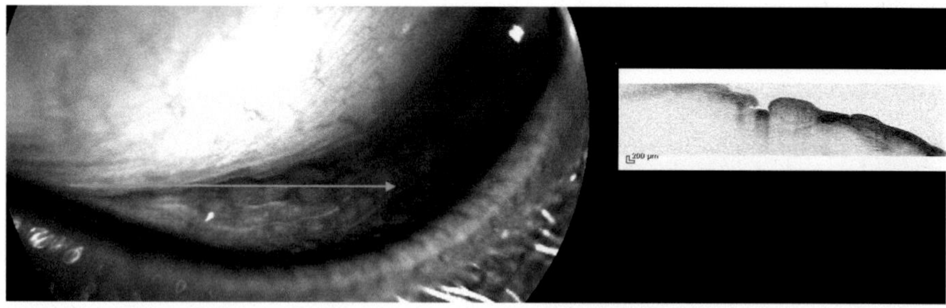

Fig. 8 Conjunctival follicles. OCT clearly shows oval to round elevations of the conjunctiva. In distinction to the conjunctival giant papillae, no central vessel can be visualized

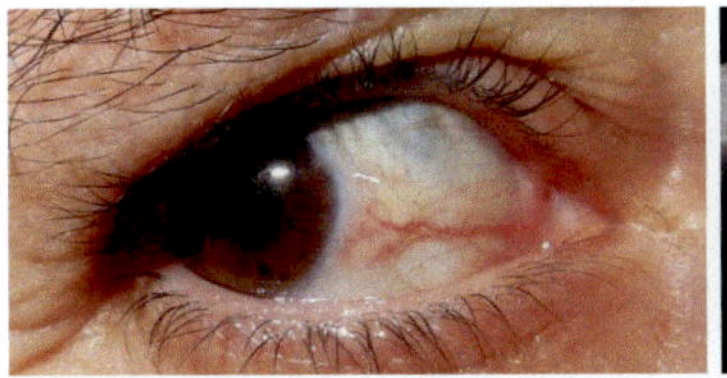
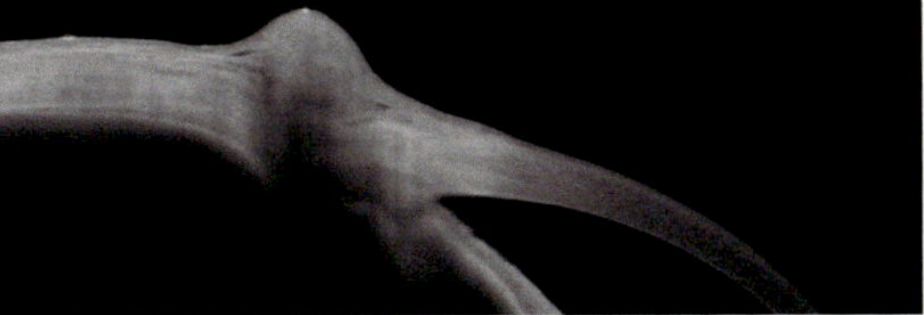

Fig. 9 Pinguecula of the conjunctiva. Clinically, a prominent, yellowish conjunctival lesion with marked, secondary inflammatory vascular injection was seen. In OCT, the pinguecula also presents as a prominent lesion with signal extinction in the scleral region. Vascular incisions can also be visualized

film. Histologically, there is marked thickening of the conjunctival stroma due to marked degeneration of the collagen fibers (Naumann 1980) (Fig. 9).

Pterygium

The Pterygium, a thickening of the conjunctiva with large-caliber vessels that grow on the cornea, is usually localized in the nasal palpebral fissure area. The most important risk factor for its development is ultraviolet radiation. Histologically, nonkeratinizing epithelium without goblet cells is found. In some cases, the multilayered keratinizing squamous epithelium also develops. The subepithelial stroma is thickened with areas of degeneration and vessels (Naumann 1980) (Fig. 10).

Dermo lipoma of the conjunctiva

Typically, dermo lipomas are located in the temporal upper quadrant between the rectus lateralis and rectus superior muscles. Extension into the orbit or on the cornea is not uncommon. Dermo lipomas usually show a reddish color and, in contrast to the adipose tissue prolapse, are not reducible and only slightly displaceable. Histologically, dermo lipomas consist predominantly of fatty tissue (Naumann 1980) (Fig. 11).

Conjunctival cyst

Conjunctival cysts due to epithelial invasion usually develop after mechanical irritation, e.g., by eye rubbing, after surgery, or trauma, and mainly affect elderly people. Histopathologically, there is usually a fluid-filled mass bordered by conjunctival stroma with an epithelial lining (Fig. 12).

Fig. 10 Pterygium of the conjunctiva. In OCT, the conjunctiva growing on the cornea is clearly hyperreflective compared to the cornea

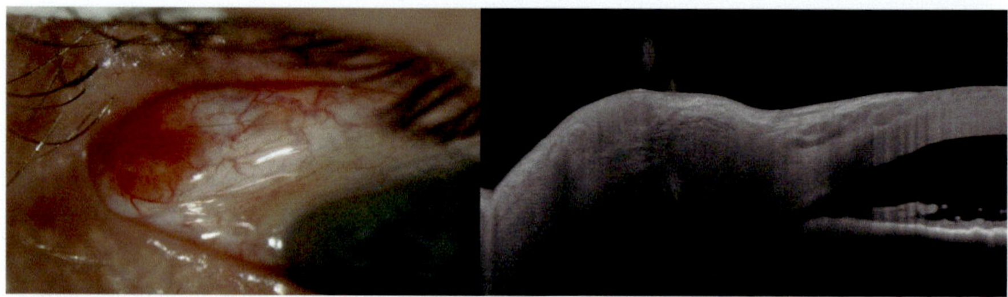

Fig. 11 Dermo lipoma of the conjunctiva in the temporal upper quadrant. OCT shows a solid mass with extension to the cornea

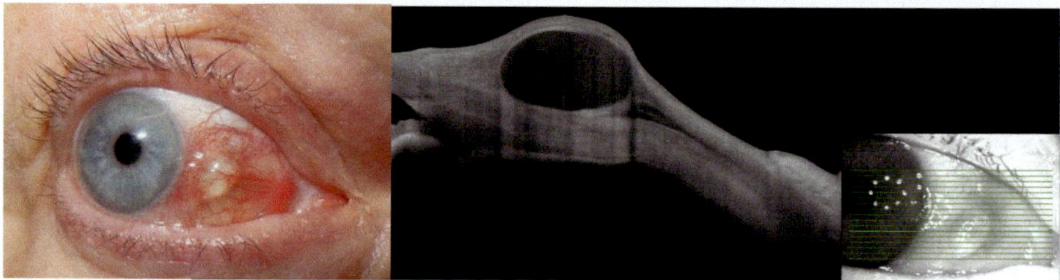

Fig. 12 Epithelial invasion cyst of the conjunctiva. Clinically, there is a prominent fluid-filled mass in the conjunctiva and a clear conjunctival injection due to inflammation. OCT shows a clearly demarcated conjunctival mass with a cystic fluid-filled space. The conjunctiva overlying the cyst presents thinned compared to the chemotic, pericystic conjunctiva. In addition, vascular incisions are delineable on OCT

Conclusions

Imaging by high-resolution OCT has not yet been established in routine clinical practice for diseases of the conjunctiva and eyelids. However, dermal OCT already provides high-resolution imaging that adds important diagnostic information to slit-lamp-only findings and may potentially find application in therapeutic decisions as well as preoperative planning. Dermal OCT will likely be routinely used in the diagnosis of periocular tumors in the next years. In perspective, the technology of OCT will be further developed and improved, e.g., by the use of nanoparticles or magnetomotive particles.

References

Berufsverband der Augenarzte Deutschlands e V, Deutsche Ophthalmologische G, Retinologische Gesellschaft e V. [Quality assurance of optical coherence tomography for diagnostics of the fundus: positional statement of the BVA, DOG and RG]. Ophthalmologe. 2017;114(7):617–24. https://doi.org/10.1007/s00347-017-0508-9.

Coleman AJ, Richardson TJ, Orchard G, Uddin A, Choi MJ, Lacy KE. Histological correlates of optical coherence tomography in non-melanoma skin cancer. Skin Res Technol. 2013;19(1):10–9. https://doi.org/10.1111/j.1600-0846.2012.00626.x.

Hou X, Rokohl AC, Ortmann M, Heindl LM. Effective treatment of locally advanced periocular basal cell carcinoma with oral hedgehog pathway inhibitor? Graefes Arch Clin Exp Ophthalmol. 2020. https://doi.org/10.1007/s00417-020-04779-5.

Kakkassery V, Heindl LM. Standard operation procedure in periorbital basal cell carcinoma. Ophthalmologe. 2020;117(2):124. https://doi.org/10.1007/s00347-019-01019-y.

Kakkassery V, Emmert S, Adamietz IA, Kovacs G, Junemann AM, Otte C, et al. Alternative treatment options for periorbital basal cell carcinoma. Ophthalmologe. 2020;117(2):113–23. https://doi.org/10.1007/s00347-019-01021-4.

Naumann GOH. Pathologie des Auges. Berlin: Springer; 1980.

Olsen J, Themstrup L, De Carvalho N, Mogensen M, Pellacani G, Jemec GB. Diagnostic accuracy of optical coherence tomography in actinic keratosis and basal cell carcinoma. Photodiagnosis Photodyn Ther. 2016;16:44–9. https://doi.org/10.1016/j.pdpdt.2016.08.004.

Pelosini L, Smith HB, Schofield JB, Meeckings A, Dhital A, Khandwala M. In vivo optical coherence tomography (OCT) in periocular basal cell carcinoma: correlations between in vivo OCT images and postoperative histology. Br J Ophthalmol. 2013;97(7):890–4. https://doi.org/10.1136/bjophthalmol-2012-303043.

Pelosini L, Smith HB, Schofield JB, Meeckings A, Dithal A, Khandwala M. A novel imaging approach to periocular basal cell carcinoma: in vivo optical coherence tomography and histological correlates. Eye (London). 2015;29(8):1092–8. https://doi.org/10.1038/eye.2015.97.

Rokohl AC, Kopecky A, Guo Y, Kakkassery V, Mor JM, Loreck N, et al. Surgical resection with ophthalmoplastic reconstruction: Gold standard in periocular basal cell carcinoma. Ophthalmologe. 2020a;117(2):95–105. https://doi.org/10.1007/s00347-019-00973-x.

Rokohl AC, Loser H, Mor JM, Loreck N, Koch KR, Heindl LM. Young male patient with unusual space-occupying lesion of the lower eyelid. Ophthalmologe. 2020b;117(1):73–7. https://doi.org/10.1007/s00347-019-00948-y.

Venkateswaran N, Mercado C, Tran AQ, Garcia A, Diaz PFM, Dubovy SR, et al. The use of high resolution anterior segment optical coherence tomography for the characterization of conjunctival lymphoma, conjunctival amyloidosis and benign reactive lymphoid hyperplasia. Eye Vis (Lond). 2019;6:17. https://doi.org/10.1186/s40662-019-0143-4.

Degenerative Corneal Disorders

Alexander Händel, Sebastian Siebelmann, and Claus Cursiefen

Degenerative corneal disorders are corneal changes that occur due to age, after injury or after (chronic) disease. Pathological changes of the curvature radii as well as opacities of the cornea can therefore lead to considerable visual impairment, changes of the visual impression (astigmatism, diplopia), photophobia or pain. The diagnostic and therapeutic possibilities have changed considerably in recent years, especially due to anterior segment OCT imaging (Ang et al. 2018). More precise diagnosis, individual therapy concepts (laser surgery (e.g. PTK), abrasion of the cornea, keratoplasty (lamellar or penetrating), vascular cauterization, local therapy (e.g. anti-VEGF (Vascular Endothelial Growth Factor)), improvement of visualization of surgical steps, as well as postoperative success control have been improved or made possible by anterior segment OCT imaging (Siebelmann et al. 2015a). In addition to patients with chronic corneal diseases such as keratoconus or with corneal scars following trauma or infection, children and infants with rare ocular anomalies or dysgenesias in particular benefit from anterior segment OCT (Siebelmann et al. 2015b).

1   Keratoconus

Keratoconus is a progressive corneal disease in which there is thinning of central and paracentral areas with concomitant irregular deformation of the cornea. Keratoconus was long considered a rare disease. However, a recent study from the Netherlands shows that the prevalence is higher than assumed in older studies

A. Händel (✉)
8001 Zürich, Switzerland
e-mail: alexander.haendel@uk-koeln.de

S. Siebelmann · C. Cursiefen
Department of Opthalmology, University Hospital of Cologne, 50937 Cologne, Germany

© The Author(s), under exclusive license to Springer Nature Switzerland AG 2022
L. M. Heindl and S. Siebelmann (eds.), *Optical Coherence Tomography of the Anterior Segment*, https://doi.org/10.1007/978-3-031-07730-2_5

(annual incidence in the Dutch population aged 10–40 years of 1:7500 or 13.3 new cases per 100 000 inhabitants; mean age at first diagnosis was 28.3 years and 60.6% of them were male) (Godefrooij et al. 2017). About 25% of affected patients suffer from a progressive course of keratoconus.

In the meantime, the spectrum of treatment options for keratoconus is very broad, so that satisfactory to very good visual acuity can be permanently achieved in most patients (Mas Tur et al. 2017). Ectasia of keratoconus progresses in stages, and the individual course is unpredictable in terms of time of onset, duration, and frequency of progression.

The following are some typical and rare findings in keratoconus patients.

2 Vogt's Striae

These are fine, vertically parallel striae in the posterior stroma and Descemet's membrane. These usually disappear when firm pressure is applied to the eyeball and reappear when pressure is removed. The presence and expression of Vogt's striae may be asymmetric depending on the degree of keratoconus. In the magnified slit-lamp photograph, the vertically extending Vogt's striae are clearly visible (Fig. 1). In anterior segment OCT (Fig. 2), Vogt's striae can be visualized as fine hyperreflective structures on the endothelium.

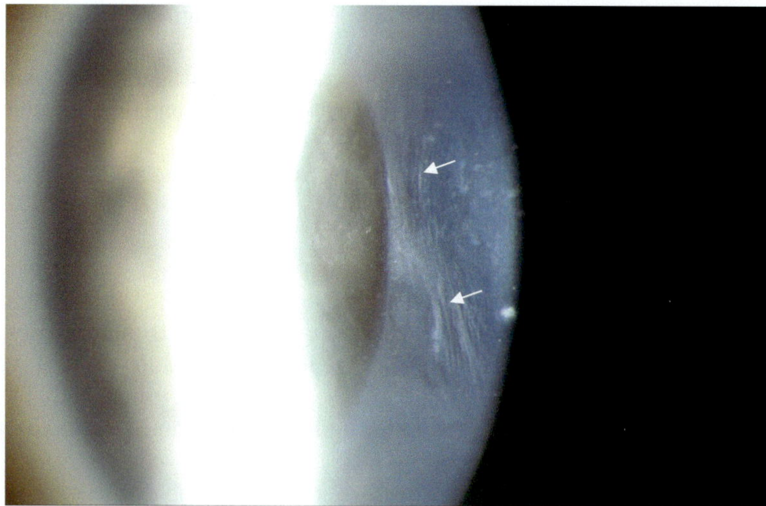

Fig. 1 Slit photograph with focus on the endothelium. Here, the vertically running Vogt's striae of a keratoconus patient can be imaged (white arrows)

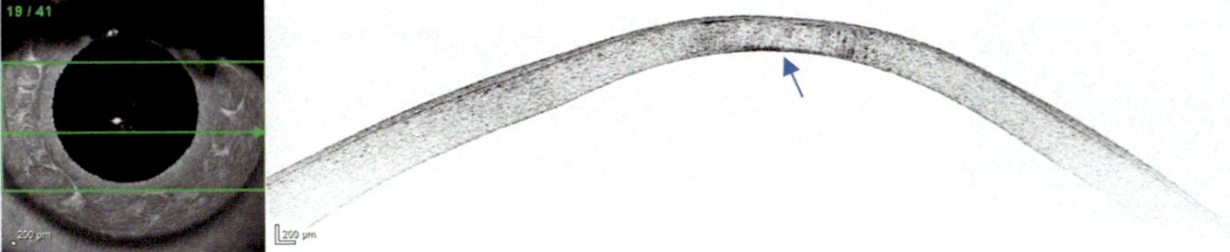

Fig. 2 Anterior segment OCT of a keratoconus patient. The Vogt's striae can be visualized on OCT as hyperreflective fine structures on the endothelium (blue arrow)

3 Corneal Ectasia

Keratoconus is a uni- or bilateral corneal ectasia characterized by central thinning and protrusion of the cornea, resulting in a cone-shaped protrusion. Slit-lamp microscopy (Fig. 3) shows corneal ectasia with a maximum keratometry (Kmax) of 120dpt. The corneal thickness at the thinnest point (blue arrow) is 151 μm in the anterior segment OCT shown here (Fig. 4) and is thus severely thinned.

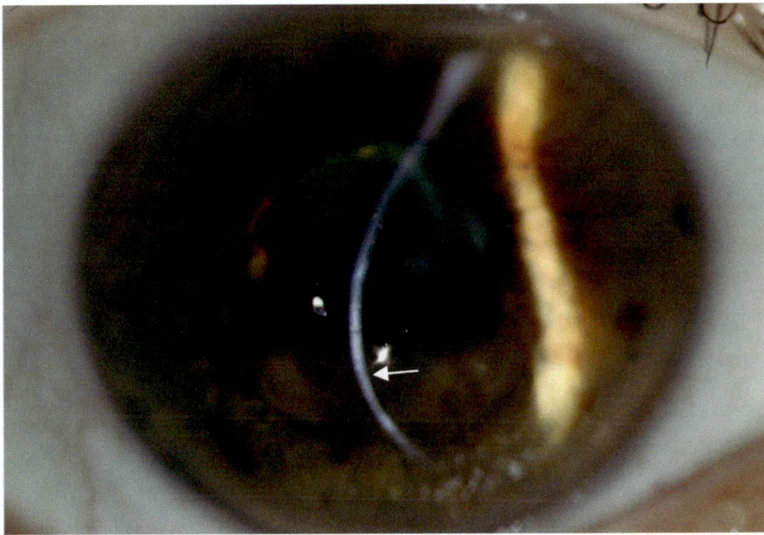

Fig. 3 Slit lamp photo of corneal ectasia in keratoconus. The cornea is strongly thinned and curved anteriorly (white arrow), the maximum keratometry (K max) here is 120dpt

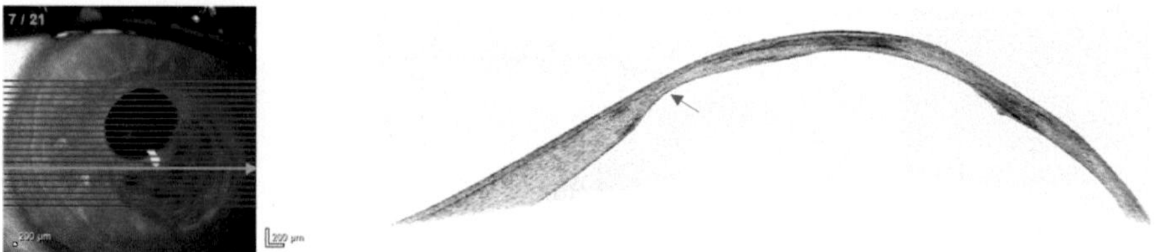

Fig. 4 Anterior segment OCT in corneal ectasia in keratoconus. The cornea is severely thinned and measures only 151 μm corneal thickness in the thinnest area (blue arrow)

4 Demarcation Line After Crosslinking

If progression can be detected based on the tomographic corneal images, it is recommended to perform UV-A riboflavin crosslinking (CXL). Collagen crosslinking with riboflavin and UV-A light is used to chemically crosslink the collagen fibers of the cornea. This increases the number of crosslinks in the cornea and thus the mechanical stability. This procedure serves to stabilize and thus reduce the progression, avoiding the need for corneal transplantation and preserving the possibility of compensation with glasses or contact lenses.

As a result of CXL treatment, a demarcation line, a transition zone between the cross-linked anterior corneal stroma and the untreated posterior corneal stroma, may develop. Using slit lamp microscopy, a fine hyperreflective line can be seen in the corneal stroma here (Fig. 5); this is the demarcation line (white arrow). In the anterior segment OCT (Fig. 6), a line is seen in the center of the corneal stroma (blue arrow, demarcation line), below which is the untreated stroma, above which is the crosslinked anterior corneal stroma after crosslinking.

5 Subepithelial Corneal Scar

When fitting rigid contact lenses, a good fit is essential. The contact lens should float on the tear film and not touch the apex. In keratoconus patients, this is a particular challenge because the cornea curves forward in a cone shape. If ill-fitting rigid contact lenses that sit on the apex are worn for an extended period of time, subepithelial scars can form. A slit-lamp photograph shows a corneal scar in the apex region (Fig. 7, white arrow), and anterior segment OCT shows the hyperreflective subepithalial scar (Fig. 8, white arrow). In addition, thinning of the epithelium is evident.

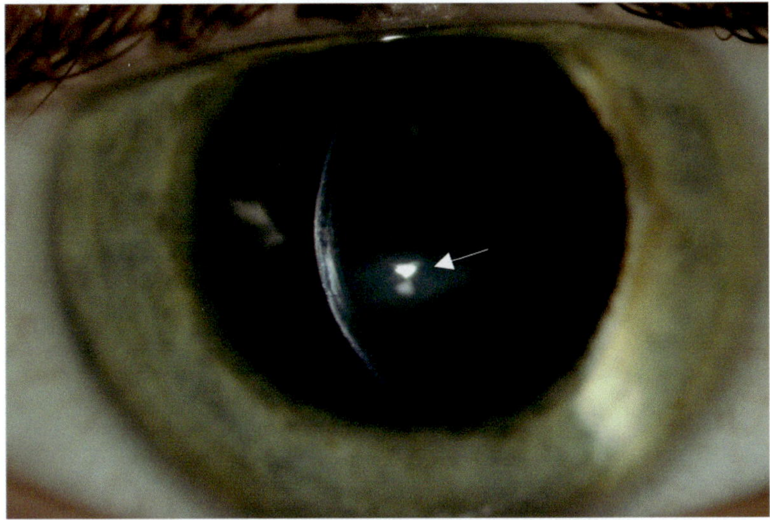

Fig. 5 Slit lamp microscopy of a patient after crosslinking. The demarcation line can be visualized in the slit in the stroma as a hyperreflective line (white arrow)

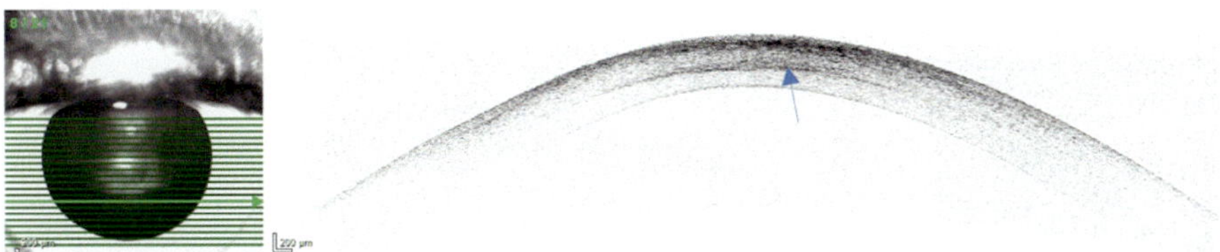

Fig. 6 Anterior segment OCT after crosslinking. In the OCT image, the demarcation line (hyperreflective line, blue arrow) demarcates the crosslinked anterior corneal stroma from the deeper, noncrosslinked stroma

6 DALK Findings Postoperatively

Deep Anterior Lamellar Keratoplasty (DALK) can be a treatment option for visual rehabilitation in cases of keratoconus, among others. The corneal endothelium of the patient is preserved and only the corneal stroma is transplanted. Accordingly, no rejection reaction against the corneal endothelium can occur with DALK, which statistically significantly increases graft survival (Hos et al. 2019). In keratoconus, DALK is an option when contact lenses do not provide sufficient visual rehabilitation.

In the slit lamp microscopy (Fig. 9), the tight double running suture can be seen, the graft is well adapted without evidence of a step and the Descemet's membrane is attached. This is confirmed on anterior segment OCT (Fig. 10), which shows that

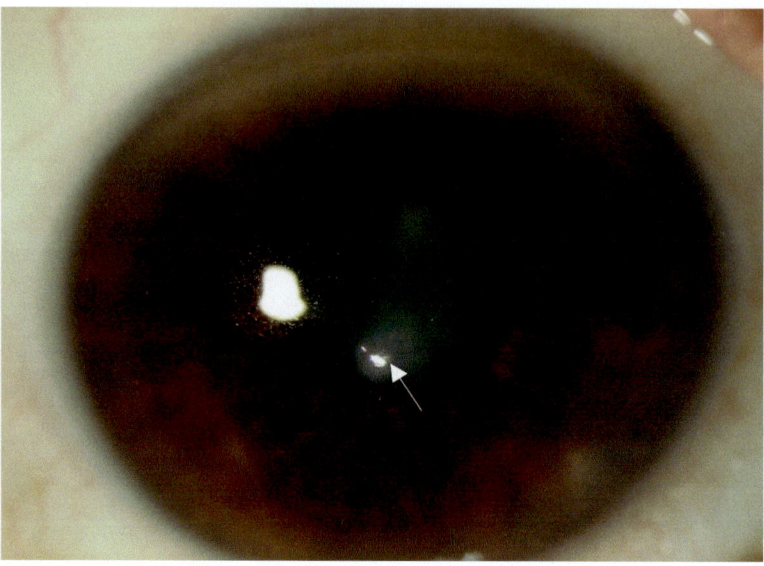

Fig. 7 Clinical photograph of a keratoconus patient with corneal scar at the apex (white arrow) due to ill-fitting rigid contact lenses

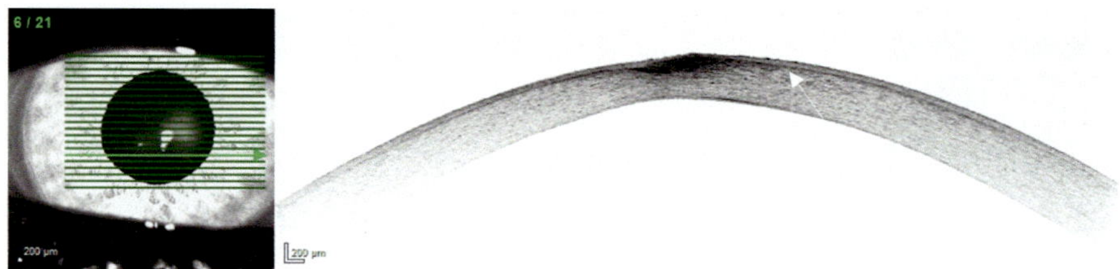

Fig. 8 Anterior segment OCT showing corneal scar at the apex (white arrow) due to ill-fitting rigid contact lenses in keratoconus. The scar extends into the anterior stromal corneal areas

the Descemet's membrane is tight throughout the graft. In the anterior segment OCT, the graft clearly demarcates from the recipient bed in the form of a vertically visible line (white arrow), the transitions are smooth and in some cases stitch channels are visible.

7 Implantation of Ring Segments

Another therapeutic option for keratoconus, which can counteract the increasing myopia and thus lead to a temporary improvement of visual acuity, is the implantation of corneal ring segments from different manufacturers.

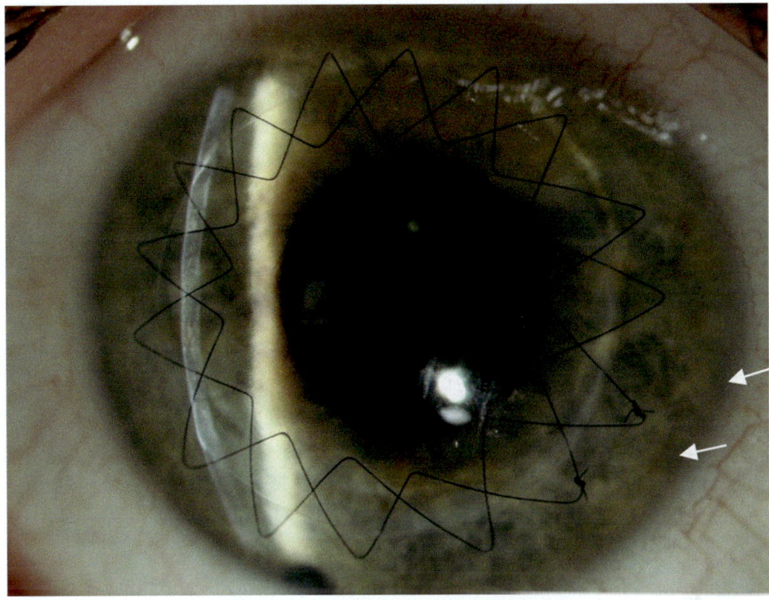

Fig. 9 Postoperative slit lamp findings after DALK with double running suture (white arrows) in keratoconus

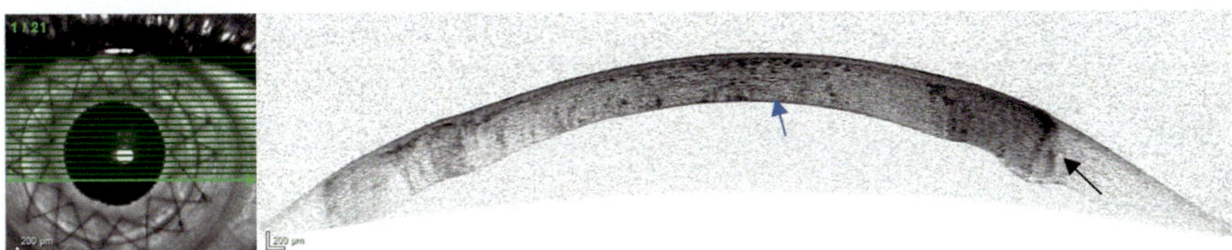

Fig. 10 Anterior segment OCT after DALK with Descemet membrane in place (blue arrow) and step-free transition between graft and recipient bed (black arrow)

By means of this method on the one hand an increased stability of the cornea is achieved and on the other hand it leads to a more even shape of the cornea and thus to a better visual performance (under certain circumstances with glasses or contact lenses). The basic requirement is that the cornea must not be below a certain thickness. In slit lamp microscopy (Fig. 11) the intracorneal implants can be seen. In the anterior segment OCT (Fig. 12) the position of the implants in the corneal stroma can be seen temporally and nasally. Of particular importance for the assessment of the correct position of the implants is the distance between the endothelium and the ring segment, as well as between the surface or epithelium and the implant.

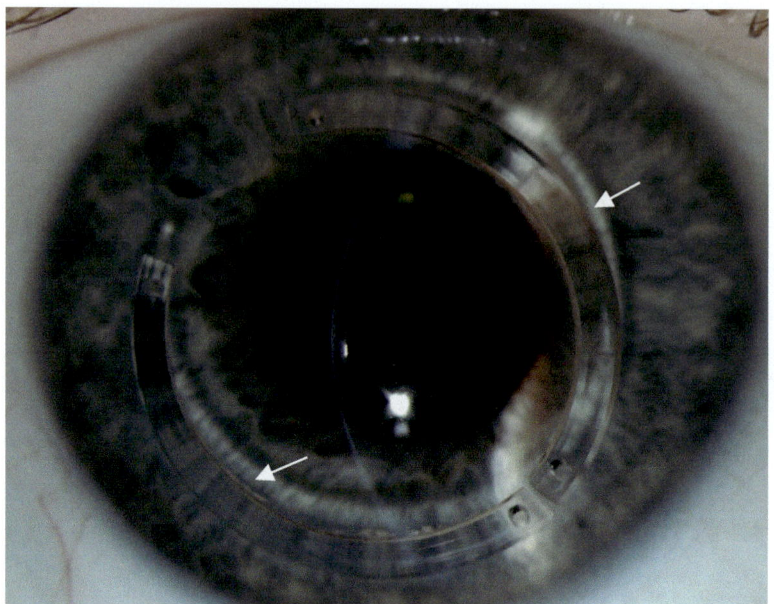

Fig. 11 Slit lamp microscopy shows the two ring segments (white arrows)

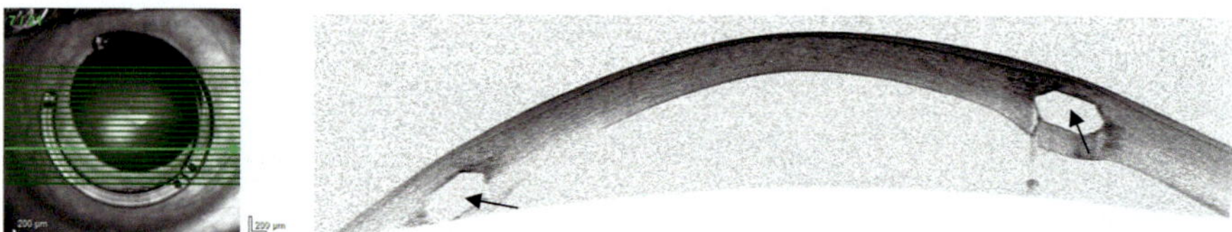

Fig. 12 Anterior segment OCT shows how the ring segments (black arrows) are located centrally in the corneal stroma

8 Krumeich Rings

The implantation of so-called Krumeich rings can be performed in keratoconus during penetrating keratoplasty (Krumeich and Duncker 2006). This rare implantation of this ring has a special alloy. This should reduce neovascularization and rejection reactions. In the slit-lamp photo (Fig. 13) you can see the silver-colored Krumeich ring, in the anterior segment OCT (Fig. 14) you can see how the Krumeich ring is positioned in the cornea.

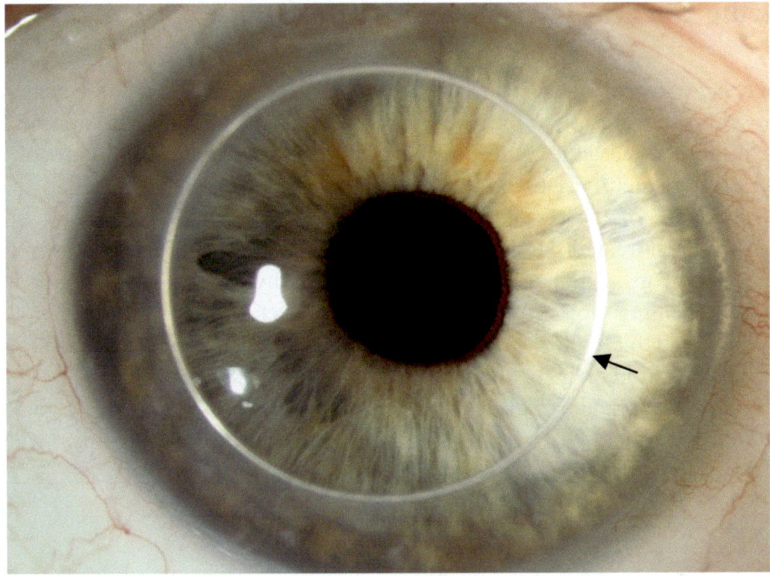

Fig. 13 Krumeich ring (black arrow) in keratoconus. This ring is designed to prevent neovascularization and rejection due to its special alloy

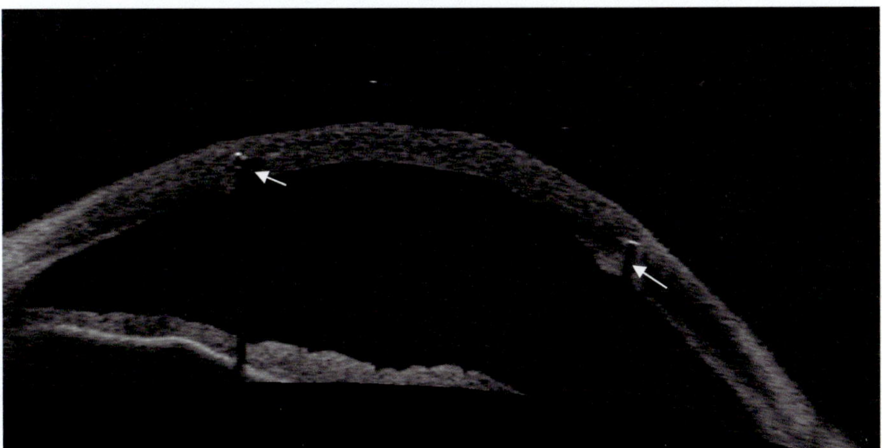

Fig. 14 Anterior segment OCT shows the depth of the ring (white arrows). Due to the nature of the ring being made of metal, the underlying corneal stroma cannot be seen

9   Acute Corneal Hydrops in Keratoconus

In progressive keratoconus, acute corneal hydrops occurs when the ectasia of the corneal stroma progresses to the point where the stiff Descemet's membrane can no longer follow the curvature and thus tears. Sudden and severe focal corneal edema then occurs. Frequently, Descemet's membrane is also partially detached from the posterior surface of the corneal stroma in this situation. This condition of acute hydrops has been treated purely conservatively with hyperosmolar and prophylactic antibiotic eye drops. The natural course after acute hydrops in keratoconus is often benign, but healing not infrequently stretches over months. There are surgical therapy options which allow a very fast dehydration of the cornea (Mini-DMEK or predescemetal sutures) (Siebelmann et al. 2019; Bachmann et al. 2019; Yahia Cherif et al. 2015; Händel et al. 2021). In addition, it is possible to apply gas only to the anterior chamber, but this does not result in as rapid a healing process as Mini-DMEK or predescemetal sutures (Panda et al. 2007).

10   Descemet's Membrane Tear

Acute hydrops in keratoconus with progressive corneal ectasia results in corneal edema due to Descemet's membrane rupture. Slit-lamp findings show focal corneal edema with marked corneal thickening and opacification (Fig. 15). In the anterior segment OCT (Fig. 16), the tear of Descemet's membrane can be seen (blue arrow), and the two ends of the DM are partially curled inward. In addition to the visible tear, Descemet's membrane is also detached from the corneal stroma (dehiscence, green arrow). The cornea is partly clearly thickened and thinned at the apex in the area of the ectasia.

11   Fluid Pockets

Due to the acute fluid inflow in corneal hydrops in keratoconus, fluid may be deposited in the cornea in the form of fluid-filled pockets or vacuoles, so-called ``fluid pockets'. In the slit lamp findings (Fig. 17) a corneal edema with opacity can be seen, the fluid pockets cannot be identified with certainty. Diagnostics with anterior segment OCT (Fig. 18) provide the possibility to determine an individual surgical procedure. Thus, these fluid pockets can be visualized during a surgical procedure using microscope-integrated OCT and can be punctured and drained (Siebelmann et al. 2019).

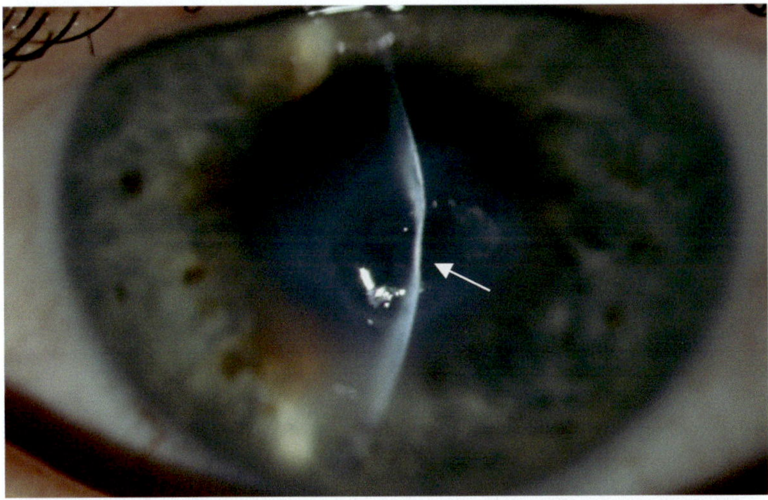

Fig. 15 Slit lamp microscopy of corneal hydrops in keratoconus. The slit shows an edema (white arrow) with intrastromal fluid deposits as well as partly clear corneal thinning and a rupture of Descemet's membrane can be guessed

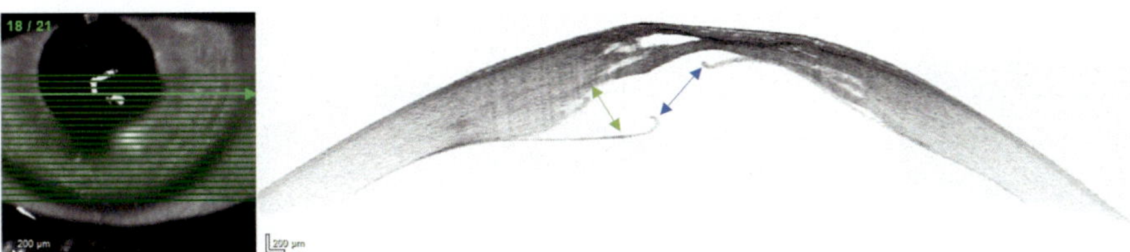

Fig. 16 Anterior segment OCT shows the severely thinned corneal stroma in the apex region with the fluid-filled stromal pockets and the rupture of Descemet's membrane (blue arrow). Descemet's membrane is partially detached from the stroma (green arrow, dehiscence)

12 Mini-DMEK

In case of acute hydrops in keratoconus there is the possibility of surgical intervention. If there is a pronounced tear of the Descemet's membrane, a Mini-DMEK can be performed. In this case, a small graft (<5 mm) is placed in the area of the defect and pressed on by means of gas. This leads to a much faster increase in visual acuity and to a much faster reduction of edema compared to a purely conservative procedure (Bachmann et al. 2019; Händel et al. 2021). Figure 19 shows the preoperative slit lamp findings and Fig. 20 shows the corresponding anterior segment OCT preoperatively with a large Descemet's membrane tear and one end of Descemet's membrane in the area of the tear (blue arrow). Using intraoperative OCT imaging, the Mini-DMEK can be visualized in the anterior chamber (Fig. 21).

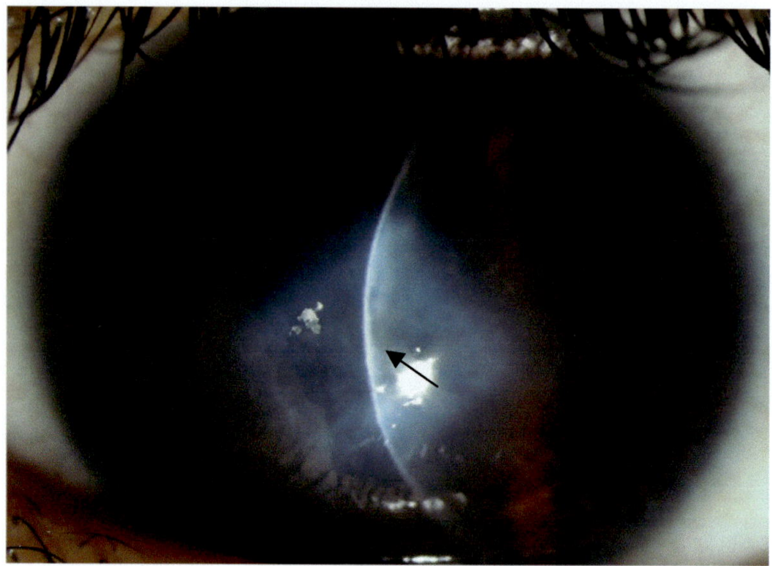

Fig. 17 Slit lamp microscopy of an acute hydrops with significant thickening of the cornea (black arrow), the view in this area is strongly reduced

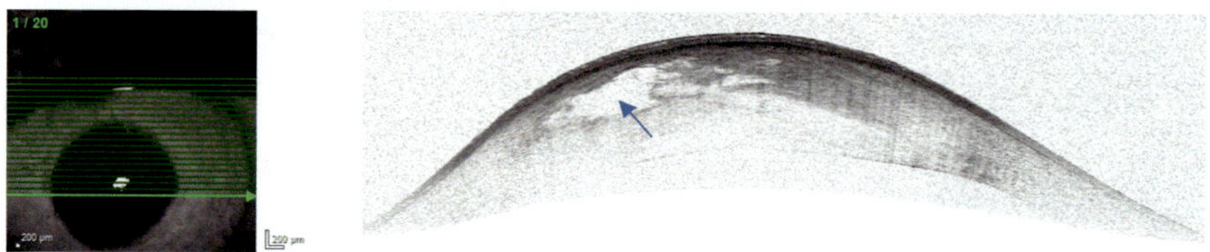

Fig. 18 Anterior segment OCT shows a large fluid-filled pocket (blue arrow) in the corneal stroma here, resulting from Descemet's membrane rupture and increasing corneal ectasia

Anterior segment OCT (Fig. 22) one month after Mini-DMEK shows a clearer cornea and an adherent Descemet's membrane without evidence of dehiscence or rupture.

13   Corneal Compression Sutures

In the case of small to medium-sized Descemet's membrane defects, it is possible to apply predescemetal sutures in the case of acute hydrops in keratoconus (Siebelmann et al. 2019; Händel et al. 2021). These cause Descemet's membrane to reattach to the corneal stroma and compress the stroma, aiding in dehydration. Preoperative slit-lamp and anterior segment OCT findings (Figs. 23 and 24) show

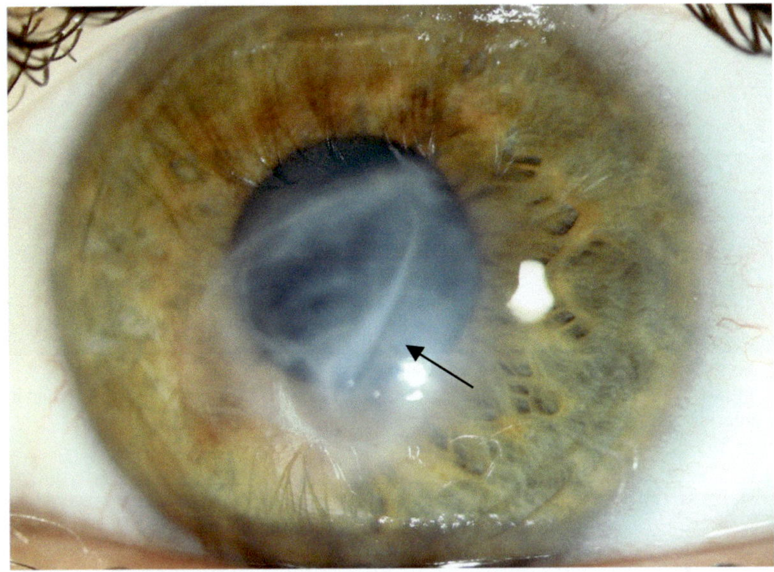

Fig. 19 Slit lamp microscopy shows the typical picture of acute hydrops in keratoconus with corneal edema (black arrow)

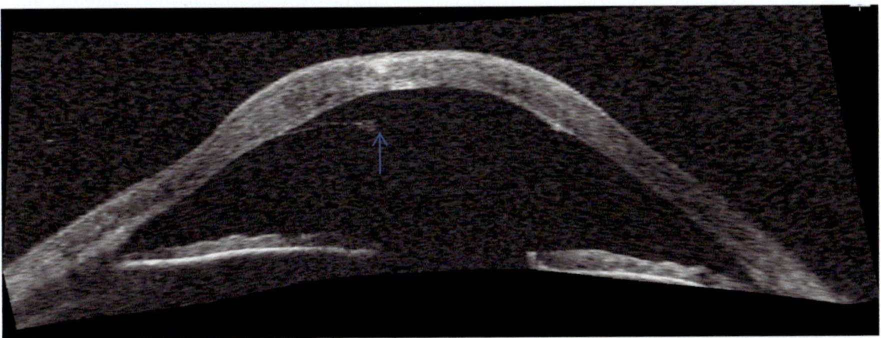

Fig. 20 Anterior segment OCT preperatively shows one end of the ruptured Descemet's membrane (blue arrow). Additionally, the thickened cornea can be seen

corneal edema and fluid pockets (blue arrows, Fig. 24) and dehiscence of Descemet's membrane. After microscope integrated OCT-guided positioning of predescemetal sutures, puncture of fluid pockets, and application of gas into the anterior chamber, the slit-lamp photograph on the first postoperative day (Fig. 25) shows a dehydrated cornea with four tight sutures, and the anterior-segment OCT (Fig. 26) shows an adherent Descemet's membrane and a dehydrated cornea.

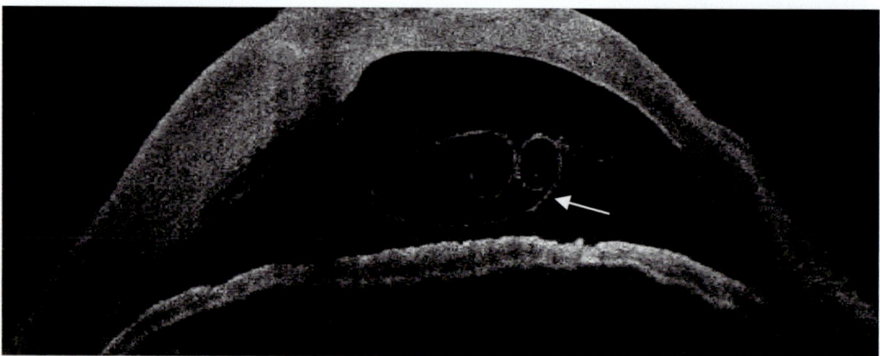

Fig. 21 Intraoperative OCT imaging shows the coiled Mini-DMEK (white arrow) after insertion into the anterior chamber using an IOL shooter

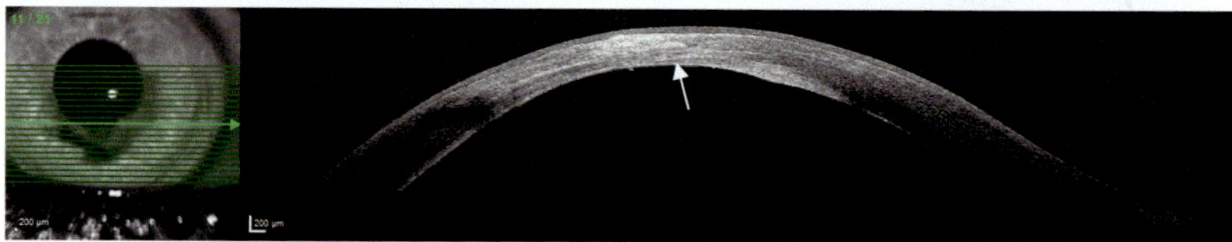

Fig. 22 After performing a Mini-DMEK, anterior segment OCT shows that the endothelium is attached in all areas (white arrow) and the corneal stroma above has dehydrated back to a normal corneal thickness

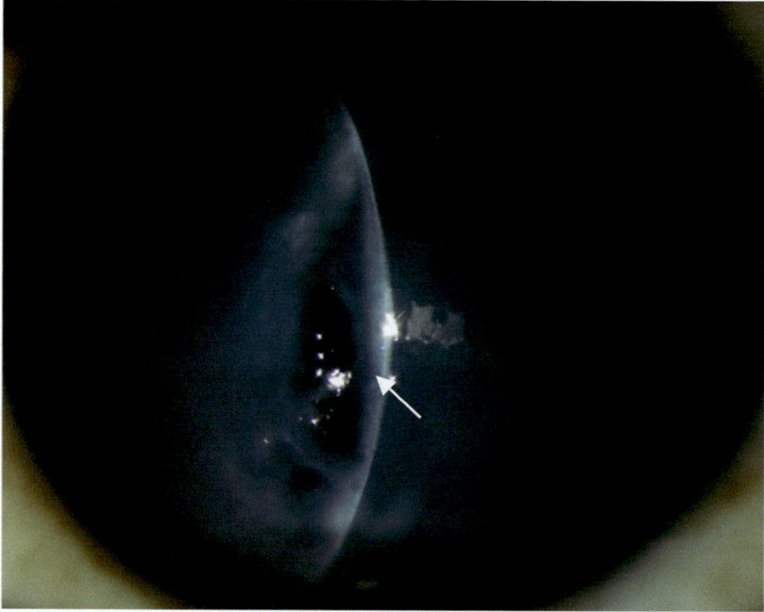

Fig. 23 This shows corneal edema in the setting of acute hydrops in keratoconus (white arrow)

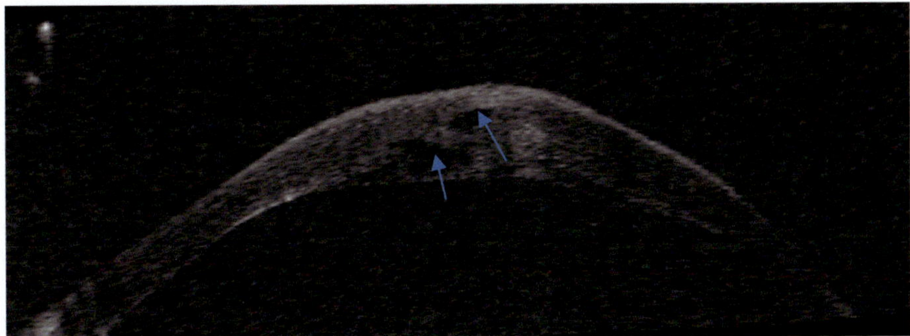

Fig. 24 Anterior segment OCT preoperatively showing fluid pockets (blue arrows) and corneal edema

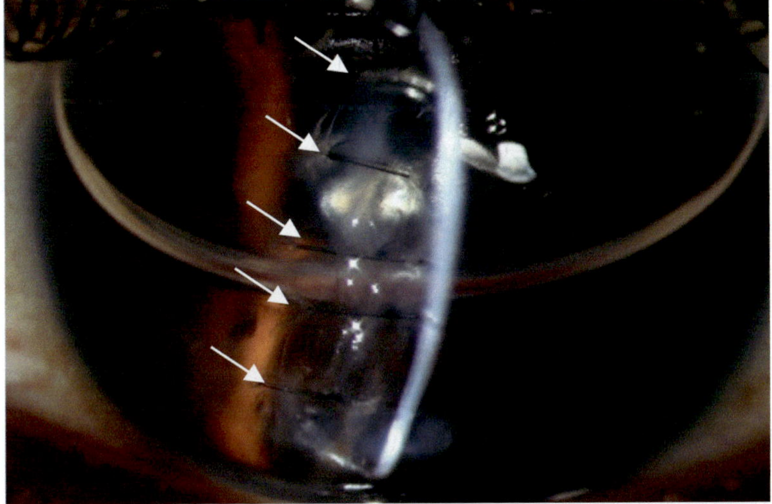

Fig. 25 After application of predescemetal sutures (white arrows) and injection of gas into the anterior chamber, clearing of the cornea is already evident on the first postoperative day

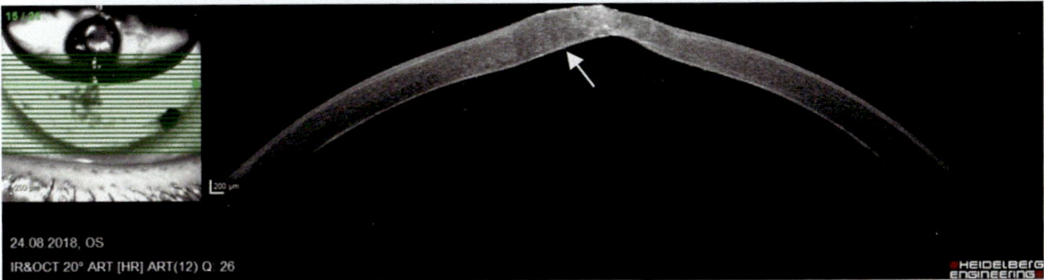

Fig. 26 Anterior segment OCT on the first postoperative day after predescemetal sutures shows a dehydrated cornea, with Descemet's membrane reattached to the corneal stroma (white arrow)

14   Contact Lenses

14.1   Rigid Contact Lenses

Rigid contact lenses can be fitted to correct refractive errors such as myopia, hyperopia (+aphakia), astigmatism and presbyopia.

In the case of keratoconus, rigid contact lenses are used when the refractive error can no longer be corrected with glasses or when the patient wishes to be free of glasses. The contact lens has no therapeutic effect on the keratoconus and serves only for visual rehabilitation. Optimal fitting is important for the further course of the disease. For example, a fitting that is too flat favors a tendency to progression as well as scarring in the apex area due to mechanical stress. In the slit-lamp photograph (Fig. 27), a well-fitted rigid contact lens can be seen that does not extend beyond the limbus and floats on the tear film. In the anterior segment OCT (Fig. 28), the rigid contact lens can be seen overlying the corneal epithelium. The tear film between the lens and the corneal epithelium cannot be seen in the anterior segment OCT. In order to check the optimal fit, staining is performed using fluorescein. The marginal area (bevel) can be very well visualized (Fig. 29, white arrow). In the anterior segment OCT, the bevel can be visualized very well as well; one can see how the contact lens is slightly tilted upwards in the peripheral area (Fig. 30, blue arrow). This ensures better sliding of the contact lens on the eye.

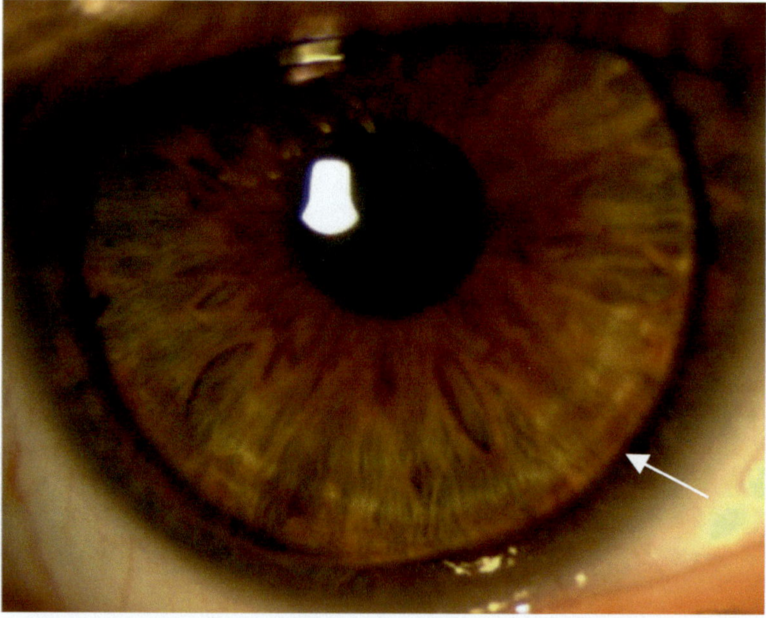

Fig. 27 Rigid contact lens in slit lamp microscopy with central fit without extending beyond the limbus (contact lens margin: white arrow)

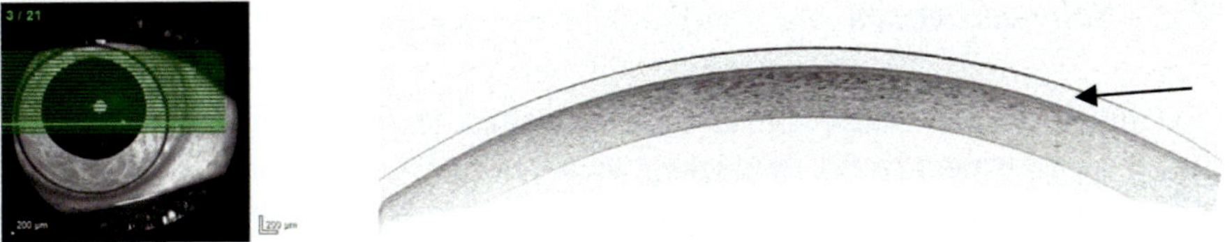

Fig. 28 Anterior segment OCT shows the rigid contact lens (black arrow) on the cornea. The tear film between the lens and the corneal epithelium is not visible in the anterior segment OCT

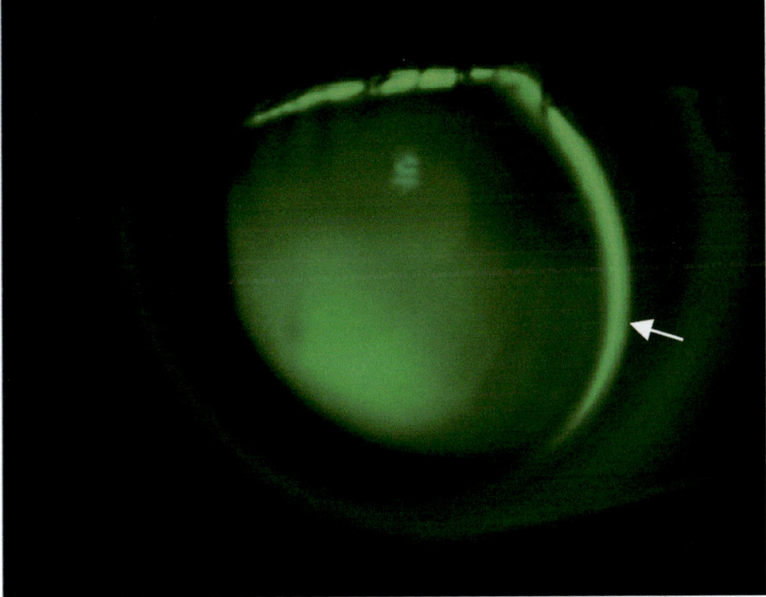

Fig. 29 Fluorescein staining shows the tear film under the lense as well as the increased accumulation of tear fluid in the marginal area (Bevel, white arrow)

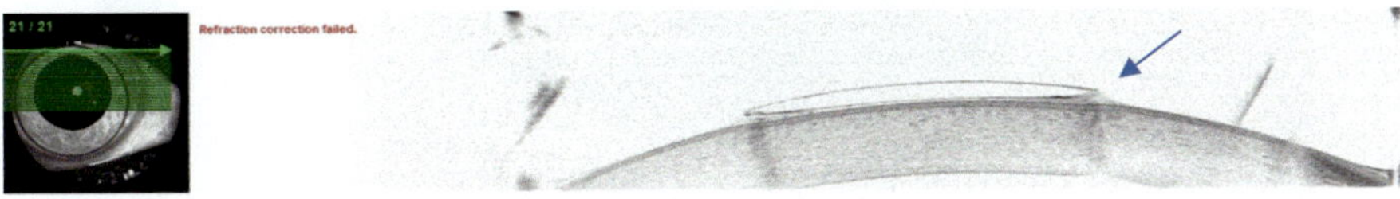

Fig. 30 Anterior segment OCT in the peripheral region. This shows how the contact lens is tilted slightly upward in the marginal area (blue arrow), ensuring better sliding of the contact lens on the eye

14.2 Scleral Lenses

If the fitting of rigid corneal contact lenses is not successful in keratoconus patients with advanced ectasia or dry eye, scleral lenses or mini-scleral lenses can often still be fitted. By resting the edge of the lens on the sclera, it is possible to bridge more advanced ectasia without touching the morphologically compromised apex. In the clinical photograph, it can be seen that the scleral lens extends well beyond the limbus and rests on the sclera (Fig. 31). Anterior segment OCT shows the already scarred apex with advanced ectasia (Fig. 32). The scleral lens does not touch the apex.

Other advantages of these lenses include low risk of loss and significantly reduced foreign body sensation. However, they remain inferior to corneal contact lenses in terms of oxygen supply to the cornea and should therefore only be considered as an alternative when, for fitting reasons or intolerance, the patient cannot be fitted with corneal contact lenses.

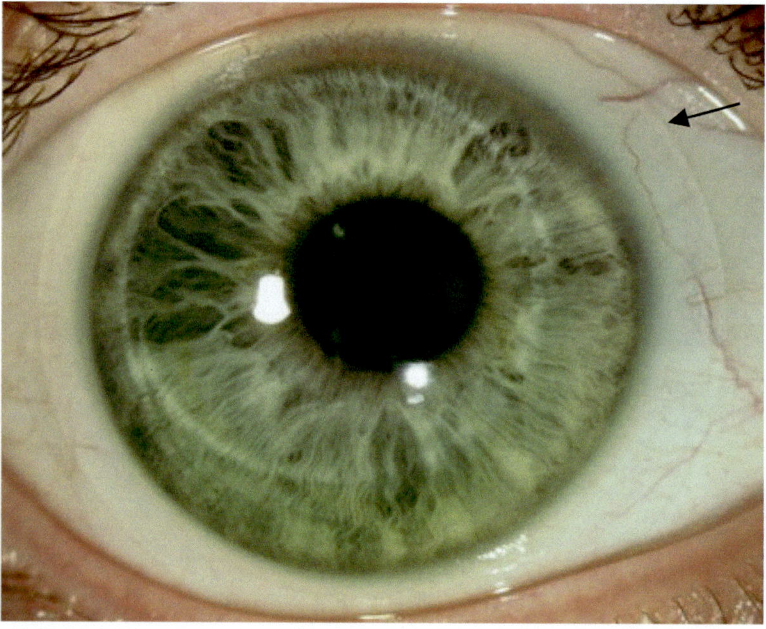

Fig. 31 Slit lamp microscopy with well-fitting scleral lens resting on the eye in the scleral region (black arrow)

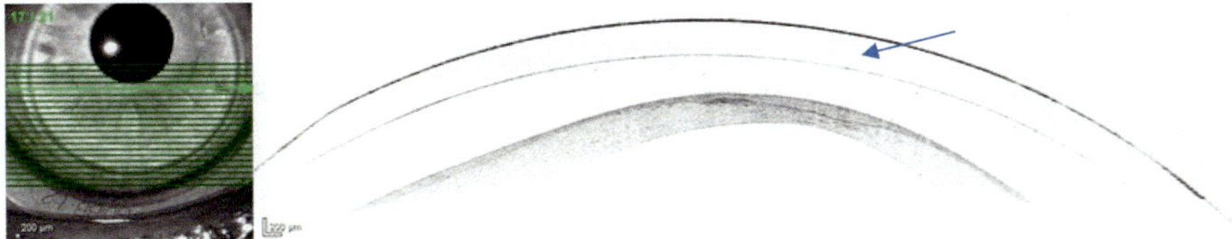

Fig. 32 Anterior segment OCT for fit control of a scleral lens (blue arrow). The cornea does not touch the scleral lens at any point, especially in the area of the apex (already scarred here)

15 Arcus Senilis

Arcus senilis usually presents opaque with gray or white annular staining in the corneal periphery, it is a deposition of lipids. The etiology is not fully understood, but there is an association with hyper-/dyslipidemia especially when occurring in younger individuals. Basically, deposition of lipids in the peripheral cornea is considered a normal aging process. It usually occurs bilaterally, unilateral arcus senilis is associated with ocular hypotony, carotid stenosis or asymmetric cranial vasculature (Naumann and Kuchle 1993). The deposition of lipids is found in the Descemet membrane and Bowman membrane (Patterson 1982) (Figs. 33 and 34).

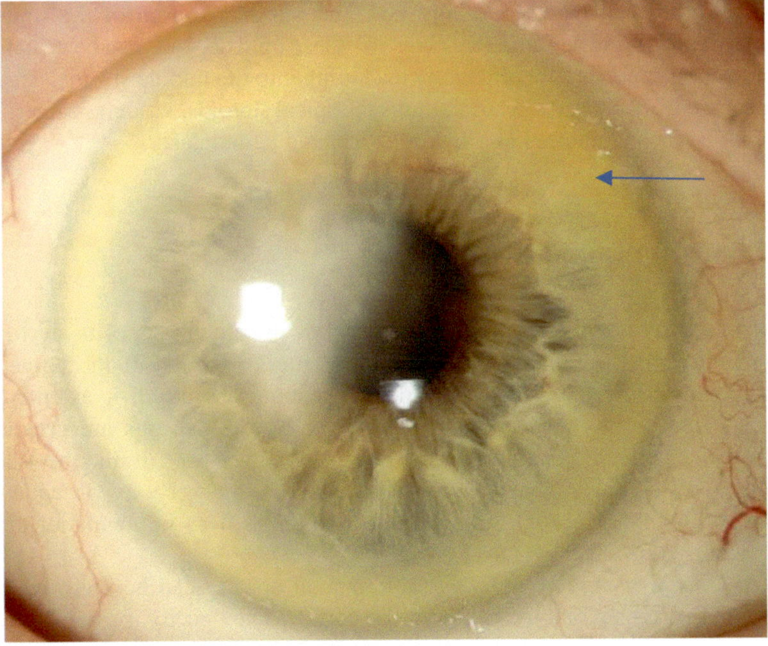

Fig. 33 Slit-lamp microscopy shows the round peripheral ring in the cornea (blue arrow). Incidentally, a central corneal scar is visible here

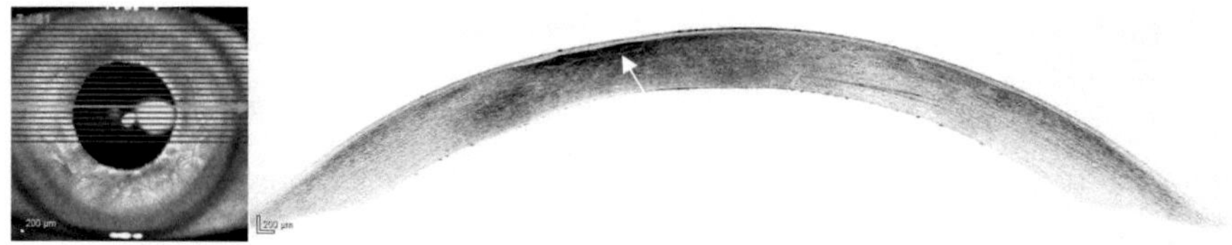

Fig. 34 In OCT imaging, an arcus senilis cannot be visualized. Here, the corneal scar can be visualized as subepithelial hpyerreflective material extending into the stroma (white arrow)

16 Lipid Keratopathy

In lipid keratopathy, as in arcus senilis, there are deposits of lipids in the cornea (stromal deposits of cholesterol and phospholipids). It may be a consequence of chronic inflammation or vascularization, or it may be idiopathic. It can be divided into primary and secondary lipid keratopathy. The primary form is not associated with elevated serum lipid levels and usually occurs bilaterally (Silva-Araujo et al. 1993). The secondary form is more common and consequence of inflammation, infection or (surgical) trauma and associated with vascularization of the cornea. It is often unilateral and serum lipid levels are usually normal. The pathomechanism is not exactly clear, accumulation of lipids by excessive production or disturbed lipid metabolism are discussed (Hall et al. 2020). In slit lamp microscopy (Fig. 35), pronounced deposits can be seen here, especially near the top and bottom of the limbus, as yellowish deposits. In OCT imaging (Fig. 36), these lipid deposits can be visualized as hyperreflective deposits subepithalially extending into the middle stroma. Treatment options range from observation of findings to topical steroids, vascular cauterization, anti-VEGF (vascular enothelial growth factor), and keratoplasty.

17 Band Keratopathy

Band keratopathy is a degenerative disease in which calcium deposits are found in the subepithelium, Bowman's membrane and anterior stroma of the cornea. The opacity begins in the marginal area and when more advanced, it extends like a horizontal band across the central cornea. Initially, the deposits are greyish, but become white as the disease progresses. The causes may vary. It may be related to systemic diseases such as autoimmune diseases, it may be a consequence of intraocular surgery or chronic intraocular diseases such as inflammation or idiopathic (Jhanji et al. 2011).

In the clinical picture (Fig. 37), the horizontal opacity can be seen, which has already progressed beyond the center of the cornea. The opacity is greyish, in some areas already chalky white. In the anterior segment OCT (Fig. 38), the subepithelial calcification is clearly visible in the form of a hyperreflective line.

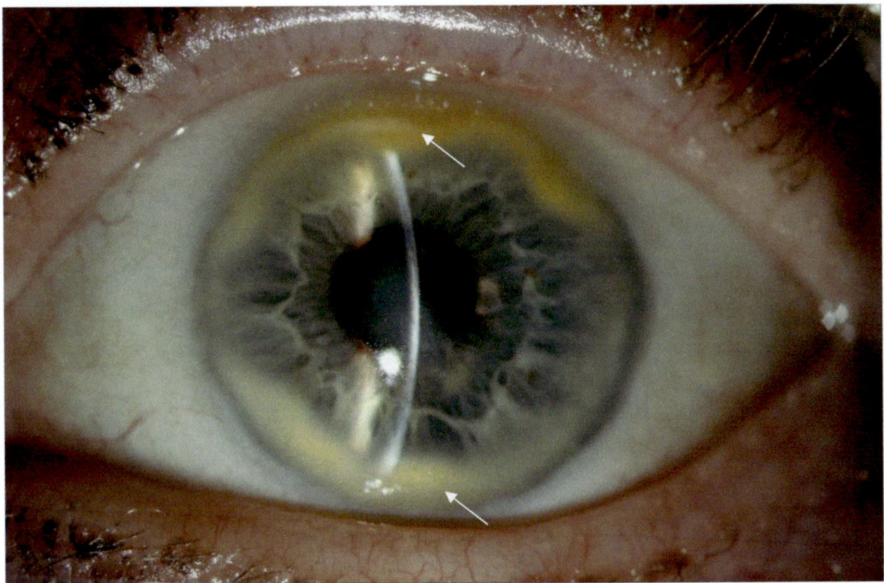

Fig. 35 Pronounced lipid keratopathy, lipid deposits with vascularization clearly visible near the limbus (white arrows)

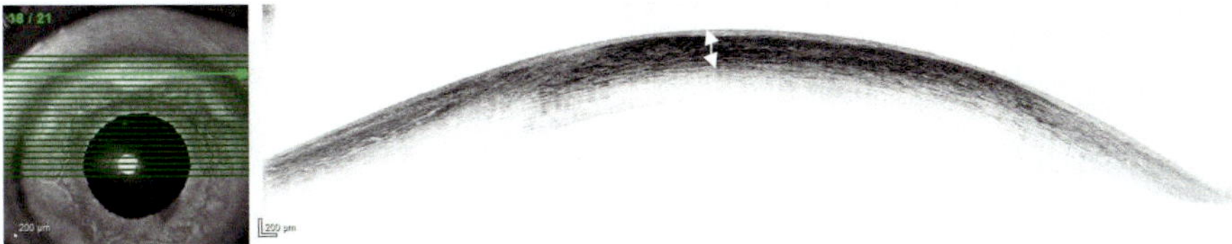

Fig. 36 In the anterior segment OCT image, the lipid inclusions can be seen as subepithelial hyperreflective areas extending into the mid-stroma (white arrow)

18   Corneal Pannus

Corneal pannus is fibrous tissue with vascular content between the corneal epithelium and Bowman's membrane. The tissue grows from the limbus onto the peripheral cornea. A distinction can be made between inflammatory and degenerative pannus. Pannus results in corneal opacity in the affected area. Pannus formation is associated with chronic hypoxia (e.g., from contact lenses) or chronic inflammatory processes. Slit lamp microscopy (Fig. 39) shows the pannus in the lower part of the cornea with corneal neovascularization. On anterior segment OCT (Fig. 40), the pannus appears as a relatively thick superimposed layer over the corneal stroma. The ocular history of this patient shows endocrine orbitopathy with exposure keratopathy and condition after corneal ulcer.

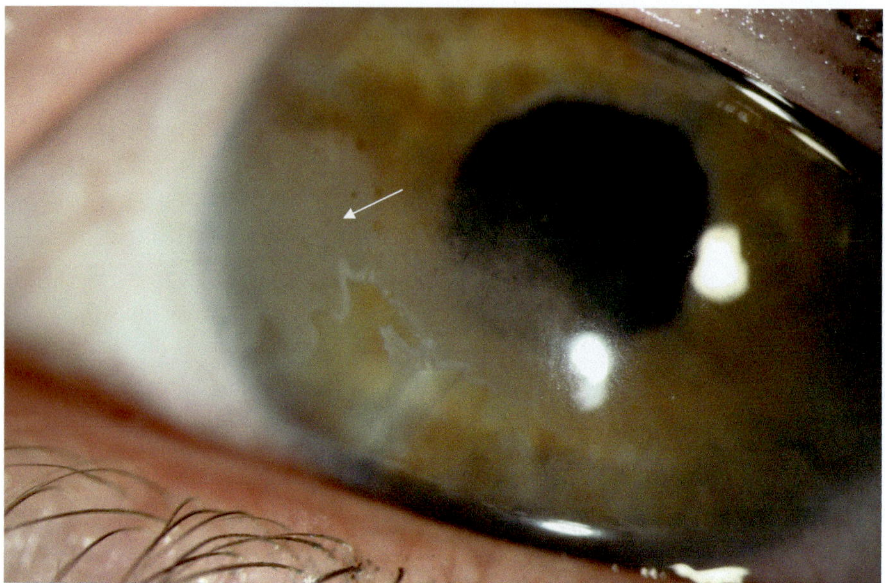

Fig. 37 Advanced band keratopathy, horizontal grayish to chalky white opacity (white arrow)

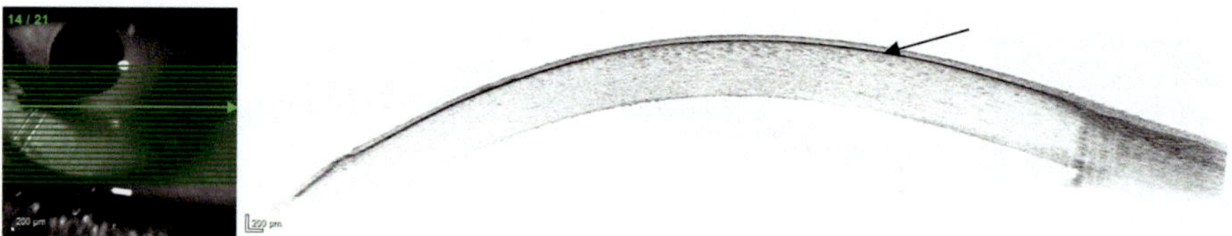

Fig. 38 In anterior segment OCT, the band-like keratopathy presents as a hyperreflective layer in the subepithelial area (black arrow)

19   Pellucidal Marginal Corneal Degeneration (PMD)

Pellucidal marginal corneal degeneration is a thinning of the corneal periphery that progresses slowly over many years. Topo- and tomographic or clinical slit-lamp findings show a crescent-shaped corneal band with thinning of the inferior cornea of about 20% of normal thickness, 1 to 2 mm high, 6 to 8 mm horizontal and 1 to 2 mm from the limbus. The central cornea is of normal thickness. In the slit photograph (Fig. 41), one can see how the cornea is thinned in the lower corneal region. In the corneal tomography (Fig. 42), it can be seen that the inferior area (shown here on the left) is clearly thinned (vertical section through the cornea) and in the color-scaled representation of the corneal thickness (bottom right), the clearly thinned crescent-shaped corneal area can be seen in the inferior cornea:

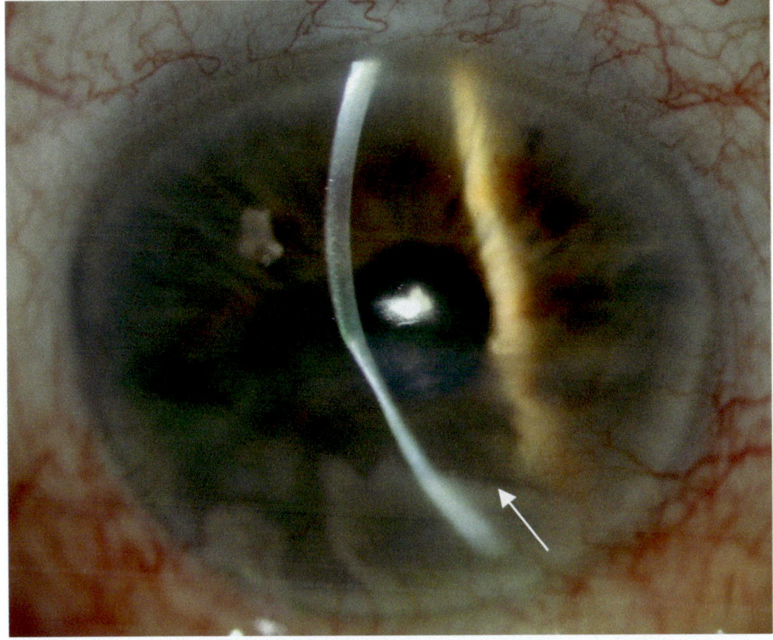

Fig. 39 Slit lamp microscopy showing corneal pannus in the lower third of the cornea (white arrow) with clear corneal neovascularization

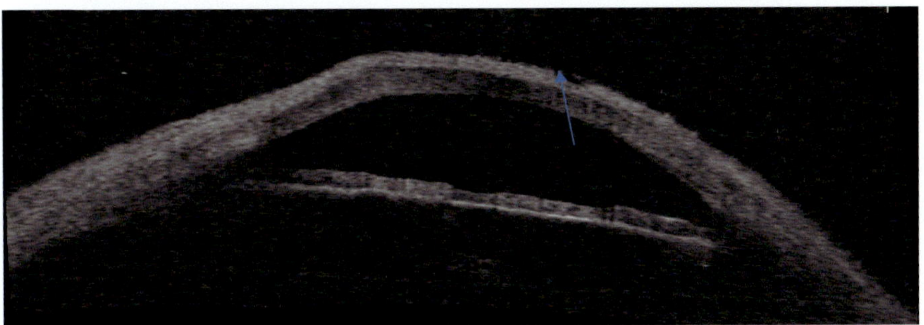

Fig. 40 Anterior segment OCT with pannus superimposed on corneal stroma (blue arrow)

20 Salzmann's Nodular Degeneration

Salzmann's nodular degeneration is a slowly progressive disease in which grayish-white to bluish nodules are seen in front of Bowman's membrane (lamina limitans anterior). The disease usually occurs bilaterally. The nodules are usually located in the midperipheral cornea or near the limbus. In the slit-lamp photograph

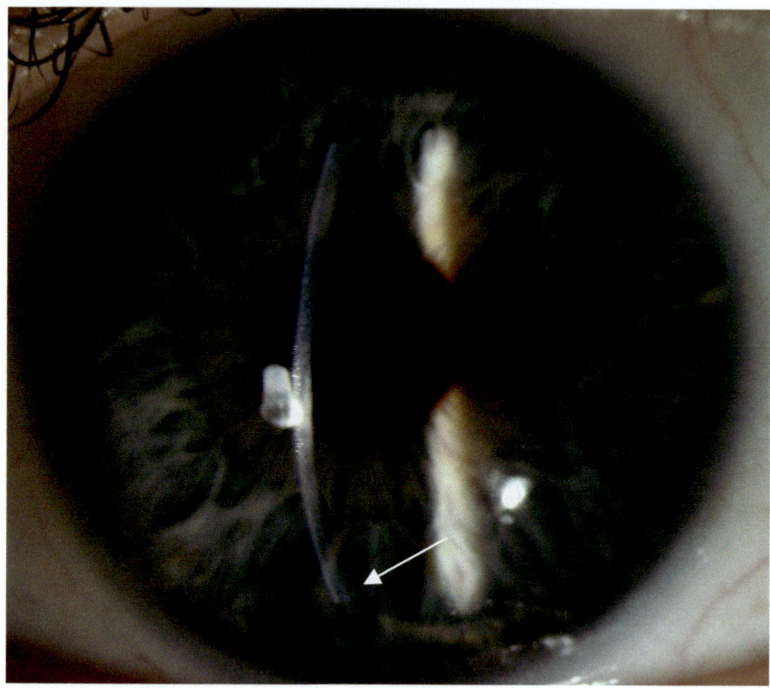

Fig. 41 Slit lamp microscopy in pellucid marginal corneal degeneration (PMD). Thinning of the cornea can be seen in the lower corneal region (white arrow)

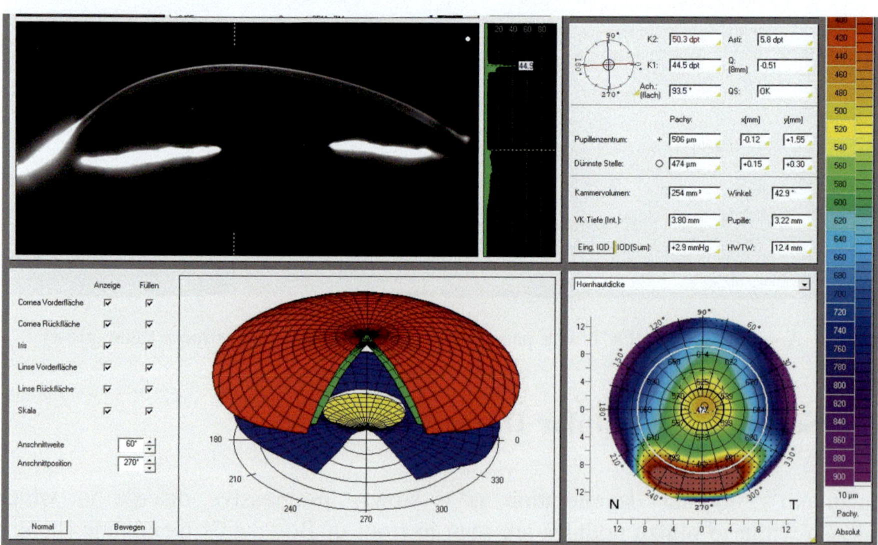

Fig. 42 In the tomographic image of the cornea, the crescent-shaped thinning of the cornea in the lower region can be seen in the color-scaled recording of the corneal thickness (lower right). In the upper left vertical image of the cornea, the thinning of the cornea in the lower region is shown (white arrow)

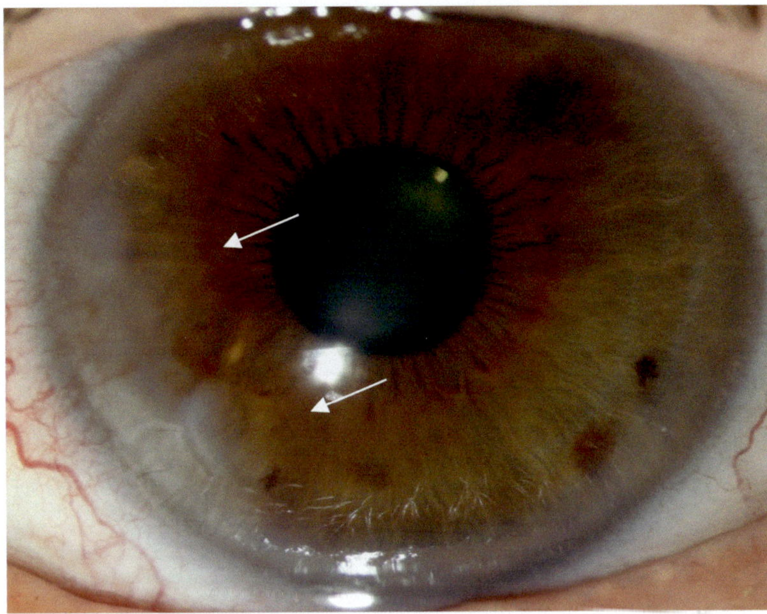

Fig. 43 Slit lamp microscopy in Salzmann's nodular degeneration. The grayish-white to bluish nodules (white arrows) appear close to the limbus nasally

(Fig. 43, white arrows), several grayish-white sometimes bluish shimmering Salzmann nodules are seen here nasally. These may cause visual acuity reduction, epiphora, photophobia, and foreign body sensation. Anterior segment OCT (Fig. 44, blue arrow) shows the hyperreflective Salzmann nodule nasally, which is located above Bowman's membrane. In case of visual impairment and chronic foreign body sensation, it is possible to ablate the nodes by PTK (see Chapter X, Refractive and Therapeutic Laser Surgery).

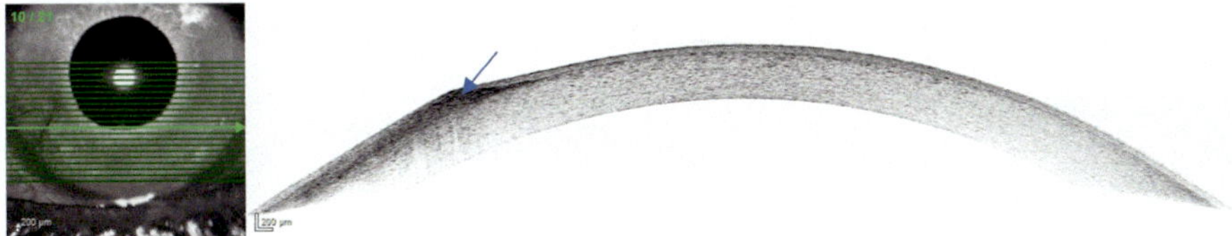

Fig. 44 In anterior segment OCT, a Salzmann node (blue arrow) presents as hyperreflective subepithelial material, here near the limbus. The Bowman membrane is respected in this case

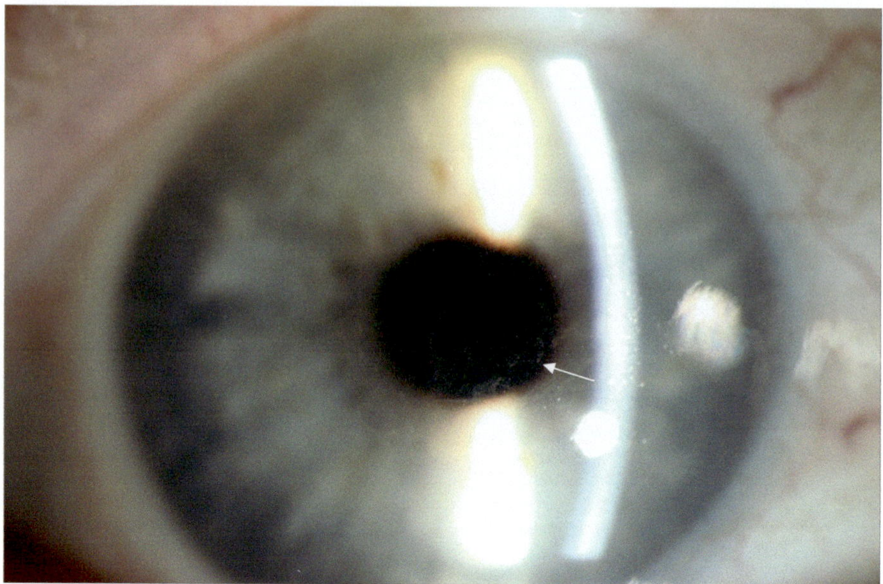

Fig. 45 Slit lamp microscopy in cornea verticillata. Vertebrally arranged opacities in the corneal epithelium in the lower corneal hemisphere can be seen (white arrow)

21 Cornea Verticillata

Vortex keratopathy (cornea verticillata) is a vortex-like opacity in the basal corneal epithelium caused by deposits (Raizman et al. 2017). These deposits are mostly found in the lower paracentral area of the cornea and can be white to brown in color. They are usually deposits of certain systemic drugs such as amiodarone, chloroquine, hydroxychloroquine, or indomethacin, but may also occur in Fabry disease. The figure (Fig. 45) shows a patient taking amiodarone regularly. Anterior segment OCT (Fig. 46) shows darkly stained deposits in the corneal epithelium.

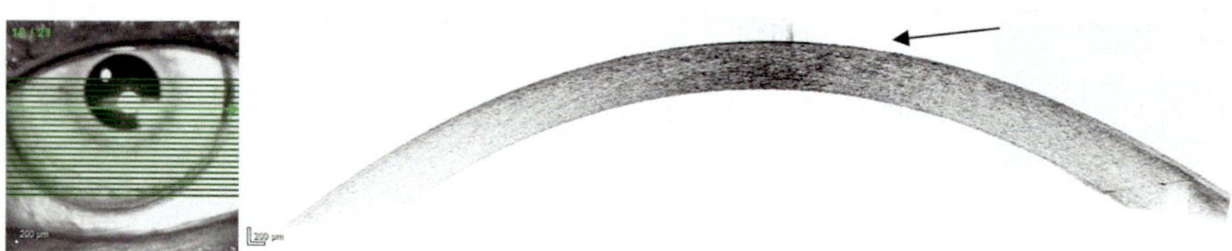

Fig. 46 Anterior segment OCT in cornea verticillata with hyperreflective inclusions in the corneal epithelium (black arrow)

22 Keratopathy in Pseudoexfoliation Syndrome

In the context of pseudoexfoliation syndrome (PEX syndrome), keratopathy may occur. PEX material is deposited retrocorneally, histopathologically there is diffuse, irregular thickening of Descemet's membrane as well as focal accumulation of PEX material on or within Descemet's membrane (Naumann and Schlotzer-Schrehardt 2000). It is usually distributed over the entire posterior surface of the cornea. This can lead to endothelial decompensation with thickening of the cornea and associated visual loss.

On the slit-lamp photograph (Fig. 47), a thickened cornea due to PEX keratopathy can be seen on the one hand. Furthermore, amorphous conglomerates of the secreted protein at the endothelium as well as its deposition at the pupillary rim can be seen. On anterior segment OCT (Fig. 48), these present as hyperreflective flakes on the endothelium. PEX keratopathy can generally be managed with endothelial keratoplasty, but is associated with a poorer prognosis due to re-deposition or deposition in the interface.

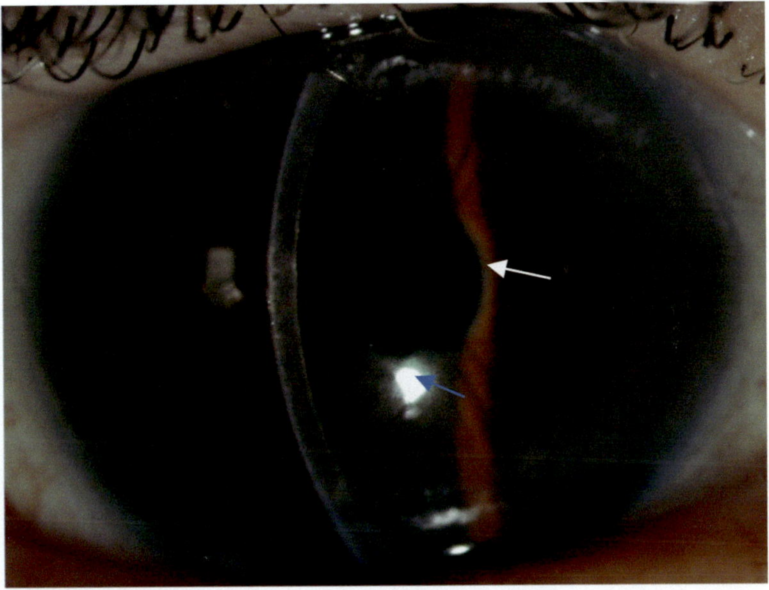

Fig. 47 Slit lamp microscopy of retrocorneal depsotions with PEX (blue arrow) as well as PEX material at the pupillary rim (white arrow)

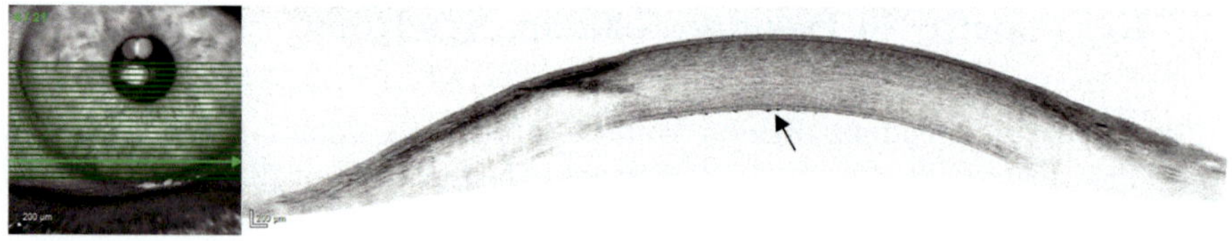

Fig. 48 In anterior segment OCT, the PEX material presents endothelially as roundish hyperreflective deposits (black arrow)

23 Degenerative, Post-Traumatic Iron Deposition of the Cornea

Corneal scars can be of very different genesis (postinflammatory, posttraumatic, degenerative). Different therapeutic options are available (abrasio corneae, PTK, keratoplasty (penetrating, lamellar)). These depend, among other things, on how deeply the scar tissue penetrates into the cornea. In these cases, an anterior segment OCT is crucial for the therapy decision. This shows a corneal scar after acanthamoebic keratitis. Slit lamp microscopy shows an iron line (Fig. 49). Using anterior segment OCT (Fig. 50), a hyperreflective line corresponding to the iron line is seen in addition to the clear demarcation of the scar. This is due to the opacity and thus the shading of the embedded iron particles (Rose and Lavin 1987). In this case, the scar tissue could be removed without complications by means of a PTK.

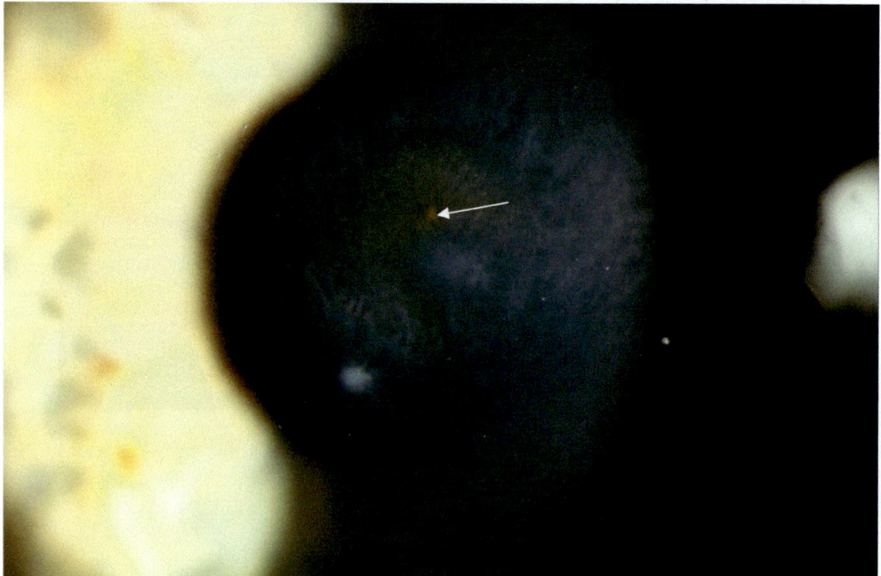

Fig. 49 Slit lamp microscopy showing a corneal scar after acanthamoeboid keratitis. Clear deposition of iron (red-brownish, white arrow) in the area of the scar

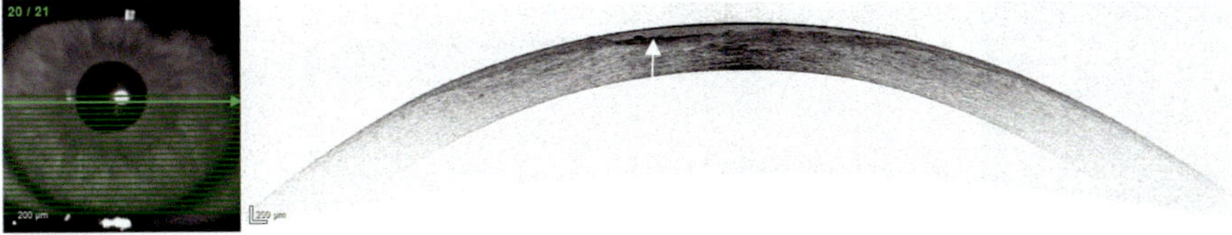

Fig. 50 In anterior segment OCT, iron incorporation corresponds to the hyperreflective line (white arrow) below the scarred area in the anterior corneal stroma

24 Haab's Striae

So-called Haab's striae are horizontal groins of Descemet's membrane. They may occur in the context of congenital glaucoma. In the slit-lamp photograph (Fig. 51) the oblique Haab's striae can be seen, in the anterior segment OCT (Fig. 52, blue arrows) the thickening in the sense of a Descemet's groin can be seen in the area of Descemet's membrane. These are endothelialized Descemet's ruptures, which usually run horizontally (Oliveira and Wilson 2020). Vertical tears of Descemet's membrane may occur in birth trauma following forceps deliveries. The cornea may decompensate in the area of Haab's striae, resulting in decreased visual acuity. Keratoplasty can lead to visual rehabilitation (Kampmeier et al. 2015; Kim et al. 2018).

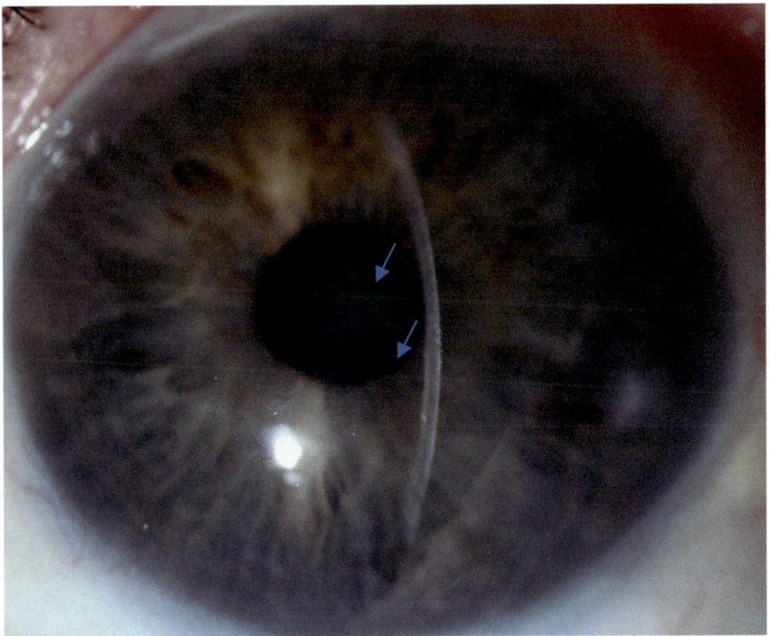

Fig. 51 Slit lamp microscopy in buphthalmos with oblique (from nasal superior to temporal inferior) Haab's striae (blue arrows)

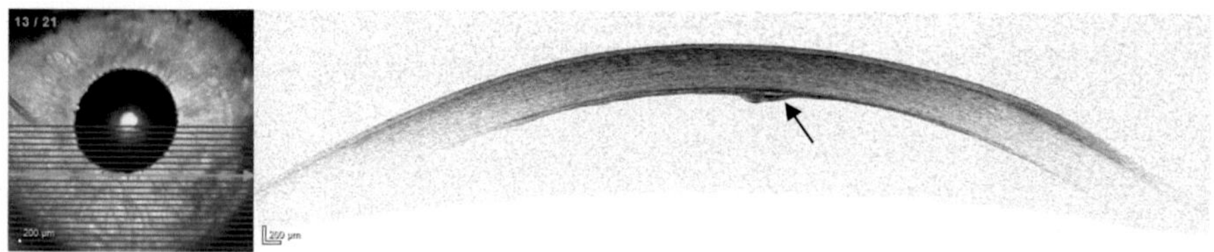

Fig. 52 On anterior segment OCT, Haab's striae appear as a thickened groin in Descemet's membrane (black arrow)

References

Ang M, Baskaran M, Werkmeister RM, et al. Anterior segment optical coherence tomography. Prog Retin Eye Res. 2018;66:132–56.

Bachmann B, Händel A, Siebelmann S, et al. Mini-descemet membrane endothelial keratoplasty for the early treatment of acute corneal hydrops in keratoconus. Cornea. 2019;38(8):1043–8.

de Oliveira RC, Wilson SE. Descemet's membrane development, structure, function and regeneration. Exp Eye Res. 2020;197: 108090.

Godefrooij DA, de Wit GA, Uiterwaal CS, et al. Age-specific incidence and prevalence of keratoconus: a nationwide registration study. Am J Ophthalmol. 2017;175:169–72.

Hall MN, Moshirfar M, Amin-Javaheri A, et al. Lipid keratopathy: a review of pathophysiology, differential diagnosis, and management. Ophthalmol Ther. 2020;9(4):833–52.

Händel A, Siebelmann S, Hos D, et al. Comparison of Mini-DMEK versus predescemetal sutures as treatment of acute hydrops in keratoconus. Acta Ophthalmol 2021.

Hos D, Matthaei M, Bock F, et al. Immune reactions after modern lamellar (DALK, DSAEK, DMEK) versus conventional penetrating corneal transplantation. Prog Retin Eye Res. 2019;73: 100768.

Jhanji V, Rapuano CJ, Vajpayee RB. Corneal calcific band keratopathy. Curr Opin Ophthalmol. 2011;22(4):283–9.

Kampmeier J, Werner JU, Wagner P, Lang GK. DMEK in a Case of Haab's Striae in Congenital Glaucoma. Klin Monbl Augenheilkd. 2015;232(12):1410–2.

Kim YJ, Jeoung JW, Kim MK, et al. Clinical features and outcome of corneal opacity associated with congenital glaucoma. BMC Ophthalmol. 2018;18(1):190.

Krumeich JH, Duncker G. Intrastromal corneal ring in penetrating keratoplasty: evidence-based update 4 years after implantation. J Cataract Refract Surg. 2006;32(6):993–8.

Mas Tur V, MacGregor C, Jayaswal R, et al. A review of keratoconus: Diagnosis, pathophysiology, and genetics. Surv Ophthalmol. 2017;62(6):770–83.

Naumann GO, Kuchle M. Unilateral corneal arcus lipoides. Lancet. 1993;342(8880):1185.

Naumann GO, Schlotzer-Schrehardt U. Keratopathy in pseudoexfoliation syndrome as a cause of corneal endothelial decompensation: a clinicopathologic study. Ophthalmology. 2000;107 (6):1111–24.

Panda A, Aggarwal A, Madhavi P, et al. Management of acute corneal hydrops secondary to keratoconus with intracameral injection of sulfur hexafluoride (SF6). Cornea. 2007;26 (9):1067–9.

Patterson L. Arcus senilis: an important forensic physical finding. Am J Forensic Med Pathol. 1982;3(2):115–8.

Raizman MB, Hamrah P, Holland EJ, et al. Drug-induced corneal epithelial changes. Surv Ophthalmol. 2017;62(3):286–301.

Rose GE, Lavin MJ. The Hudson-Stahli line. III: Observations on morphology, a critical review of aetiology and a unified theory for the formation of iron lines of the corneal epithelium. Eye (Lond) 1987;1 (Pt 4):475–9.

Siebelmann S, Steven P, Cursiefen C. Intraoperative optical coherence tomography: ocular surgery on a higher level or just nice pictures? JAMA Ophthalmol. 2015a;133(10):1133–4.

Siebelmann S, Hermann M, Dietlein T, et al. Intraoperative Optical Coherence Tomography in Children with Anterior Segment Anomalies. Ophthalmology. 2015b;122(12):2582–4.

Siebelmann S, Händel A, Matthaei M, et al. Microscope-integrated optical coherence tomography-guided drainage of acute corneal hydrops in keratoconus combined with suturing and gas-aided reattachment of descemet membrane. Cornea. 2019;38(8):1058–61.

Silva-Araujo A, Tavares MA, Lemos MM, et al. Primary lipid keratopathy: a morphological and biochemical assessment. Br J Ophthalmol. 1993;77(4):248–50.

Yahia Cherif H, Gueudry J, Afriat M, et al. Efficacy and safety of pre-descemet's membrane sutures for the management of acute corneal hydrops in keratoconus. Br J Ophthalmol. 2015;99 (6):773–7.

Epithelial Mapping

Maya Müller and Theo G. Seiler

1 The Corneal Epithelium

The corneal epithelium is a multi-layered non-keratinized squamous epithelium with a central thickness of approximately 50 to 60 μm. The epithelial stem cells are mainly located at the limbus and have a high mitotic rate, whereas differentiated epithelial cells in the healthy cornea move from the peripheral limbus to the center. This lateral migration allows epithelial defects (erosions) to be closed in a very short time.

The recurrent blink, with an average of 300 to 1500 blinks per hour, constantly "planes" the superficial layer and small irregularities, which can normally result in a very smooth surface. This mechanism also allows deeper stromal irregularities or stromal substance defects to be filled and topographically masked. Conversely, epithelial thinning over raised stroma is also possible through this mechanism. However, such a natural compensatory effect can also deceive the refractive surgeon and lead to surgical surprises such as a "vertical gas breakthrough". In anterior stromal defects (e.g. foreign body defect with subsequent epithelial filling), the cavitation gas generated by fs laser application breaks through the weak epithelial layer and leads to incision errors.

Previously, the available methods OCT, confocal microscopy and ultrasound pachymetry only gave single thickness measurements of epithelium and corneal

M. Müller (✉) · T. G. Seiler
Institute for Refractive and Ophthalmic Surgery, IROC, Stockerstrasse 37, 8704 Zuerich, Switzerland
e-mail: maya.mueller@iroc.ch

T. G. Seiler
e-mail: theo.seiler@med.uni-duesseldorf.de

T. G. Seiler
Department of Ophthalmology, University Hospital of Duesseldorf, Moorenstrasse 5, 40225 Duesseldorf, Germany

L. M. Heindl and S. Siebelmann (eds.), *Optical Coherence Tomography of the Anterior Segment*, https://doi.org/10.1007/978-3-031-07730-2_6

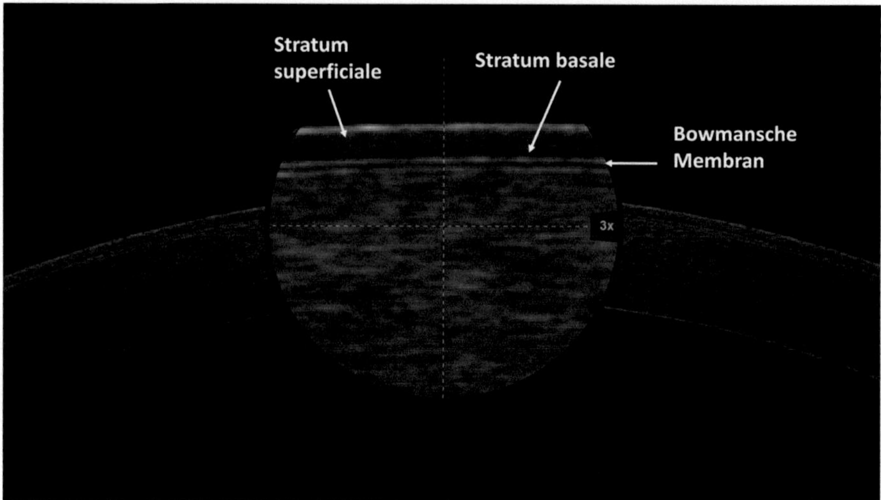

Fig. 1 High-resolution OCT of a cornea with magnification of the epithelium

stroma. However, profiles are much more useful for characterizing epithelial changes, such as after refractive surgery. New high-resolution anterior segment OCTs (axial resolution approx. 5 μm) generate contact-free epithelial thickness profiles from multiple cross-sections of the cornea (Fig. 1) and allow conclusions to be drawn from specific, sometimes even pathognomonic epithelial tomographies.

The physiological epithelial thickness distribution of 53.4 ± 4.6 μm centrally is known from measurements on healthy subjects. The epithelium is 5.7 μm thicker inferiorly than superiorly and 1.2 μm thicker temporally than nasally (Reinstein et al. 2008), which is probably due to the constant blinking of the eyelids. Thus, epithelial mapping can provide a decisive diagnostic clue in uncertain cases or prevent some surprises when planning refractive surgery. Especially in transepithelial refractive procedures, the precision of the intervention can be significantly increased by precisely determining the epithelial thickness.

2 Epithelial Thickness Profile in Corneal Diseases

2.1 *Keratoconus*

From histopathological examinations of corneas with keratoconus, it is known that there is epithelial thinning above the ectasia. Haque et al. were able to confirm this using OCT (Haque et al. 2006). The epithelium is thinnest over the steepest part (apex) and thickened in a ring around it (doughnut profile). This can again be explained by the mechanical component of the blink, which causes modelling of the epithelium and thus regularization with masking of the even steeper Bowman's membrane.

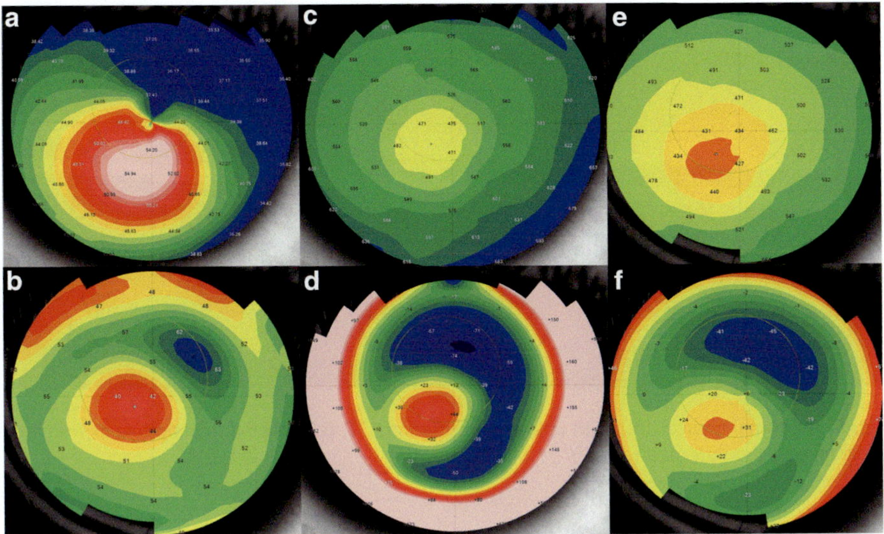

Fig. 2 Typical keratoconus: **a** Sagittal anterior curvature map with superior-inferior asymmetry; **b** Epithelial thickness map with epithelial thinning over the apex and surrounding epithelial thickening (doughnut profile); **c** Corneal thickness map with focal thinning; **d** Posterior height map (BFS of inner 8 mm) with focal protrusion; **e** Stromal thickness map also with focal thinning; **f** Stromal height map (BFS of inner 8 mm) with stromal protrusion corresponding to epithelial thinning

Thus, the characteristic epithelial thickness profile with thinning over the apex can be interpreted as an early sign of keratoconus, even if the anterior height and curvature map is still normal and posterior ectasia is not yet pronounced (Reinstein et al. 2009a). Recently, this can also be shown by means of a stromal height and thickness map (Fig. 2e and f). In advanced state, keratoconus presents characteristically with apical epithelial thinning, surrounding annular epithelial thickening, posterior protrusion and superior-inferior asymmetry (Fig. 2).

Conversely, if the inferior epithelium is normal or even thickened, an underlying ectasia is less likely even with inferior steepening in the curvature map. Thus, changes in the cornea, such as a contact lens "warpage" can imitate keratoconus at first glance. Only after checking all relevant parameters, and especially the epithelial thickness measurement, the diagnosis of keratoconus should be confirmed or rejected.

2.2 Corneal Scars

Due to the compensatory and rapidly proliferative properties of the epithelium, epithelial closures can be observed within a short time even in the case of deeper

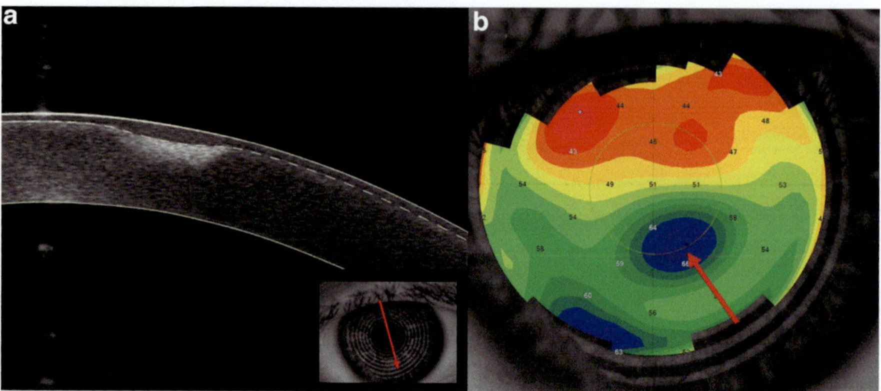

Fig. 3 **a** Stromal corneal scar with epithelial filling in OCT; **b** Epithelial thickness map with focal thickening in the scar area (arrow)

stromal injuries, in which the epithelium fills the stromal defect accordingly (Fig. 3). Thus, even corneal topographies can appear normal again.

2.3 Epithelial Changes After Refractive Surgery

After refractive surgery, epithelial thickness changes occur from the first postoperative day. With LASIK, these changes are usually completed 3 months postoperatively. After PRK, such epithelial modelling can be observed for much longer, which is probably due to a possible interaction of epithelial cells and keratocytes. Thus, according to the laser ablation profile, characteristic epithelial changes appear, which attempt to compensate for the resulting stromal deficit. In myopic LASIK with a central deficit (also after intrastromal lenticule extraction or RK) and consecutive flattening (Fig. 4a), a clear central epithelial thickening is seen in the postoperative course (Fig. 4b). In the case of hyperopic ablation (Fig. 4c), the situation is exactly the opposite. There is peripheral epithelial filling over the groove-like ablation surface and simultaneous central thinning (Fig. 4d). Part of the regression that occurs in corneal refractive procedures is due to these epithelial adaptations or this compensation mechanism, which is also considered in modern nomograms. This is one of the reasons why a slight overcorrection is always measurable, especially with high corrections in the early postoperative phase.

With the evolution of epithelial mapping, modern refractive surgery will continue to benefit. For example, recently developed epithelial wavefronts can further increase the accuracy of re-operations (Khamar et al. 2020; Zhou et al. 2019).

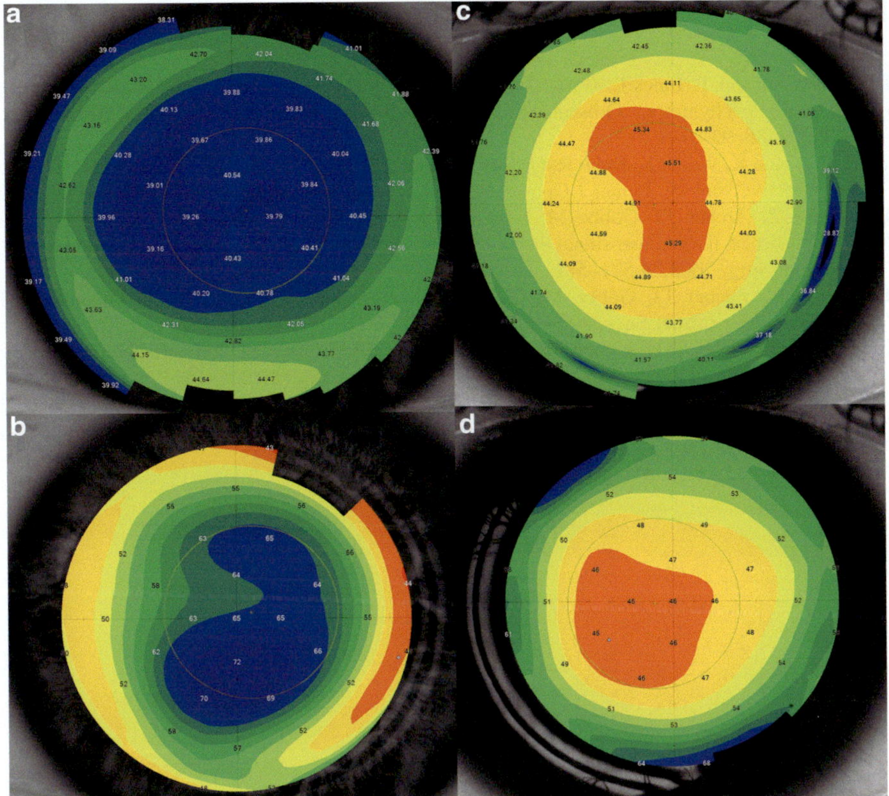

Fig. 4 Epithelial changes after refractive surgery: **a** Sagittal curvature map and **b** Epithelial thickness map with central thickening after myopic correction; **c** Sagittal curvature map and **d** Epithelial thickness map with central epithelial thinning and annular thickening after hyperopic correction

Contact lens practitioners also take advantage of the "flexible" properties of the epithelium. In Ortho-K contact lenses (rigid night lenses), most of the refractive effect can be attributed to changes in the epithelial thickness profile (Reinstein et al. 2019b).

In summary, it should be emphasized that the corneal epithelium balances the surface and models and compensates for stromal irregularities by means of mechanical stress from the blink.

References

Haque S, Simpson T, Jones L. Corneal and epithelial thickness in keratoconus: a comparison of ultrasonic pachymetry, Orbscan and optical coherence tomography. J Refract Surg. 2006;22:486–93.

Khamar P, Rao K, Wadia K, Dalai R, Grover T, Versaci F, Gupta K. Advanced epithelial mapping for refractive surgery. Indian J Ophthalmol. 2020;68(12):2819–30.

Reinstein DZ, Archer TJ, Gobbe M, Silverman RH, Coleman DJ. Epithelial thickness in the normal cornea: three-dimensional display with Artemis very high -frequency digital ultrasound. J Refract Surg. 2008;24:571–581.

Reinstein DZ, Archer TJ, Gobbe M. Corneal epithelial thickness profile in the diagnosis of keratoconus. J Refract Surg. 2009a;25(7):604–10.

Reinstein DZ, Gobbe M, Archer TJ, Bloom B. Epithelial, stromal, and corneal pachymetry changes during orthokeratology. Optom Vis Sci. 2009b; 86(8):E1006–14.

Zhou W, Reinstein DZ, Chen X, Shen S, Xu Y, Utheim TP, Stojanovic A. Transepithelial topography-guided ablation assisted by epithelial thickness mapping for treatment of regression after myopic refractive surgery. J Refract Surg. 2019;35(8):525–33.

Inflammatory Corneal Diseases

Inflammatory Corneal Diseases in the Clinical Picture and by Anterior Segment- and Slit Lamp-Adapted Anterior Segment (SL)-Optical Coherence Tomography (OCT)

Simona Schlereth

1 Infectious Corneal Diseases

Infectious keratitis, usually caused by bacteria, fungi, viruses or protozoa, usually begins with a punctiform lesion in the corneal epithelium, which, due to the inflammation, can spread to a corneal ulceration with destruction of the collagen fibers. Healing induces the formation of scars, neovascularizations and usually a significant reduction in vision. The etiology and frequency of microbial keratitis varies geographically. Worldwide, bacterial keratitis is the second most common cause of blindness after cataract (Al-Mujaini et al. 2009).

1.1 *Pseudomonas Aeruginosa Induced Corneal Ulcer*

The bacterial keratitis is mostly caused by Staphylococcus aureus, Streptococcus spp., Pseudomonas aeruginosa, coagulase-negative staphylococci or Enterobacteriaceae (Stapleton and Carnt 2012). In contact lens-associated keratitis, P. aeruginosa is the most frequently detected pathogen (Saeed et al. 2009; Stapleton et al. 2017). P. aeruginosa is a gram-negative bacterium that occurs ubiquitously and can cause severe keratitis. It is one of the leading causes of vision-threatening keratitis in otherwise healthy contact lens wearers (Yildiz et al. 2012; Ng et al. 2015).

The clinical and SL-OCT picture shows a corneal ulcer due to infection with Pseudomonas aeruginosa in a 23-year-old healthy contact lens wearer. Local and intraocular antibiotic therapy were applied, as well as antibacterial crosslinking twice. The clinical picture and the anterior segment OCT show the extensive

S. Schlereth (✉)
Department of Opthalmology, University Hospital of Cologne, Cologne, Germany
e-mail: simona.schlereth@uk-koeln.de

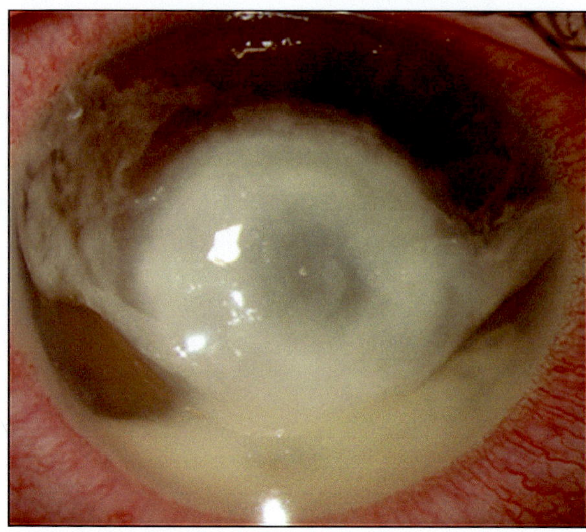

Fig. 1 A fulminant corneal ulcer with melting and hypopyon due to Pseudomonas aeruginosa infection is seen. Datei: Fig. 1_Pseudomonas.Ulkus.tif. Abb.-Typ: Strich-Abb. Farbigkeit (IST): 1c. Farbigkeit (SOLL): 1c. Bildrechte: [Urheberrecht beim Autor]. Abdruckrechte: Nicht notwendig. Hinweise Verlag/Setzerei

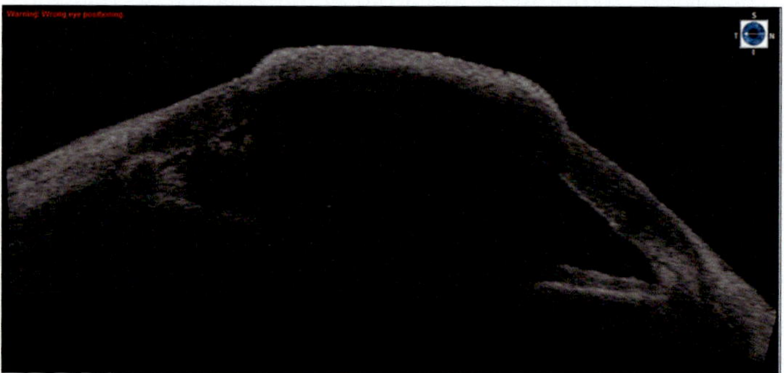

Fig. 2 Visualization of infectious corneal ulcer in anterior segment OCT: The hypopyon is visible in the anterior segment OCT on the left side of the image as a condensation in the anterior chamber. Details in the cornea can only be seen far anteriorly due to the opacity. Behind the anterior corneal opacity, like a sound shadow, no further details are visible. Datei: Fig. 2 Pseudomonas-ulkus.tif. Abb.-Typ: Strich-Abb. Farbigkeit (IST): 1c. Farbigkeit (SOLL): 1c. Bildrechte: [Urheberrecht beim Autor]. Abdruckrechte: Nicht notwendig. Hinweise Verlag/Setzerei

infection with swollen cornea, with significantly reduced view into the anterior chamber in the photo, as well as the anterior segment OCT (compare Figs. 1 and 2).

In the course of the disease a small perforation occurred, which was treated twice with an amniotic membrane in multilayer technique. The extension of the findings

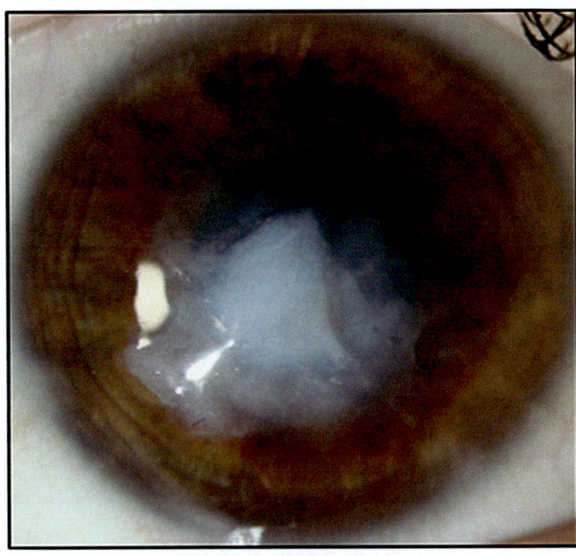

Fig. 3 Clinical picture of a sutured amniotic membrane using the multilayer technique in the infection-free interval due to perforation after infectious corneal ulcer with Pseudomonas aeruginosa. Datei: Fig. 3-amn1.tif. Abb.-Typ: Strich-Abb. Farbigkeit (IST): 1c. Farbigkeit (SOLL): 1c. Bildrechte: [Urheberrecht beim Autor]. Abdruckrechte: Nicht notwendig. Hinweise Verlag/Setzerei

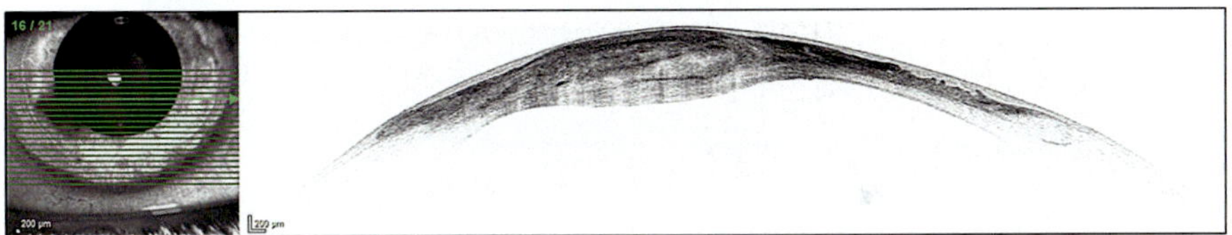

Fig. 4 Visualization of the multilayer amniotic membranes in anterior segment OCT. The extension into the depth as well as the representation of the amniotic membrane layers can be seen well here. Datei: Fig. 4-AMN.tif. Abb.-Typ: Strich-Abb. Farbigkeit (IST): 1c. Farbigkeit (SOLL): 1c. Bildrechte: [Urheberrecht beim Autor]. Abdruckrechte: Nicht notwendig. Hinweise Verlag/ Setzerei

into the depth can be visualized particularly well in the anterior segment OCT (compare Figs. 3 and 4).

Following healing of the corneal infection and after vascular cauterization of several corneal neovascularizations, penetrating keratoplasty was performed for visual rehabilitation. In the meantime, with residual astigmatism of −4dpt, a visual acuity of 0.8 was achieved. Unfortunately, central keratitis developed again on the penetrating keratoplasty, possibly contact lens-associated again. The last visual acuity was corrected 0.2 (compare Figs. 5, 6 and 7, the arrow shows the infiltrate in all images).

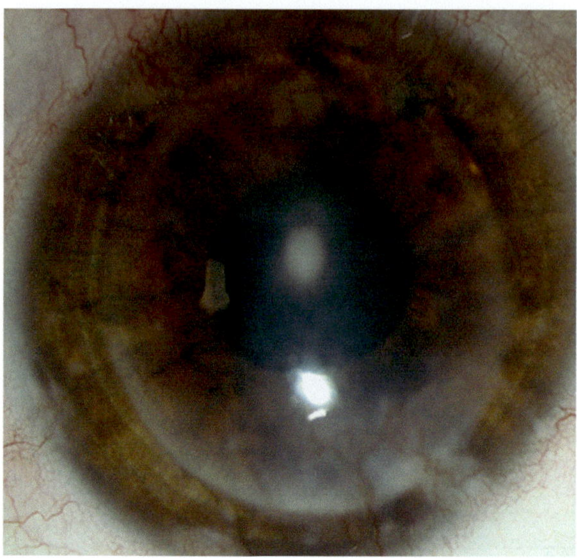

Fig. 5 Clinical picture of penetrating keratoplasty with central infectious localized keratitis, and inferior neovascularizations on the graft. Datei: Fig. 5_keratitis.tif. Abb.-Typ: Strich-Abb. Farbigkeit (IST): 1c. Farbigkeit (SOLL): 1c. Bildrechte: [Urheberrecht beim Autor]. Abdruckrechte: Nicht notwendig. Hinweise Verlag/Setzerei

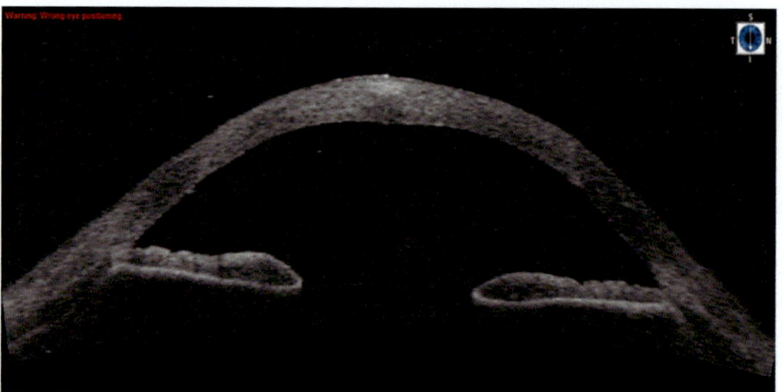

Fig. 6 Slit-lamp-adapted anterior segment OCT (SL-OCT) shows keratitis as a superficial hyperreflective opacity centrally. The transition from donor graft to recipient cornea is visible peripherally. Datei: Fig. 6-Auto Biometry.tif. Abb.-Typ: Strich-Abb. Farbigkeit (IST): 1c. Farbigkeit (SOLL): 1c. Bildrechte: [Urheberrecht beim Autor]. Abdruckrechte: Nicht notwendig. Hinweise Verlag/Setzerei

The next picture shows a corneal scar of a 24-year-old patient, after expired pseudomonas keratitis. This was treated intensively and early with antibiotics, as well as Lavasept and Brolene, because initially an acanthamoeba keratitis was also considered as a differential diagnosis. The infection healed, leaving a round central corneal scar. The depth extent is easily visualized on anterior segment-OCT

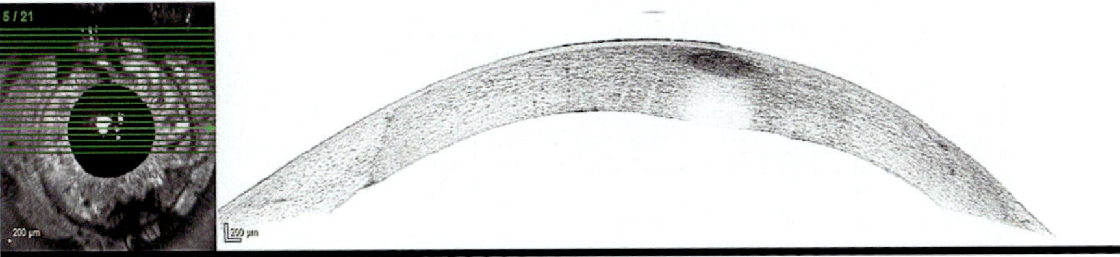

Fig. 7 Anterior segment OCT also shows the superficial infection with localized edema of the cornea. The transition from the recipient cornea to the graft is peripherally visible as a fine line. Datei: Fig. 7_OCT.tif. Abb.-Typ: Strich-Abb. Farbigkeit (IST): 1c. Farbigkeit (SOLL): 1c. Bildrechte: [Urheberrecht beim Autor]. Abdruckrechte: Nicht notwendig. Hinweise Verlag/ Setzerei:

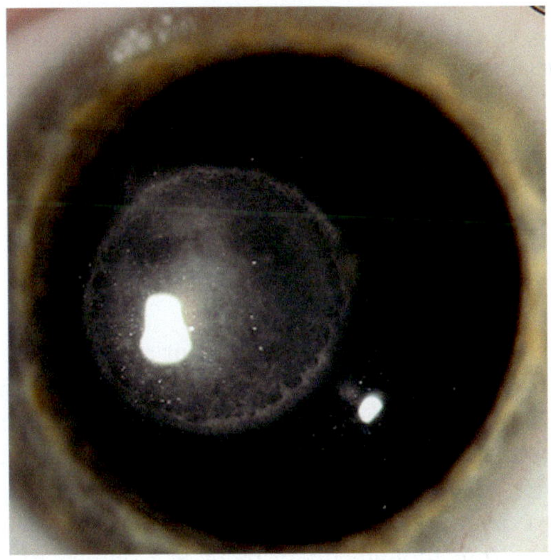

Fig. 8 Clinical picture of a round corneal scar in a 24-year-old patient, after expired pseudomonas keratitis. Datei: Fig. 8-pseudomonas narbe.tif. Abb.-Typ: Strich-Abb. Farbigkeit (IST): 1c. Farbigkeit (SOLL): 1c. Bildrechte: [Urheberrecht beim Autor]. Abdruckrechte: Nicht notwendig. Hinweise Verlag/Setzerei

(compare Figs. 8 and 9). This may help in determining whether phototherapeutic keratectomy (PTK) is useful to restore vision. In this patient, the findings are too deep stromal for PTK because more than half of the stroma is affected by the scar. In general, anterior corneal opacities are thought to be well treated by PTK. The patient's visual acuity has increased from initial hand movement to 0.5. Lamellar keratoplasty, in terms of Deep Anterior Lamellar Keratoplasty (DALK) could be considered for further visual improvement.

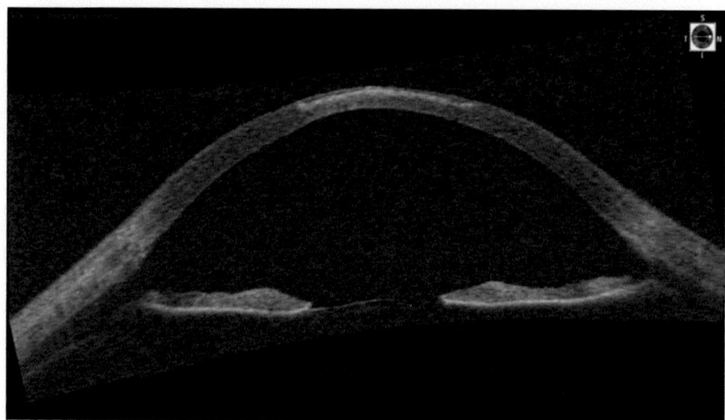

Fig. 9 SL-OCT shows the corneal scar to be extended anteriorly into the middle stroma. Here, a measurement of the total corneal thickness, as well as the scar, can be made (compare Fig. 13), which may be helpful for the decision of further interventions, like PTK. Datei: Fig. 9-pseudomonas narbe.tif. Abb.-Typ: Strich-Abb. Farbigkeit (IST): 1c. Farbigkeit (SOLL): 1c. Bildrechte: [Urheberrecht beim Autor]. Abdruckrechte: Nicht notwendig. Hinweise Verlag/Setzerei

1.2 Corneal Ulcer in Acanthamoeboid Keratitis

Acanthamoebae are ubiquitous protozoa that occur as active trophozoites or in the dormant cyst form. Acanthamoebic keratitis is a potentially visually threatening infection with an often poor prognosis. This is often due to late diagnosis but also in the lack of effective therapies. This infection is associated with contact lens wear. Other risk factors are poor hygiene or contact with contaminated water (Maycock and Jayaswal 2016). Diagnostic testing is performed using corneal sharp smears, which are examined histopathologically or by PCR. Confocal microscopy is used to detect cysts in the cornea. Therapy includes topical biguanides, diamidines, or steroids. Antibiotics are also given to eliminate bacteria, especially Escherichia coli, which serve as food for the acanthamoebae. Surgically, amniotic membranes or penetrating or lamellar keratoplasty may be considered.

The following image shows an expired acanthamoeboid keratitis. This patient is a 20-year-old contact lens wearer who required the contact lenses due to bilateral aphakia associated with juvenile cataract. With early and intensive therapy, the acanthamoeboid keratitis was controlled. A scar has developed and the cornea has thinned significantly. In this case, the additional function of anterior segment OCT with pachymetry may be helpful (Figs. 10, 11, 12 and 13). The last visual acuity was 0.5. The therapy with Brolene, antiseptics as well as phasic steroids was continued for 1 year.

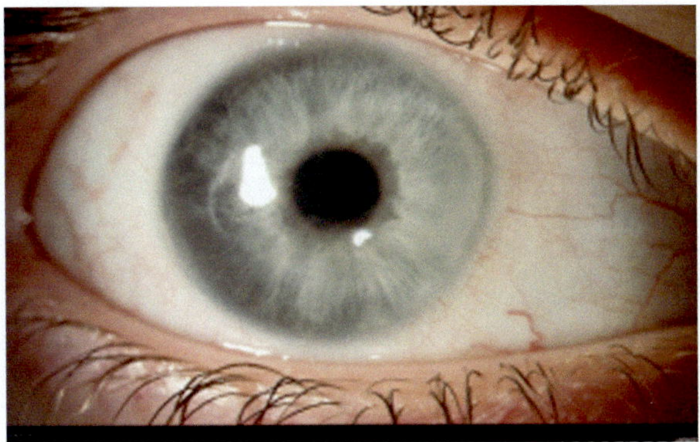

Fig. 10 Clinical picture of a corneal scar after expired acanthamoebic keratitis in overview. A fine roundish scar is visible centrally. Datei: Fig. 10.tif. Abb.-Typ: Strich-Abb. Farbigkeit (IST): 1c. Farbigkeit (SOLL): 1c. Bildrechte: [Urheberrecht beim Autor]. Abdruckrechte: Nicht notwendig. Hinweise Verlag/Setzerei

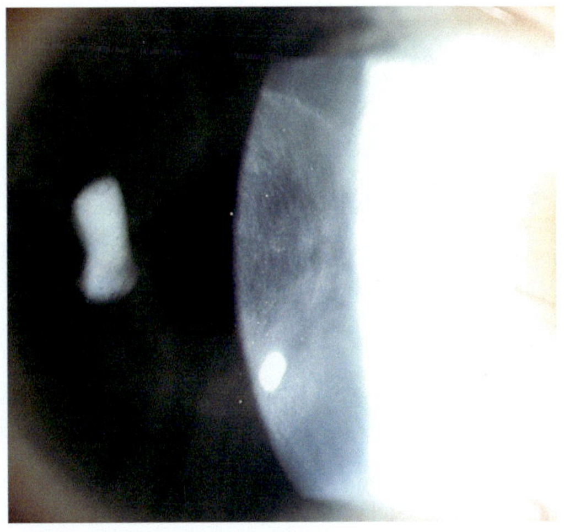

Fig. 11 Enlarged clinical view of corneal scar after expired acanthamoeboid keratitis. Datei: Fig. 11, alte Akanthm.narbe.tif. Abb.-Typ: Strich-Abb. Farbigkeit (IST): 1c. Farbigkeit (SOLL): 1c. Bildrechte: [Urheberrecht beim Autor]. Abdruckrechte: Nicht notwendig. Hinweise Verlag/ Setzerei

1.3 Crystalline Keratitis

The infectious crystalline keratopathy is a rare corneal disease. It affects mainly patients after keratoplasty, as well as after long applied topical glucocorticoid therapy. The disease is usually not painful, as the epithelium is normally closed. The most common pathogen detected is. S. viridans (Ormerod et al. 1991). Fungi

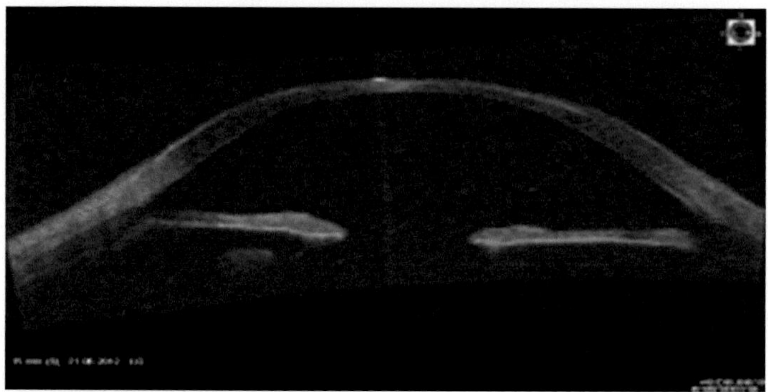

Fig. 12 Visualization of corneal scar caused by acanthamoeboid keratitis using SL-OCT. Superficially, the hyperreflective corneal scar is shown with thinning of the cornea. Datei: Fig. 12_SL OCT Akant.narbe.tif. Abb.-Typ: Strich-Abb. Farbigkeit (IST): 1c. Farbigkeit (SOLL): 1c. Bildrechte: [Urheberrecht beim Autor]. Abdruckrechte: Nicht notwendig. Hinweise Verlag/ Setzerei

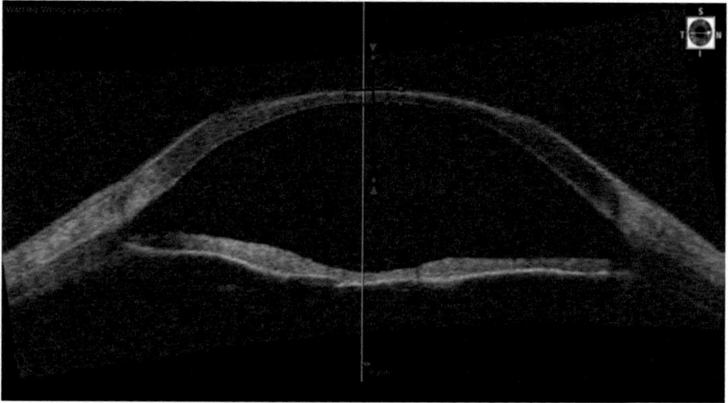

Fig. 13 Illustration of the pachymetry function in SL-OCT. Here, corneal thinning due to acanthamoeboid keratitis with subsequent scarring can be quantified to approximately 285 μm. Datei: Fig. 13-Interactive Pachymetry.tif. Abb.-Typ: Strich-Abb. Farbigkeit (IST): 1c. Farbigkeit (SOLL): 1c. Bildrechte: [Urheberrecht beim Autor]. Abdruckrechte: Nicht notwendig. Hinweise Verlag/Setzerei

are also possible pathogens. As visible in the clinical picture (Fig. 14), a slowly progressive whitish-branched crystalline stromal opacity is often found. The 69-year-old patient shown here developed the crystalline keratitis approximately 1 year after penetrating keratoplasty. OCT imaging shows the extension in the depth of the stroma with closed epithelium very well (arrow marks inflammation localized deep in the stroma). The visual acuity was partly due to a glaucoma fera

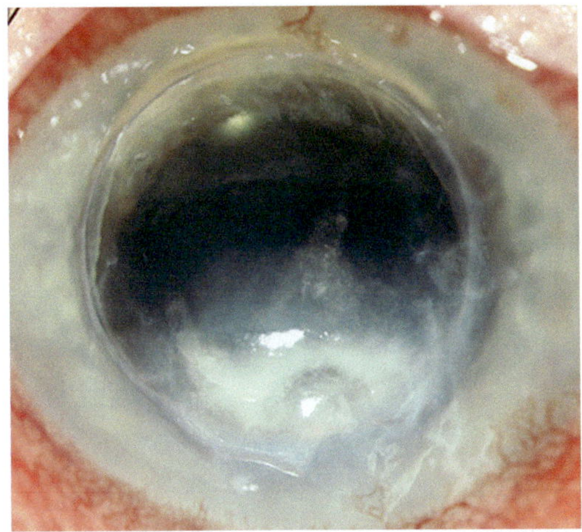

Fig. 14 Clinical picture of crystalline keratitis on the ground of keratoplasty. The lower third of the cornea shows a whitish, branched, partly crystalline stromal opacity. Datei: Fig. 14 Keratitis nach pKPL.tif. Abb.-Typ: Strich-Abb. Farbigkeit (IST): 1c. Farbigkeit (SOLL): 1c. Bildrechte: [Urheberrecht beim Autor]. Abdruckrechte: Nicht notwendig. Hinweise Verlag/Setzerei

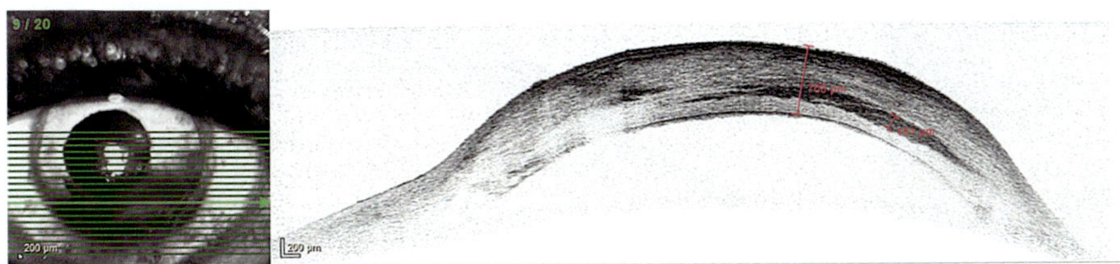

Fig. 15 In anterior segment OCT, the relatively limited keratitis in the depth of the stroma with closed epithelium presents as a hyperreflective structure (marked with arrow). This cross-sectional visualization on OCT can be applied supportively to decide whether to perform a corneal biopsy or a sharp smear. In this example, the sharp smear does not appear to be useful due to the deep stromal location. Datei: Fig. 15 mit pachy.tif. Abb.-Typ: Strich-Abb. Farbigkeit (IST): 1c. Farbigkeit (SOLL): 1c. Bildrechte: [Urheberrecht beim Autor]. Abdruckrechte: Nicht notwendig. Hinweise Verlag/Setzerei

absolutum at hand movements. A sharp swab or corneal biopsy is recommended for diagnosis. The decision whether a swab or a corneal biopsy is more appropriate can be supported by anterior segment-OCT. Therapy is performed by application of local antibiotics over several weeks.

Under antibiotic therapy the findings improved clinically and are also seen in anterior segment-OCT. In anterior segment-OCT the improvement is seen by a decreasing hyperreflectivity in the area of the cornea (arrow) (compare Figs. 16 and 17).

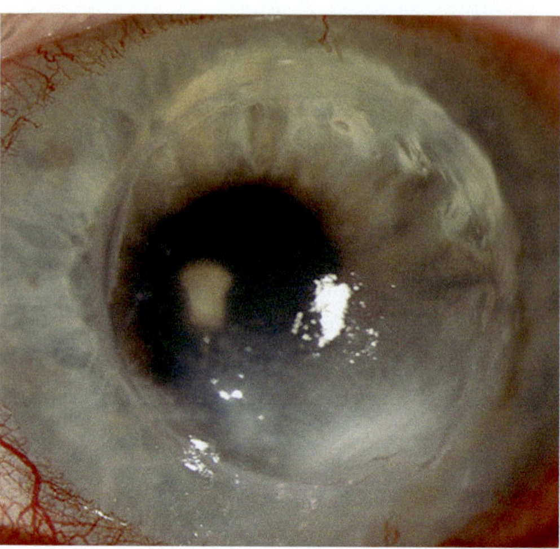

Fig. 16 Clinical picture of crystalline keratitis under local antibiotic therapy. The inflamed area becomes smaller and the graft clears up again. Datei: Fig. 16.tif. Abb.-Typ: Strich-Abb. Farbigkeit (IST): 1c. Farbigkeit (SOLL): 1c. Bildrechte: [Urheberrecht beim Autor]. Abdruckrechte: Nicht notwendig. Hinweise Verlag/Setzerei

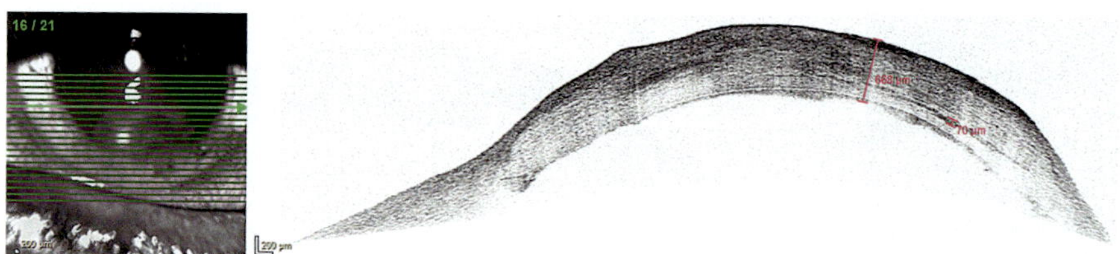

Fig. 17 Anterior segment-OCT image of crystalline keratitis under antibiotic therapy. The previously large deep-stromal keratitis area has now already become much smaller. In cross-section, the hyperreflective area is much flatter and smaller in horizontal extent. Also the corneal edema decreases. Shown in both images is also the thickness measurement in the anterior segment OCT. Thus, corneal thickness decreased from 708 μm to 668 μm under therapy and infiltrate height decreased from 151 μm to 70 μm. Thus, corneal changes can be quantified and compared over time and can thus be helpful in therapy decisions. Datei: Fig. 17.tif. Abb.-Typ: Strich-Abb. Farbigkeit (IST): 1c. Farbigkeit (SOLL): 1c. Bildrechte: [Urheberrecht beim Autor]. Abdruckrechte: Nicht notwendig. Hinweise Verlag/Setzerei

1.4 Herpetic Keratitis

Herpes simplex virus (HSV), usually type 1 is a common causative pathogen of ocular infections. Primary infection involves the eyelids in form of a vesicular blepharitis, but recurrences mostly occur in the cornea. Furthermore, conjunctiva, uvea, sclera and retina may be involved. In herpetic keratitis, the corneal epithelium, stroma, and endothelium may be affected. Metaherpetic keratopathy may develop due to damage of the corneal nerves. HSV lesions can recur throughout life and often lead to progressive corneal scarring, in many cases with neovascularization and corresponding visual loss. Therapy consists of antiviral medications, supplemented by steroids in stromal or endothelial forms. Examples of herpetic keratitis on clinical and OCT images are shown below.

The 8-year-old patient developed a paracentral 0.3 mm subepithelial infiltrate under cyclosporine eye drops, with a 3 mm endothelial annular lesion and localized stromal edema. In this case, the diagnosis was herpetic keratitis with endothelial involvement. The epithelium was already closed at presentation. With local and systemic antiviral therapy, the findings improved rapidly, and the clinical and OCT pictures show the findings after 6 days of therapy. OCT imaging still clearly shows hyperreflective spots in the anterior to mid stroma, presumably immune cells in the setting of inflammation. Visual acuity recovered from 0.1 to 0.6.

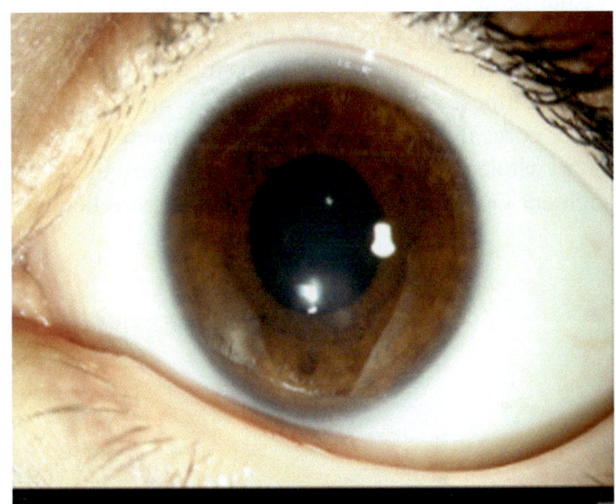

Fig. 18 Clinical picture of herpes keratitis in healing with already closed epithelium. Datei: Fig. 18_herpes.tif. Abb.-Typ: Strich-Abb. Farbigkeit (IST): 1c. Farbigkeit (SOLL): 1c. Bildrechte: [Urheberrecht beim Autor]. Abdruckrechte: Nicht notwendig. Hinweise Verlag/Setzerei

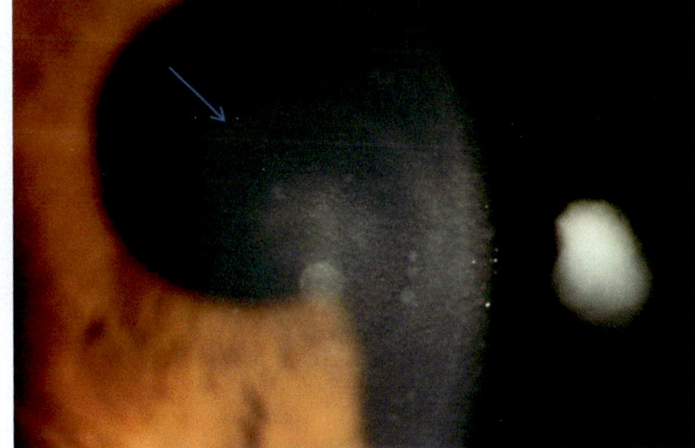

Fig. 19 Enlarged view of Fig. 18. An annular change close to the endothelium is seen, as well as a fine diffuse stromal opacity. Datei: Fig. 19_endotheliiit.tif. Abb.-Typ: Strich-Abb. Farbigkeit (IST): 1c. Farbigkeit (SOLL): 1c. Bildrechte: [Urheberrecht beim Autor]. Abdruckrechte: Nicht notwendig. Hinweise Verlag/Setzerei

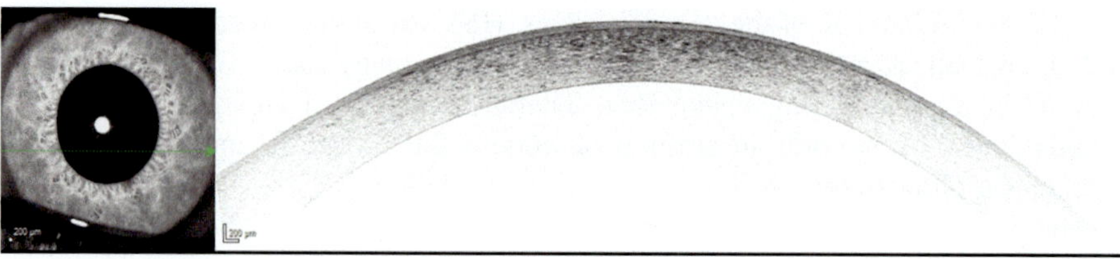

Fig. 20 Anterior segment OCT shows diffuse central compaction with hyperreflective spots, presumably immune cells. Datei: Fig. 20-herpeskeratisis.tif. Abb.-Typ: Strich-Abb. Farbigkeit (IST): 1c. Farbigkeit (SOLL): 1c. Bildrechte: [Urheberrecht beim Autor]. Abdruckrechte: Nicht notwendig. Hinweise Verlag/Setzerei

The following 37 year old patient suffered from metaherpetic keratopathy with significant stromal thinning and marked scarring, as well as neovascularization. Visual acuity was 0.05. There was a history of corneal ulceration in metaherpetic keratopathy, which explains the roundish corneal scar. There had been multiple vascular cauterizations and Avastin applications, as well as amniotic membrane grafts 5 times. Anterior segment-OCT shows two localizations in the cornea. In the upper corneal region, lateral stromal thinning is seen, and paracentrally, the cornea as a whole is clearly thinned and scarred. The scar appears in the anterior segment-OCT as a two-dimensional, hyperreflective structure.

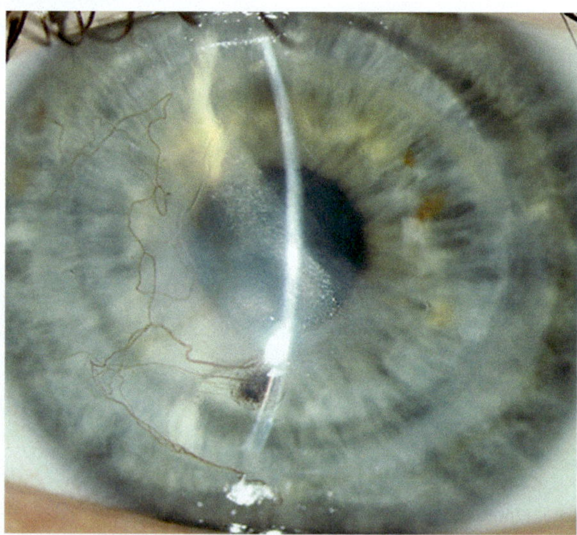

Fig. 21 Clinical picture of metaherpetic keratitis. The scar extending to the optic center, and neovascularizations from nasal inferior and superior are noticeable. Datei: Fig. 21-metaher..tif. Abb.-Typ: Strich-Abb. Farbigkeit (IST): 1c. Farbigkeit (SOLL): 1c. Bildrechte: [Urheberrecht beim Autor]. Abdruckrechte: Nicht notwendig. Hinweise Verlag/Setzerei

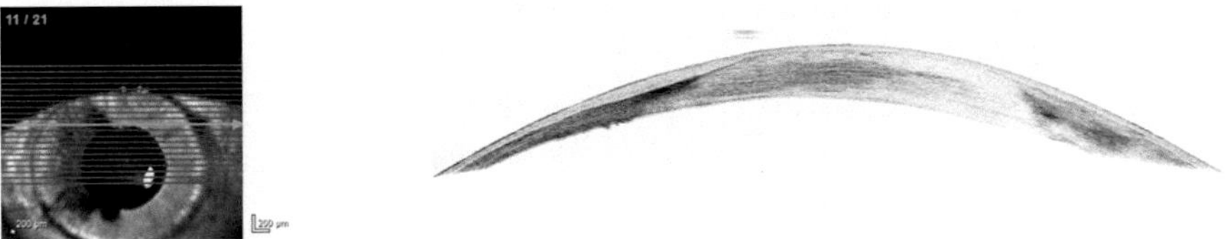

Fig. 22 Visualization of the metaherpetic corneal scar in the anterior segment OCT. In the overview image it can be seen that this cross-section was made in the upper third of the cornea. The irregular cornea with areas of different thickness is shown. Nasally, the cornea is clearly thinned. The scars are hyperreflective areas coming from the nasal as well as from the temporal side. Abb.-Typ: Strich-Abb. Farbigkeit (IST): 1c. Farbigkeit (SOLL): 1c. Bildrechte: [Urheberrecht beim Autor]. Abdruckrechte: Nicht notwendig. Hinweise Verlag/Setzerei: Datei: Fig. 22.tif

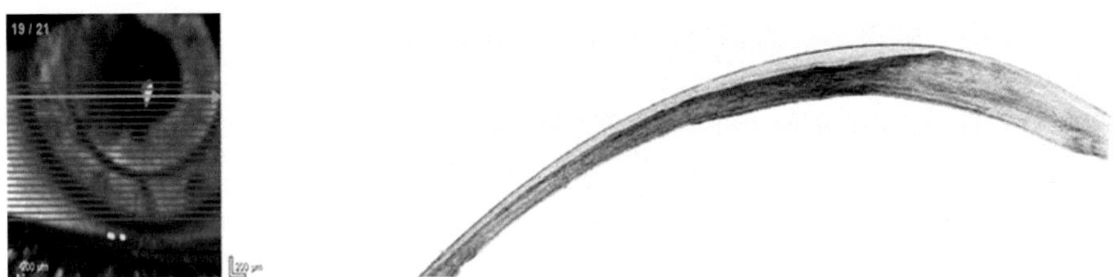

Fig. 23 Anterior segment OCT of a metaherpetic corneal scar. In the overview image at the left margin, it can be seen that this picture is localized just below the optic axis. The scar and the distinct thinning of the cornea extend far peripherally. The central cornea is also affected by the scar, recognizable by the dark hyperreflective areas centrally. The epithelium may partially compensate for the different corneal thicknesses in the transition area, visible by the overlying epithelial layer, which is thicker over the scar and rather thinner in the healthy cornea. Abb.-Typ: Strich-Abb. Datei: Fig. 23.tif. Farbigkeit (IST): 1c. Farbigkeit (SOLL): 1c. Bildrechte: [Urheberrecht beim Autor]. Abdruckrechte: Nicht notwendig. Hinweise Verlag/Setzerei

Penetrating typed keratoplasty with Avastin and repeated vascular cautery was performed. (Figs. 24 and 25) Visual acuity was 0.5 with corneal sutures still in place.

The next 79-year-old patient presented with epithelial herpes keratitis at 9 o'clock (compare Figs. 25 and 26). Visual acuity was 0.8. Herpes infection could be detected by laboratory analysis. Anterior segment-OCT showed localized epithelial thickening around the epithelial defect with marked cell thickening in the area in terms of inflammation.

1.5   Interstitial Keratitis

Interstitial keratitis is a non-ulcerating, non-purulent inflammation of the cornea associated with vascularization in the corneal stroma. The corneal lesions are caused by bacteria (mainly syphilis, borrelia, tuberculosis), viruses (about 40% of

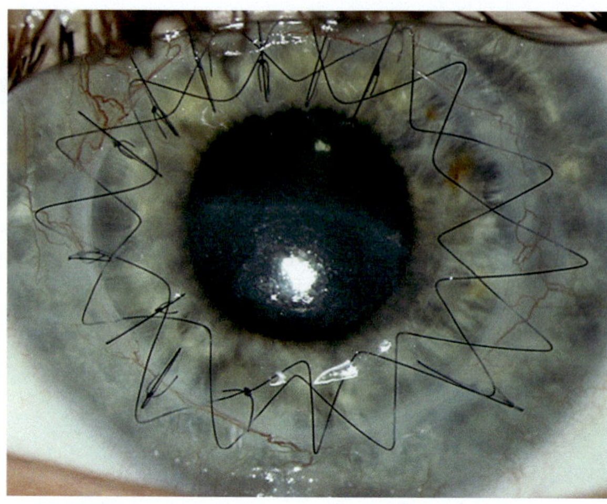

Fig. 24 Clinical picture after penetrating typified keratoplasty on the floor of a metaherpetic corneal scar. The double continuous stellate suture, single single knot sutures, and a central epithelial closure are visible. The neovascularizations were cauterized preoperatively, but are again in the interface. Datei: Fig. 24, nach typ.kP.tif. Abb.-Typ: Strich-Abb. Farbigkeit (IST): 1c. Farbigkeit (SOLL): 1c. Bildrechte: [Urheberrecht beim Autor]. Abdruckrechte: Nicht notwendig. Hinweise Verlag/Setzerei

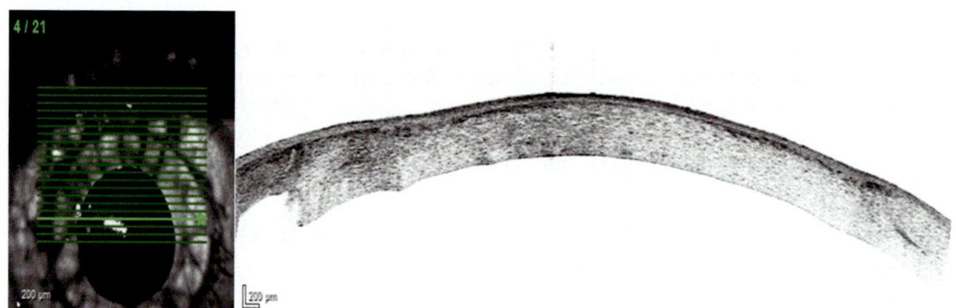

Fig. 25 Anterior segment OCT of a penetrating keratoplasty in a patient with a thinned metaherpetic corneal scar. In the interface area on the left side of the image, the transition between the thin recipient cornea and the graft with an internal step is clearly visible. On the right side of the picture a lying corneal suture in the stroma can be seen peripherally. Datei: Fig. 25, nach typ. kp.tif. Abb.-Typ: Strich-Abb. Farbigkeit (IST): 1c. Farbigkeit (SOLL): 1c. Bildrechte: [Urheberrecht beim Autor]. Abdruckrechte: Nicht notwendig. Hinweise Verlag/Setzerei

cases, mainly HSV; EBV, measles, rubella, mups, influenza), parasites (e.g. malaria, leischmaniasis) or autoimmune diseases (1% of cases, e.g. sarcoidosis, Hodgkins disease, Cogan's syndrome) (Gauthier et al. 2019). A distinction is made between two phases: the active phase and the scarring phase. In the scarring phase, the vessels may present as ghost vessels. Since the disease may be accompanied by

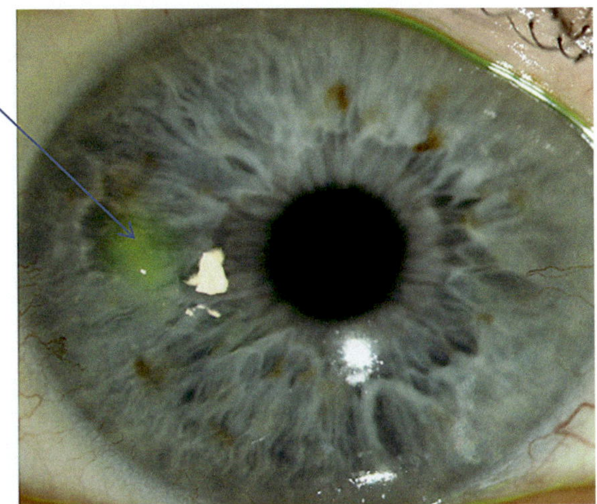

Fig. 26 Clinical picture of epithelial punctate keratitis. The lesion stains yellow with fluorescein. The optic axis is not affected. Datei: Fig. 26-Herpeskeratitis.tif. Abb.-Typ: Strich-Abb. Farbigkeit (IST): 1c. Farbigkeit (SOLL): 1c. Bildrechte: [Urheberrecht beim Autor]. Abdruckrechte: Nicht notwendig. Hinweise Verlag/Setzerei

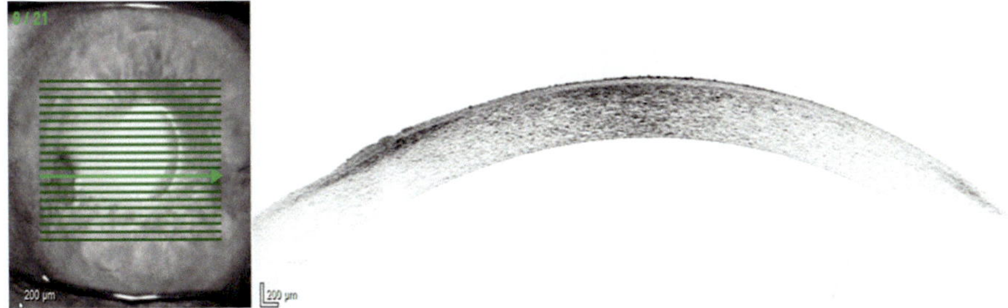

Fig. 27 Anterior segment OCT image through a herpetic epithelial corneal lesion. Localized epithelial thickening in the temporal region of the cornea is seen with marked hyperreflectivity here due to inflammation. Datei: Fig. 27-Herpeskeratitis.tif. Abb.-Typ: Strich-Abb. Farbigkeit (IST): 1c. Farbigkeit (SOLL): 1c. Bildrechte: [Urheberrecht beim Autor]. Abdruckrechte: Nicht notwendig. Hinweise Verlag/Setzerei

systemic infections such as sarcoidosis or syphilis, early diagnosis with appropriate systemic treatment, if necessary, is essential not only for vision.

Two examples of interstitial keratitis are shown below.

The first 32-year-old patient presented with bilateral findings: deep stromal ghost vessels were seen limbally at 6 o'clock, an infiltrate was seen superiorly limbally at 12 o'clock, and the epithelium was closed. On the fellow eye, the findings were similar but milder. In the first image block, the finding in the right eye is shown superiorly. Anterior segment-OCT shows a rather high stromal extension of the interstial keratitis. In the second image block, the finding is shown at 5–6 o'clock with distinct ghost vessels. Here, a low-stromal location is more apparent. Scrolling through the OCT slice images in the volume scan, the course of these vessels, which are no longer perfused, can be partially traced. The diagnosis for Lues and Borrelia was negative, the patient did not show up for the control appointments, which is why the cause of the interstitial keratitis could not be clarified in this case.

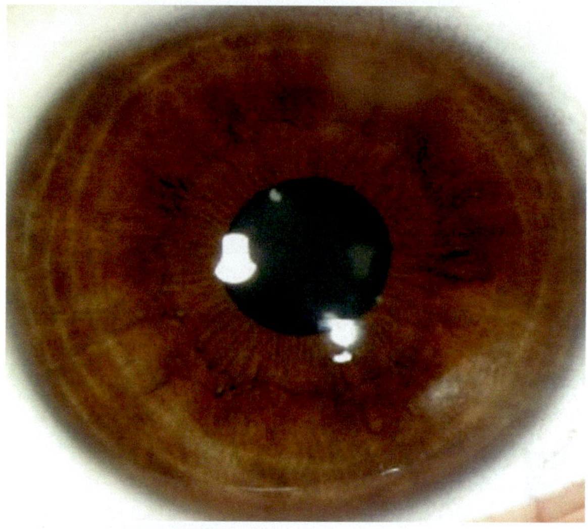

Fig. 28 Interstitial keratitis in the overview. Datei: Fig. 28, interst. Keratitis RA.tif. Abb.-Typ: Strich-Abb. Farbigkeit (IST): 1c. Bildrechte: [Urheberrecht beim Autor]. Abdruckrechte: Nicht notwendig. Hinweise Verlag/Setzerei

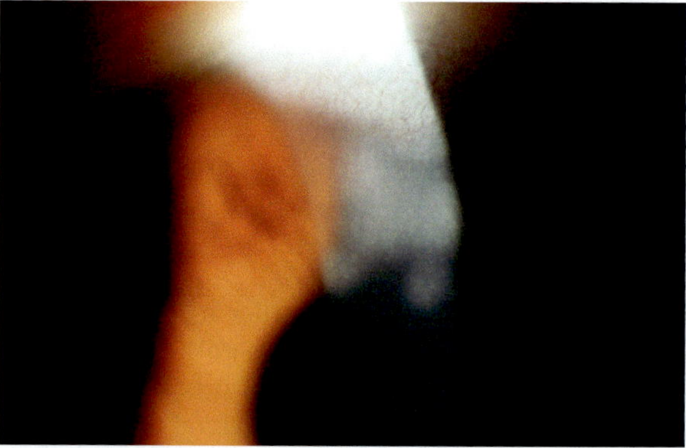

Fig. 29 Interstitial keratitis in higher magnification: there is an infiltrate limbally at 12 o'clock, the epithelium is closed. Datei: Fig. 29 interst. Keratitis RA sup oben.tif. Abb.-Typ: Strich-Abb. Farbigkeit (IST): 1c. Farbigkeit (SOLL): 1c. Bildrechte: [Urheberrecht beim Autor]. Abdruckrechte: Nicht notwendig

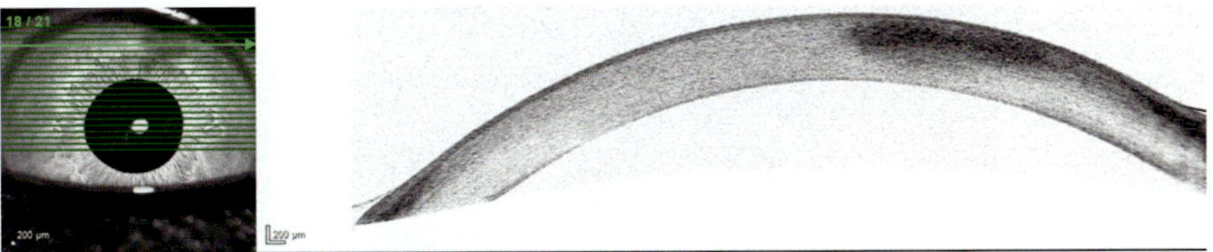

Fig. 30 Interstitial keratitis on anterior segment OCT: anterior to mid stroma shows hyperreflective areas with closed epithelium and regular endothelium and posterior stroma. Datei: Fig. 30, interst. Keratitis RA.tif. Farbigkeit (IST): 1c. Farbigkeit (SOLL): 1c. Bildrechte: [Urheberrecht beim Autor]. Abdruckrechte: Nicht notwendig. Hinweise Verlag/Setzerei

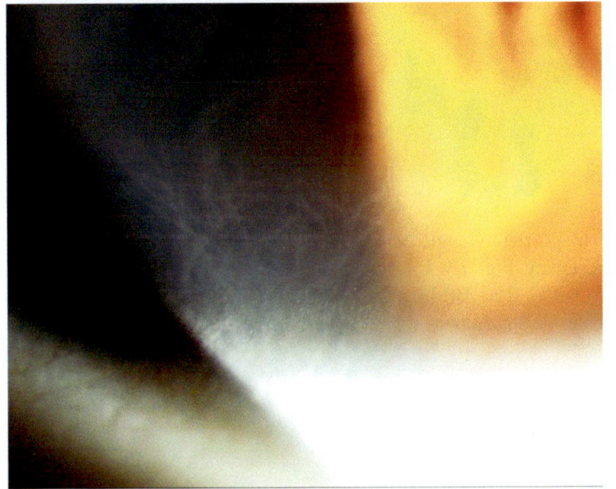

Fig. 31 Clinical image of ghost vessels originating from the limbus at 6 o'clock in magnification. Datei: Fig. 31, ghost vessels.tif. Abb.-Typ: Strich-Abb. Farbigkeit (IST): 1c. Farbigkeit (SOLL): 1c. Bildrechte: [Urheberrecht beim Autor]. Abdruckrechte: Nicht notwendig. Hinweise Verlag/ Setzerei

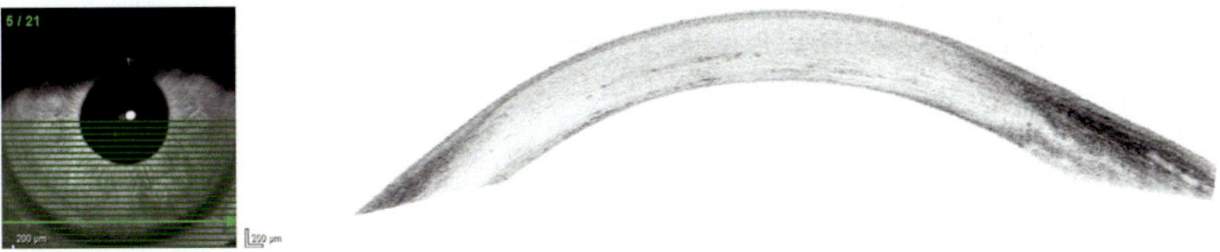

Fig. 32 Visualization of ghost vessels on anterior segment OCT. The ghost vessels are shown as hyperreflective spots localized in the posterior to mid stroma. Datei: Fig. 32_ghost vesssels.tif. Abb.-Typ: Strich-Abb. Farbigkeit (IST): 1c. Farbigkeit (SOLL): 1c. Bildrechte: [Urheberrecht beim Autor]. Abdruckrechte: Nicht notwendig. Hinweise Verlag/Setzerei

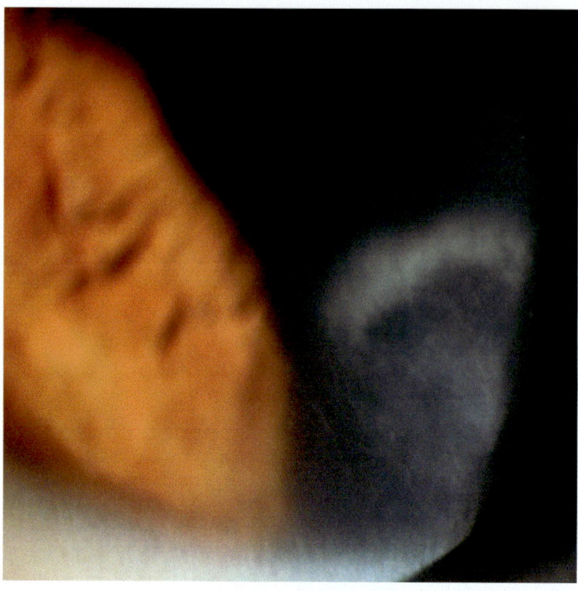

Fig. 33 Clinical magnified image of inferior peripheral corneal scar with ghost vessels in interstitial keratitis. Datei: Fig. 33, LA interst. Kerat,.tif. Abb.-Typ: Strich-Abb. Farbigkeit (IST): 1c. Farbigkeit (SOLL): 1c. Bildrechte: [Urheberrecht beim Autor]. Abdruckrechte: Nicht notwendig. Hinweise Verlag/Setzerei

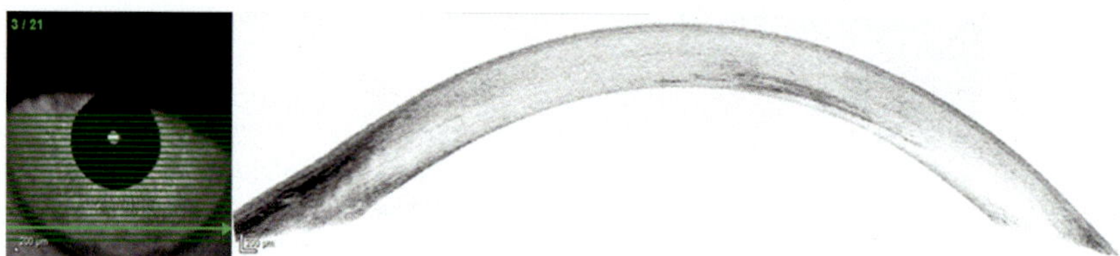

Fig. 34 Visualization of ghost vessels in interstitial keratitis in anterior segment OCT: here, the ghost vessels are recognizable as hyperreflective spots. Their location is again deep to middle stromal. Datei: Fig. 34, interst. Kerati, LA.tif. Abb.-Typ: Strich-Abb. Bildrechte: [Urheberrecht beim Autor]. Abdruckrechte: Nicht notwendig. Hinweise Verlag/Setzerei

The left eye also showed ghost vessels with stromal scars.

The second case shows a 30-year-old woman with interstitial bilateral keratitis, induced by a borrellia infection. Visual acuity was 0.6 and 0.8. Diffuse opacities were seen in the superficial stroma, with only isolated deep stromal areas.

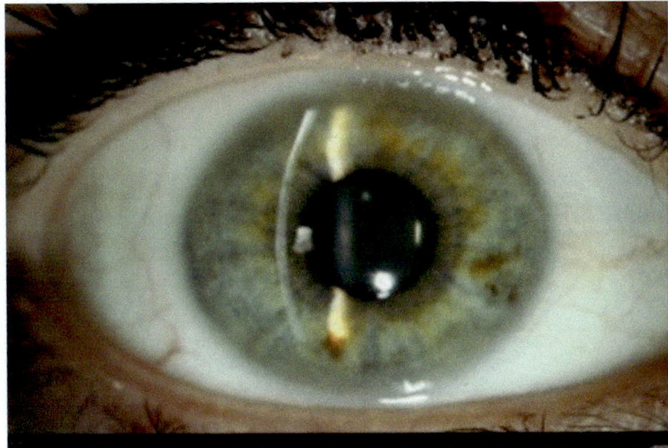

Fig. 35 Clinical overview of a patient with interstitial keratitis caused by a Borrelia infection. Datei: Fig. 35, IK.tif. Abb.-Typ: Strich-Abb. Farbigkeit (IST): 1c. Farbigkeit (SOLL): 1c. Bildrechte: [Urheberrecht beim Autor]. Abdruckrechte: Nicht notwendig. Hinweise Verlag/Setzerei

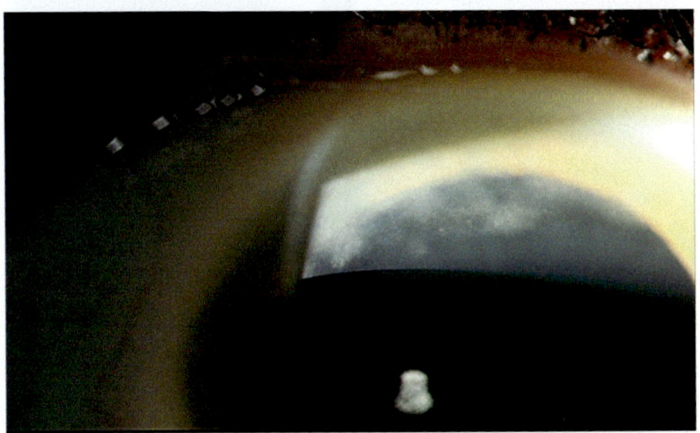

Fig. 36 Magnification shows the superficial partly patchy opacity of the cornea coming from the limbus at 12 o'clock. Datei: Fig. 36, IK.tif. Abb.-Typ: Strich-Abb. Farbigkeit (IST): 1c. Farbigkeit (SOLL): 1c. Bildrechte: [Urheberrecht beim Autor]. Abdruckrechte: Nicht notwendig. Hinweise Verlag/Setzerei

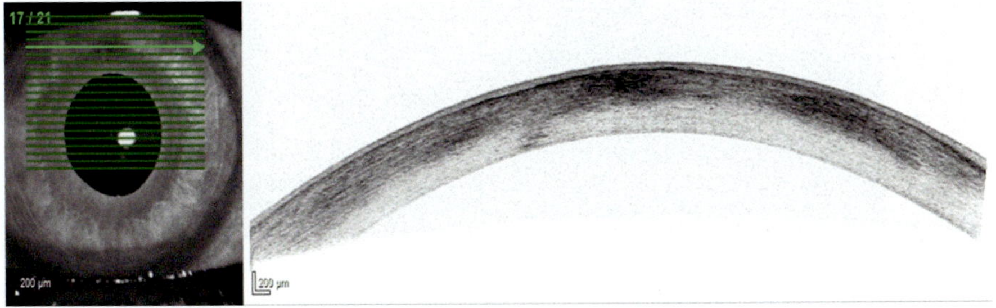

Fig. 37 Interstitial borrelia-related keratitis on anterior segment OCT. The corneal opacities are mainly located in the anterior and middle stroma, only occasionally they extend to the deep stroma. Datei: Fig. 37, IK.tif. Abb.-Typ: Strich Abb. Farbigkeit (IST): 1c. Farbigkeit (SOLL): 1c. Bildrechte: [Urheberrecht beim Autor]. Abdruckrechte: Nicht notwendig. Hinweise Verlag/Setzerei

1.6 Corneal Involvement in Scleromalacia

A 43-year-old patient came in with the findings shown in Figs. 38 and 39. More than 20 years ago he had suffered from autoimmune scleritis with corneal involvement. Since that time, this corneal finding presented with significantly swollen stroma and, in some cases, markedly thinned areas. Visual acuity was 0.1. There was a high irregular astigmatism.

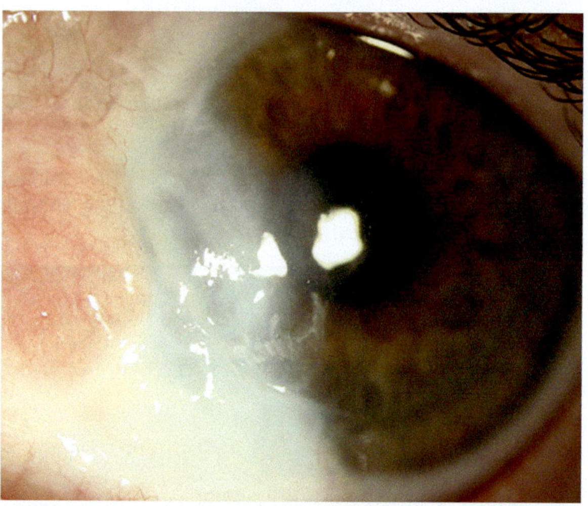

Fig. 38 Clinical picture of a patient with corneal involvement in scleromalacia. The cornea from nasal is scarred and appears odematous. Datei: Fig. 38_Skleromalazie.tif. Abb.-Typ: Strich-Abb. Farbigkeit (IST): 1c. Farbigkeit (SOLL): 1c. Bildrechte: [Urheberrecht beim Autor]. Abdruckrechte: Nicht notwendig. Hinweise Verlag/Setzerei

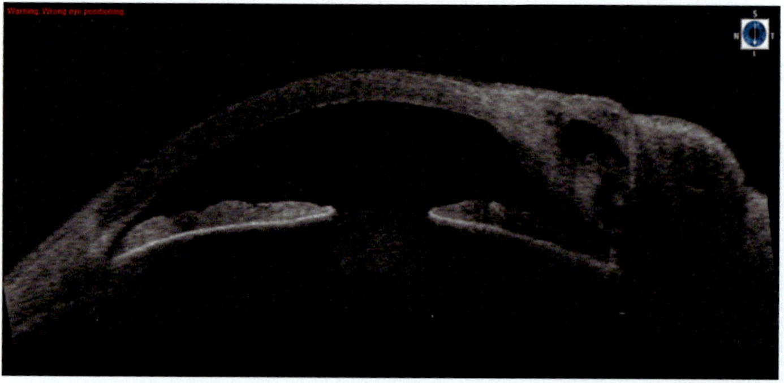

Fig. 39 SL-OCT of corneal involvement in scleromalacia. The cornea is clearly thickened in the affected area. A cystic structure is visible under the epithelium. Datei: Fig. 39-Auto Biometry.tif. Abb.-Typ: Strich-Abb. Farbigkeit (IST): 1c. Farbigkeit (SOLL): 1c. Bildrechte: [Urheberrecht beim Autor]. Abdruckrechte: Nicht notwendig. Hinweise Verlag/Setzerei

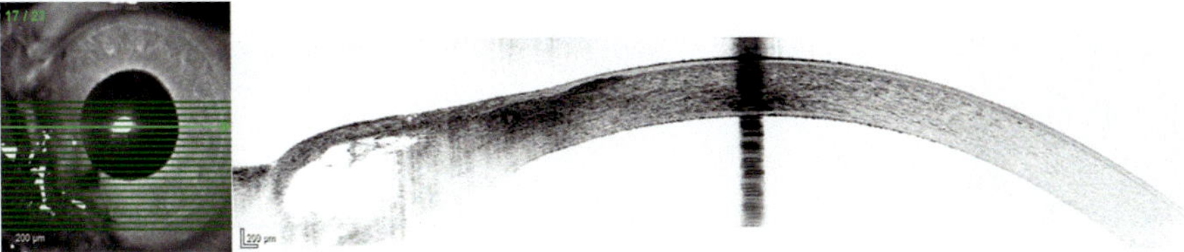

Fig. 40 Corneal involvement in scleromalacia on anterior segment OCT: here, the cystic structure arises in nasal detail. Next to it, the corneal scar presents as a dense relatively homogeneous hyperreflective layer. Datei: Fig. 40-oct.tif. Abb.-Typ: Strich-Abb. Farbigkeit (IST): 1c. Farbigkeit (SOLL): 1c. Bildrechte: [Urheberrecht beim Autor]. Abdruckrechte: Nicht notwendig. Hinweise Verlag/Setzerei

SL- and anterior segment-OCT show the cystically altered limbal area with marked thickening of cornea and sclera in this case.

1.7 Autoimmune Corneal Ulcer with Descemetocele

A 41-year-old female patient presented with visual deterioration in the right eye for 3 years. There was a localized almost complete stromal melting of the cornea with descemetocele (Figs. 41, 42, 43 and 44). Anterior segment OCT and SL-OCT each clearly show the stromal melting in cross-section. This allows, for example,

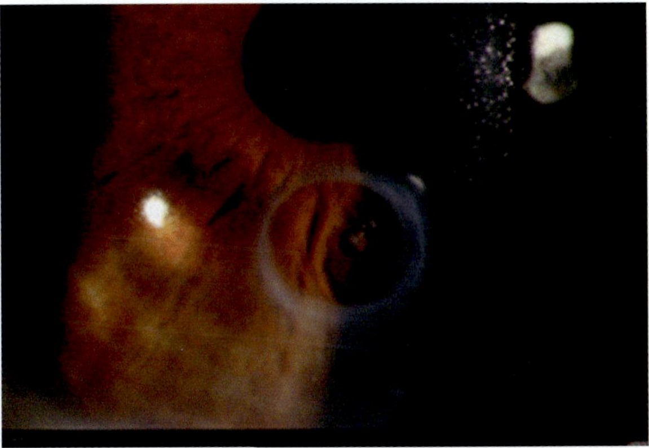

Fig. 41 Clinical picture of autoimmune corneal melting with descemetocele. Datei: Fig. 41, autoimmun ulkus.tif. Abb.-Typ: Strich-Abb. Farbigkeit (IST): 1c. Farbigkeit (SOLL): 1c. Bildrechte: [Urheberrecht beim Autor]. **a**: Enlarged image of autoimmune corneal melting with descemetocele. Datei: Fig. 41a, autoimmun ulkus.tif. Abb.-Typ: Strich-Abb. Farbigkeit (IST): 1c. Farbigkeit (SOLL): 1c. Bildrechte: [Urheberrecht beim Autor]. Abdruckrechte: Nicht notwendig. Hinweise Verlag/Setzerei

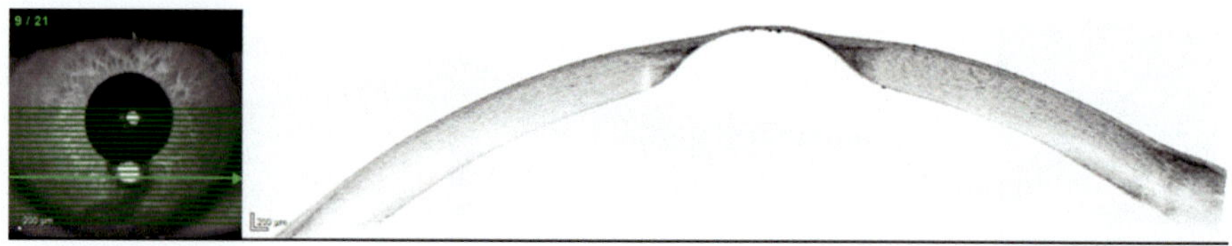

Fig. 42 Visualization of the descemetocele in the anterior segment OCT. The marked stromal melting is visible, as well as fine pigment coatings on the endothelium. Directly adjacent to the descemetocele there is increased hyperreflectivity, in the sense of increased inflammation here. Datei: autoimmun ulkus OCT Fig. 42.tif. Abb.-Typ: Strich-Abb. Farbigkeit (IST): 1c. Farbigkeit (SOLL): 1c. Bildrechte: [Urheberrecht beim Autor]. Abdruckrechte: Nicht notwendig. Hinweise Verlag/Setzerei

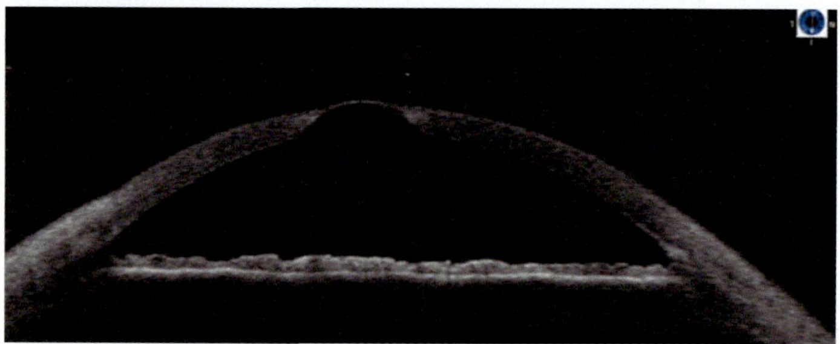

Fig. 43 (Fig. 45) Illustration of the decemetocele in SL-OCT. This also clearly shows the pronounced stromal melting, as well as a better overview of the entire anterior chamber, but less detail in the cornea. Datei: Fig. 43 oct.tif. Abb.-Typ: Strich-Abb. Farbigkeit (IST): 1c. Farbigkeit (SOLL): 1c. Bildrechte: [Urheberrecht beim Autor]. Abdruckrechte: Nicht notwendig. Hinweise Verlag/Setzerei

measurement of the residual corneal thickness, which in this patient was 58 μm (image of measurement not shown). Anterior segment and SL-OCT show hyperreflective areas in addition to the descemetocele, presumably due to increased inflammation. Also visible on anterior segment OCT are fine pigmentary coatings on the endothelium. Due to the paracentral location, visual acuity was still at 0.6. She developed sectorial anterior scleritis during the course. The examination of rheumatologic or infectious causes was unremarkable, so that an idiopathic scleritis with autoimmunologic corneal melting with descemetocele was assumed. The finding remained unchanged for 2 years and was treated with cortisone in descending dosage to a low systemic maintenance dose (5 mg) and locally 1 drop of cortisone daily. Furthermore, a bandage lens was applied. However, due to trauma, perforation then occurred and the descemetocele was treated with mini-keratoplasty. Visual acuity 4 weeks postoperatively was 0.3. A further increase is expected in the course after removal of the sutures.

Fig. 44 Clinical picture after perforating mini-keratoplasty on the base of a perforation of the descemetocele. The cornea is supplied with a bandage lens. Datei: Fig. 44, mini KPL.tif. Abb.-Typ: Strich-Abb. Farbigkeit (IST): 1c. Farbigkeit (SOLL): 1c. Bildrechte: [Urheberrecht beim Autor]. Abdruckrechte: Nicht notwendig. Hinweise Verlag/Setzerei

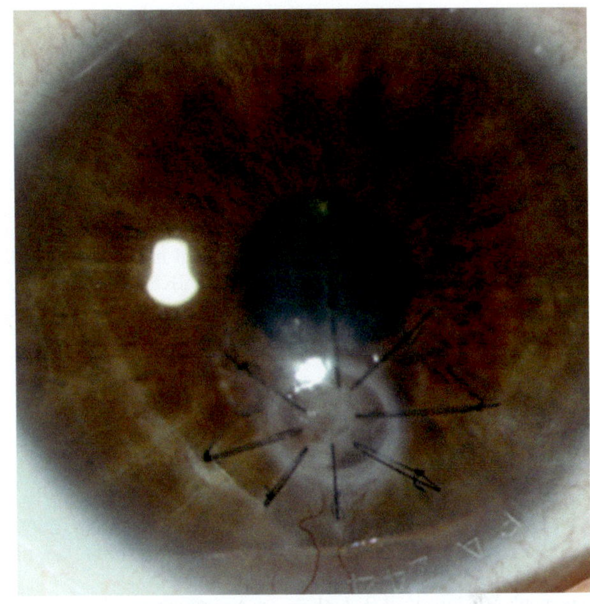

Fig. 45 Enlarged view of penetrating mini-keratoplasty with single knot sutures. Inferiorly, neovascularization is already visible up to the graft margin. Datei: Fig. 45, mini kpl.tif. Abb.-Typ: Strich-Abb. Farbigkeit (IST): 1c. Farbigkeit (SOLL): 1c. Bildrechte: [Urheberrecht beim Autor]. Abdruckrechte: Nicht notwendig. Hinweise Verlag/Setzerei

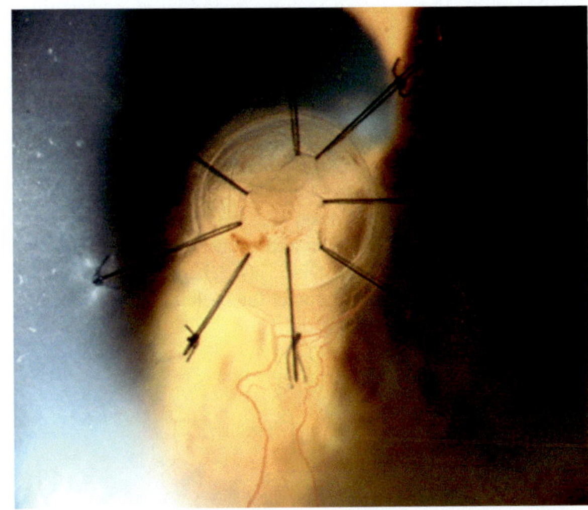

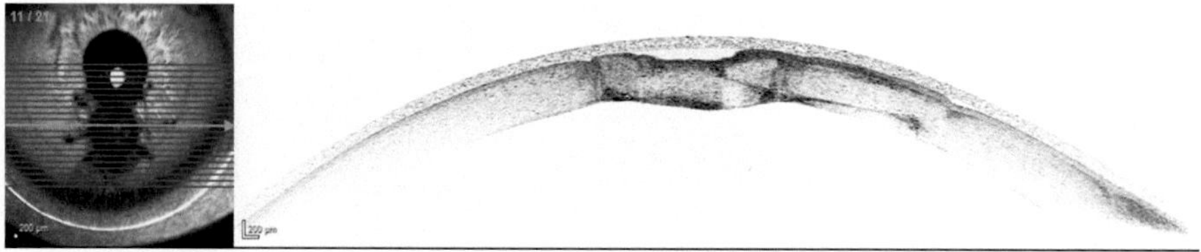

Fig. 46 Visualization of penetrating mini-keratoplasty in anterior segment OCT. The image is taken 4 weeks postoperatively; the graft still has wrinkles and appears slightly wavy. Overlying shows the bandage lens. Datei: Fig. 46, miniKPL.tif. Abb.-Typ: Strich-Abb. Farbigkeit (IST): 1c. Farbigkeit (SOLL): 1c. Bildrechte: [Urheberrecht beim Autor]. Abdruckrechte: Nicht notwendig. Hinweise Verlag/Setzerei

References

Al-Mujaini A, et al. Bacterial keratitis: perspective on epidemiology, clinico-pathogenesis, diagnosis and treatment. Sultan Qaboos Univ Med J. 2009;9(2):184–95.

Gauthier AS, Noureddine S, Delbosc B. Interstitial keratitis diagnosis and treatment. J Fr Ophtalmol. 2019;42(6):e229–37.

Maycock NJ, Jayaswal R. Update on Acanthamoeba keratitis: diagnosis, treatment, and outcomes. Cornea. 2016;35(5):713–20.

Ng AL, et al. Predisposing factors, microbial characteristics, and clinical outcome of microbial keratitis in a tertiary centre in Hong Kong: a 10-year experience. J Ophthalmol. 2015;2015: 769436.

Ormerod LD et al. Infectious crystalline keratopathy. Role of nutritionally variant streptococci and other bacterial factors. Ophthalmology. 1991;98(2):159–69.

Saeed A, et al. Risk factors, microbiological findings, and clinical outcomes in cases of microbial keratitis admitted to a tertiary referral center in Ireland. Cornea. 2009;28(3):285–92.

Stapleton F, Carnt N. Contact lens-related microbial keratitis: how have epidemiology and genetics helped us with pathogenesis and prophylaxis. Eye (London). 2012;26(2):185–93.

Stapleton F, et al. Risk factors and causative organisms in microbial keratitis in daily disposable contact lens wear. PLoS ONE. 2017;12(8): e0181343.

Yildiz EH, et al. Trends in contact lens-related corneal ulcers at a tertiary referral center. Cornea. 2012;31(10):1097–102.

Optical Coherence Tomography in Corneal Dystrophies

Sebastian Siebelmann, Simon Sonnenschein, Takahiko Hayashi, Mario Matthaei, Ludwig M. Heindl, Claus Cursiefen, Oscar Gris, and José Güell

The term corneal dystrophy was initially introduced in 1890 by Groenouw on the basis of two patients with macular and granular corneal dystrophy and was subsequently used by various other authors such as Biber or Fuchs. Corneal dystrophies are hereditary diseases of the cornea associated with different deposits in different layers of the cornea. Currently, corneal dystrophies are divided into 22 different dystrophies according to the IC3D classification. In general, the subtypes (a) epithelial-subepithelial, (b) epithelial-stromal TGFBI, (c) stromal and (d) endothelial dystrophies are distinguished (Weiss et al. 2015).

Depending on the affected layer, patients usually suffer from symptoms such as a reduction in visual acuity, irritative phenomena such as foreign body sensation, redness or burning, and even recurrent erosions. Corneal dystrophies are usually diagnosed directly by a trained examiner using a slit lamp microscope. Nevertheless, the differential diagnosis of different corneal dystrophies is a challenge and is technically performed by different illumination variations of the slit lamp, especially by means of illumination in retroillumination. The diagnosis is then made as an interplay of anamnesis and typical, pattern-shaped distribution of deposits in the cornea. The depth of the deposits within the cornea also plays an important role. This is not only decisive for the diagnosis, but in times of laser surgery and lamellar corneal transplants, it is especially important for the following surgical therapy and the prognosis of the disease. For example, in the case of superficial deposits in the cornea, an excimer laser phototherapeutic keratectomy

S. Siebelmann (✉) · S. Sonnenschein · M. Matthaei · L. M. Heindl · C. Cursiefen
Department of Ophthalmology, University Hospital of Cologne, Cologne, Germany
e-mail: s.siebelmann@googlemail.com

T. Hayashi
Division of Ophthalmology, Department of Visual Sciences, Nihon University School of Medicine, Itabashi, Tokyo, Japan

O. Gris · J. Güell
Instituto Microcirugia Ocular (IMO), IMO, Barcelona, Spain

L. M. Heindl and S. Siebelmann (eds.), *Optical Coherence Tomography of the Anterior Segment*, https://doi.org/10.1007/978-3-031-07730-2_8

(PTK) or an anterior lamellar keratoplasty (ALK) can be a good treatment for the patient (Hong et al. 2010). On the other hand, for medium depth deposits that do not affect the Descemet membrane, a deep anterior lamellar keratoplasty (DALK) should be performed. This has the advantage that the patients experience a faster visual rehabilitation on the one hand and on the other hand no endothelial rejection reactions occur, because the eye is not opened and the recipient Descemet's membrane with endothelium remains intact. Due to these significant advantages, the evaluation and examination of corneal dystrophies by means of Optical Coherence Tomography (OCT) is gaining more and more importance. In fact, not only can it help to establish the correct diagnosis, but it can also be of great importance in the planning of the subsequent surgical procedure and, if necessary, even prevent complications and improve the safety profile of the surgery. In particular, the possibility of visualizing all corneal layers by means of optical coherence tomography and of distinguishing, for example, between deep-stromal and endothelial pathologies, and subepithelial and anterior stromal deposits, is of great value. The increasing resolution in anterior segment OCT in recent years, as well as the developments in automatic image data analysis, especially by means of artificial intelligence (AI), as well as volume calculation and three-dimensional representation of specific structures, will increasingly put OCT in the focus of diagnostics and treatment planning in patients with corneal dystrophies in the coming years. In addition, even after lamellar or penetrating keratoplasty, the success of the operation and the postoperative course can be analysed by OCT and evaluated in an outpatient setting (see Chap. 10 "Corneal Transplantion"). In addition, microscope-integrated intraoperative MI-OCT is becoming more and more important in the treatment of corneal dystrophies, especially when the view into the anterior chamber is reduced or very thin or transparent structures are to be transplanted, as in Descemet Membrane Endothelial Keratoplasty (DMEK) and Descemet Stripping Automated Endothelial Keratoplasty (DSAEK) (Siebelmann et al. 2016). In the following, an overview of the findings visible in anterior segment OCT for different corneal dystrophies will be given. If available, a clinical image will always be placed next to an exemplary OCT image. In this context, OCT can be used to display high-resolution and cross-sectional characteristics for the individual corneal dystrophies. The OCT image describes with a good correlation the structural and morphological changes of the underlying dystrophies. Also depth, extent, size and position of the respective morphology can be displayed.

This combination of a microscopic view using a slit lamp on the one hand and an almost histological cross-sectional view using OCT on the other is particularly helpful and attractive.

The following chapter will give an overview of typical OCT findings in different corneal dystrophies. These are listed according to the IC3D classification and, if possible, a slit lamp image is compared to the OCT image. So far, however, no data exist for the Fleck Corneal Dystrophy (FCD), the Subepithelial Mucinous Corneal Dystrophy (SMCD), the Posterior Amorphous Corneal Dystrophy (PACD) and the X-chromosomal Endothelial Corneal Dystrophy (XECD).

INFOBOX: Intraoperative OCT for Anaesthetic Examinations of Children Newborns and infants, as well as patients with mental or physical disabilities, often cannot be placed in front of a normal, ambulant OCT devices and examined with it. For this group of patients, microscope-integrated, intraoperative OCT offers a great advantage. In MI-OCT, an OCT is technically integrated into a surgical microscope, so that patients who require examination under general anaesthesia can be examined simultaneously with the high magnification surgical microscope and simultaneously with high-resolution OCT (Geerling et al. 2005). This examination is particularly important in the case of congenital or juvenile corneal opacities. On the one hand, a Peters anomaly can be distinguished from a sclerocornea, other dysgenesis of the anterior segment of the eye or a simple superficial corneal scars (Siebelmann et al. 2015a). On the other hand, the depth of the respective changes can be shown. As described above, this is decisive for the following treatment, which can then range from a simple lamellar keratectomy, an excimer laser phototherapeutic keratectomy to a lamellar or complete or autorotation keratoplasty, depending on the examination findings (Siebelmann et al. 2015a, 2018a). In addition, when examining children with congenital glaucoma or retinal diseases, it is also possible to visualize the optic nerve head in the sense of a optic nerve head OCT or to search the macula, e.g. to exclude macular edema (Siebelmann et al. 2018a). However, the limitations of this technology to date are still insufficient intraoperative measurement tools, e.g. for measuring corneal thickness, the depth of corneal scars or the depth of the anterior chamber. Furthermore, the devices are still quite expensive and are usually replaced by newer devices after a short time, so that there is still a lot of potential for development (Siebelmann et al. 2015b).

(1) Epithelial Basement Membrane Dystrophy (EBMD)

Epithelial Basement Membrane Dystrophy (EBMD) is also generally known as Map-Dot-Fingerprint Dystrophy. This name already describes the classical findings visible at the slit lamp. In this context, intraepithelial maps, Cogan dots, and fingerprint lines that resemble fingerprints are conspicuous at the slit lamp. In addition, microcystic patterns combined with Cogan dots may also be conspicuous, as well as epithelial double folds, or blisters, which sometimes lead to recurrent corneal erosions (Rodrigues et al. 1974).

OCT findings: All findings that can also be detected by slit lamp are to be visualized by OCT. Both the histologically described irregularities and fractures of the Bowman's layer with fragments that partly even protrude into the corneal epithelium are noticeable. Furthermore, intraepithelial and subepithelial inclusions are visible, which correlate with the dots in the slit-lamp findings. Furthermore, the epithelium is very irregular with thinned, but also thickened and bulging regions. Furthermore, focal epithelial detachments or doublings in the sense of the vesicles seen at the slit lamp are visible. Thickenings caused by maps, dots and fingerprint-like deposits are hyperreflective in the OCT image. These only affect the epithelium and subepithelial areas. In addition, the Bowman's layer and superficial, stromal areas of the cornea are affected. Deeper deposits are not visible (Wu et al. 2013) (Figs. 1, 2, 3 and 4).

(2) Epithelial Recurrent Erosion Dystrophy (ERED)

Patients with a dystrophy of recurrent corneal erosion, or with recurrent corneal erosion syndrome (Epithelial Recurrent Erosion Dystrophy, ERED) suffer from multiple and recurrent phases of corneal erosion, as already included in the name of dystrophy. In the acute phase these are naturally recognizable by the slit lamp, in the symptom-free interval only subtle epithelial condensations, a focal subepithelial fibrosis or raised and loose epithelial bullae are visible (Goldman et al. 1969).

OCT findings: Using optical coherence tomography, patients suffering from this dystrophy are often easily identifiable. Often localized irregularities as well as fractures or protrusions of the corneal epithelium are visible. In some cases whole, coherent epithelial dehiscences are visible which are not noticeable at the slit lamp. Also, intraepithelial and hyperreflective lines and foci below the Bowman's layer may be visible. Fractures in the Bowman's layer are also visible (Diez-Feijóo and Durán 2015) (Fig. 5).

(3) Subepithelial Mucinous Corneal Dystrophy (SMCD)

No image data are available for subepithelial, mucinous corneal dystrophy.

(4) Meesmann Corneal Dystrophy (MECD)

The diagnosis of Meesmann's corneal dystrophy is particularly facilitated by retroillumination using a slit lamp. Intraepithelial cysts are particularly noticeable. In addition, whitish opacities of the cornea and roundish, mostly transparent, small intraepithelial inclusions are noticeable (Patel et al. 2005).

OCT findings: With the help of anterior segment OCT, slit-lamp findings in particular can be traced very well in retrograde illumination. In this respect, the

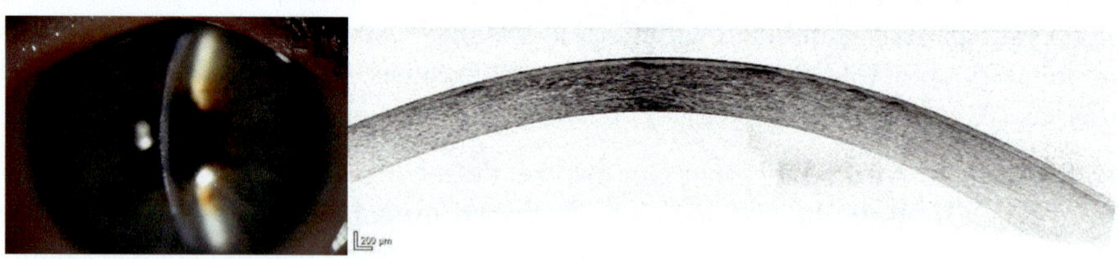

Fig. 1 Epithelial Basement Membrane Dystrophy (EBMD). OCT imaging reveals epithelial flare, hyperreflective areas, and a disrupted and raised Bowman's layer

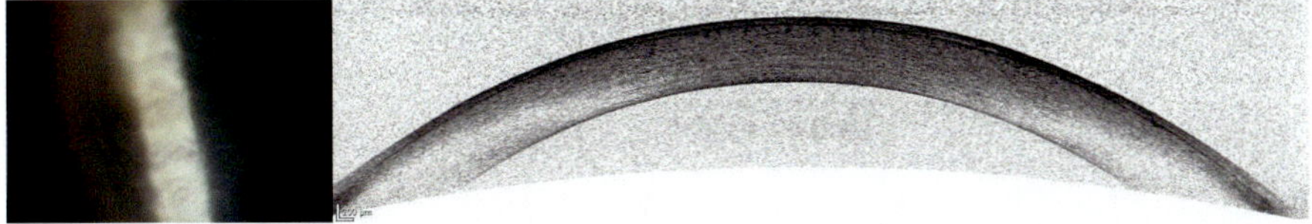

Fig. 2 Epithelial Basement Membrane Dystrophy (EBMD). While a normal corneal image can be seen at the slit lamp, OCT imaging can show an area where the epithelium is lamellarly detached. This patient probably has an increased risk for corneal erosion. However, there are no studies that investigate whether treatment, such as therapeutic contact lenses or hyperosmolar eye drops in this case, should be based on OCT findings alone

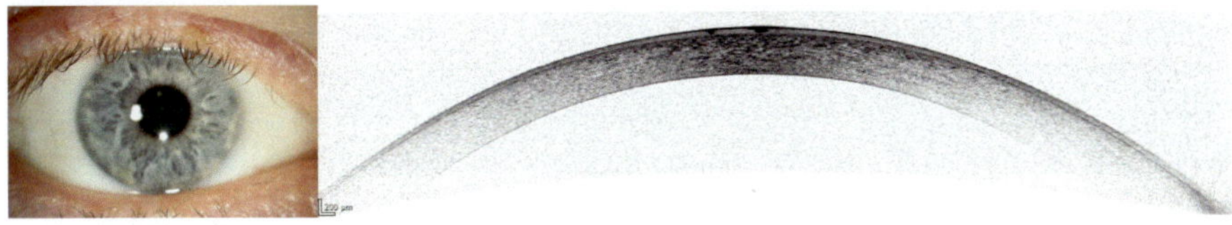

Fig. 3 Epithelial Basement Membrane Dystrophy (EBMD). This image shows hyperreflective epithelial inclusions in OCT imaging. The Bowman's layer is irregular but not clearly prominent. The epithelial inclusions also lead to slight epithelial elevations

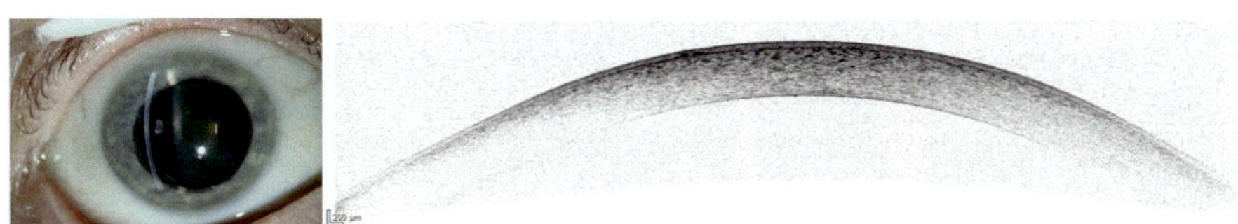

Fig. 4 Epithelial Basement Membrane Dystrophy (EBMD). In this OCT image both epithelial and subepithelial inclusions are visible. The Bowmwn's layer is partly completely interrupted and partly thickened. The epithelium is also clearly raised, but in some areas extremely thinned

characteristic intraepithelial cysts of the slit lamp are shown in the OCT image as disseminated and rather hyporeflective cysts within the epithelium. Furthermore, a thickening of the basement membrane is visible (Vajzovic et al. 2011) (Fig. 6).

(5) Lisch Epithelial Corneal Dystrophy (LECD)

Typical slit-lamp findings in epithelial corneal dystrophy, named after Prof. Lisch, are focal, vertebral opacities in the epithelium, some of which form grayish radial, feathery or club-shaped formations. Epithelial cysts are also noticeable in regressive light (Lisch et al. 1992).

OCT findings: By means of OCT, clear compressions can be seen, especially in the epithelium. However, the epithelium itself is not thickened. Nevertheless, subepithelial shading is visible due to the epithelial, hyperreflective thickening (Alvarez-Fischer et al. 2005) (Fig. 7).

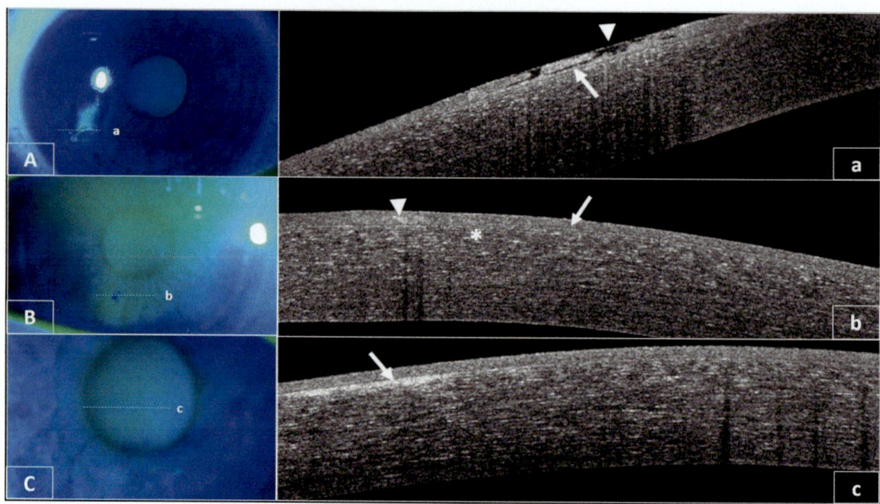

Fig. 5 Epithelial Recurrent Erosion Dystrophy. **A + a** Imaging shows breaks and localized detachments in the epithelium. **B + b** There are also isolated hyperreflective areas in the epithelium and subepithelial epithelium. **C + c** Also distinct hyperreflective areas are visible subepithelially. (From Diez-Feijóo and Durán 2015)

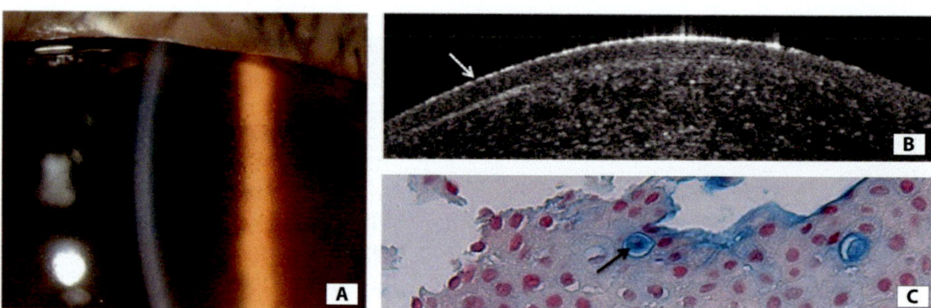

Fig. 6 Meesmann's Corneal Dystrophy. **A** Clinical slit lamp findings. **B** In Meesmann's Corneal Dystrophy, OCT imaging shows mainly intraepithelial microcysts which can be visualized as hyporeflective. Also a clear thickening of the basement membrane can be seen very well. **C** Histologically, intraepithelial microcysts which are Alcian blue positive can be found (from Vajzovic et al. 2011)

(6) Gelatinous Drop-like Corneal Dystrophy (GDLD)

Gelatinous Drop-like Corneal Dystrophy presents itself at the slit lamp mostly in the form of subepithelial, gel-like drop-shaped lesions. These can be stained with fluorescein. In addition, small nodules are usually conspicuous, which often show superficial vascularization (Tsujikawa 2012).

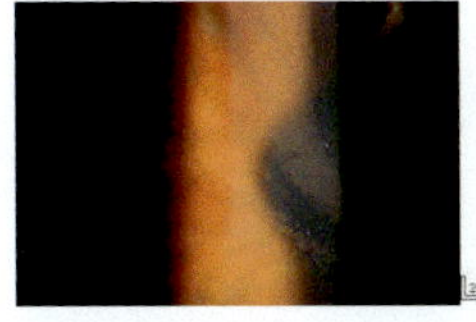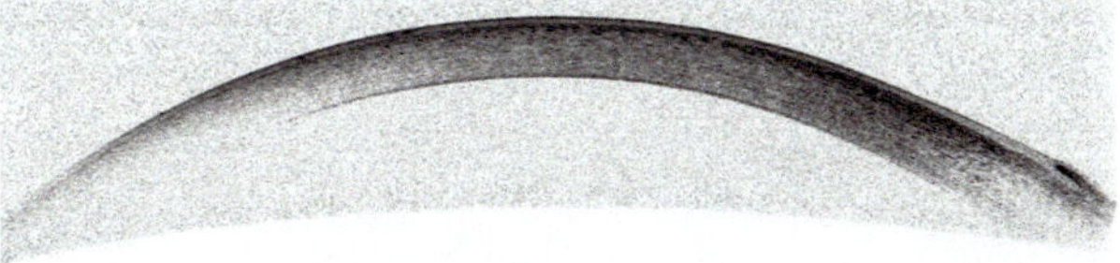

Fig. 7 Lisch Epithelial Corneal Dystrophy. The Lisch corneal dystrophy is conspicuous at the slit lamp by vortex-like, focal opacities in the epithelium. These can be detected by OCT as epithelial, hyperreflective condensations, but without the epithelium itself being thickened or raised

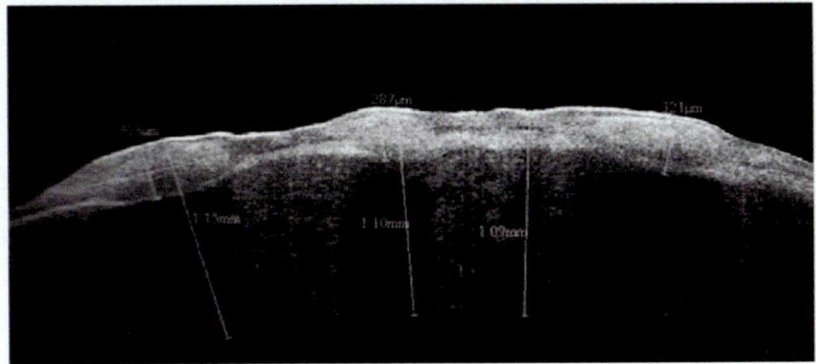

Fig. 8 Gelatinous Drop-like Corneal Dystrophy. In Gelatinous Drop-like Corneal Dystrophy, large, hyperreflective nodules in the anterior corneal stroma are impressive. These are located at the level of the basal epithelial cell layer. In addition, the epithelium is very irregular and smaller nodules with neovascularizations are also found. (from Magalhães et al. 2012)

OCT findings: Using anterior segment OCT, the gel-like nodes can be visualized as dense, hyperreflective formations on the level of the basal epithelial cell layer. In addition, the anterior chamber of the eye can also often be well visualized, even if it is not visible at the slit lamp. The epithelium also shows distinct irregularities and is often interrupted, while the basement membrane is usually shown to be intact (Magalhães et al. 2012) (Fig. 8).

1   Epithelial-Stromal TGFBI Dystrophies

(1) Reis-Bückler's Corneal Dystrophy (RBCD)

Reis-Bückler`s Corneal Dystrophy impresses at the slit lamp mostly in the form of disseminated greyish opacities which are restricted to the superficial corneal stroma. Mostly the Bowman's layer is also affected in places (Kobayashi and Sugiyama 2007; Liang et al. 2014).

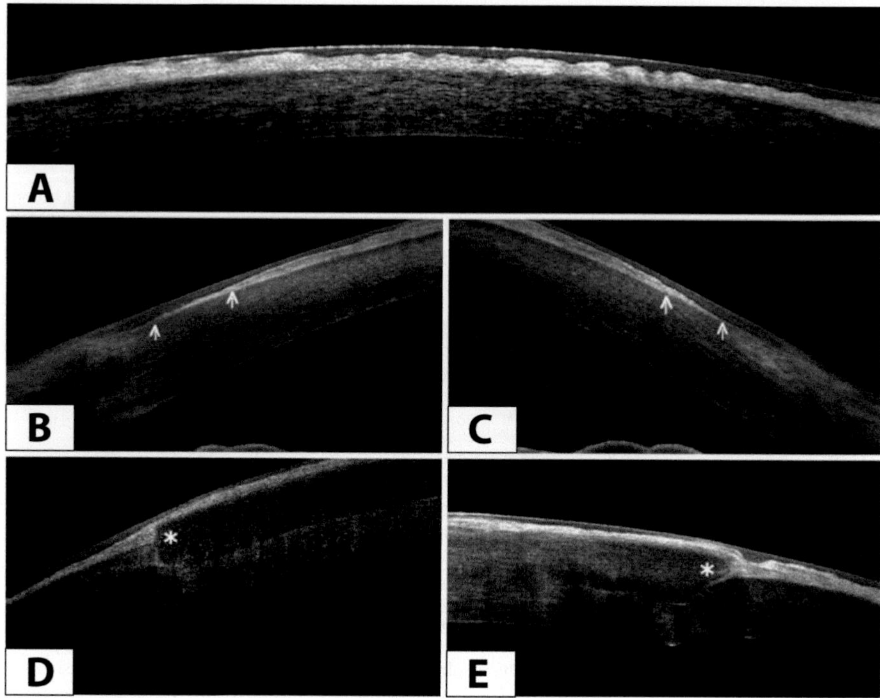

Fig. 9 Reis-Bückler's Corneal Dystrophy. **A** OCT imaging reveals dense deposits at the level of the Bowman's layer, which (**B + C**) dilute towards the periphery. **D + E** show a recurrence after anterior lamellar keratoplasty. (From Liang et al. 2014)

OCT findings: OCT reveals dense and hyperreflective deposits, especially at the level of the Bowman's layer. These are more pronounced centrally than in the periphery. In addition, the deposits are limited to the epithelium. The anterior stroma is usually not affected and the limbal border is respected (Liang et al. 2014) (Fig. 9).

(2) Thiel-Behnke Corneal Dystrophy (TBCD).

In Thiel-Behnke Corneal Dystrophy the slit lamp shows rather irregular, also grayish opacities at the level of Bowman's layer. In addition, subepithelial honeycomb-like opacities are prominent. The corneal center is affected whereas the periphery is not affected in Thiel-Behnke Corneal Dystrophy. In addition, epithelial irregularities are often visible (Kobayashi et al. 2003).

OCT findings: OCT imaging reveals characteristic hyperreflective, sawtooth-shaped deposits at the level of the Bowman's layer, which protrude into the epithelium. The anterior corneal stroma is usually clear and not affected by the deposits (Vajzovic et al. 2011) (Fig. 10).

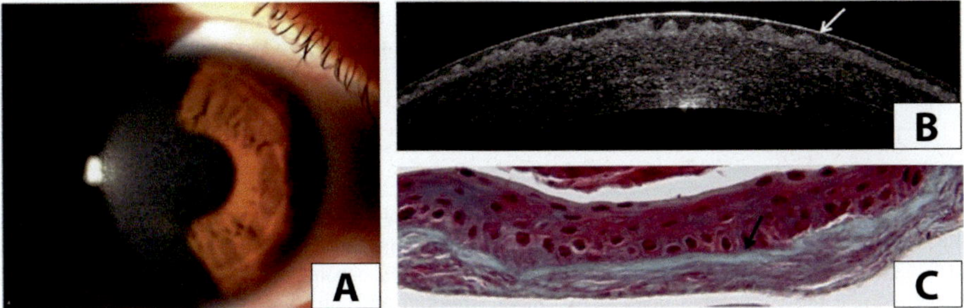

Fig. 10 Thiel-Behnke Corneal Dystrophy. Thiel-Behnke Corneal Dystrophy in slit-lamp findings, OCT image and histology. The OCT image (**B**) shows typical sawtooth-shaped deposits at the level of the Bowman's layer. These protrude into the epithelium, the anterior corneal stroma is not involved. In addition, the epithelium is usually not protruding. **C** Histologically, the Masson Trichrome staining shows fibrotic material above the Bowman's layer (Vajzovic et al. 2011)

(3) Lattice Corneal Dystrophy (LCD)

In the case of Lattice Corneal Dystrophy, slit-lamp findings show in particular central, subepithelial, lattice-like opacities of the cornea which partly extend into the anterior stroma. These grid lines are particularly well visible in regredient light. In most cases, the lines begin in the center of the cornea and extend to the periphery. The epithelium may also be irregular and thickened or thinned in places (Lanier et al. 1976).

OCT findings: Using OCT imaging, the deposits in the cornea can be detected at the level of the Bowman's layer up to the anterior stroma. In addition, the grid lines can be tracked as hyperreflective deposits in cross section as well as in longitudinal section. In most cases the Bowman's layer is missing or interrupted, the epithelium is also irregular in OCT (Ghouali et al. 2015) (Fig. 11).

(4) Granular Corneal Dystrophy Type 1 (GCD1)

Granular Corneal Dystrophy Type 1 is visible by slit-lamp through vortex-shaped, brownish, crumbly deposits at the level of the Bowman's layer. In regressing light, multiple, small, punctiform deposits can be seen, the limbus and the periphery of

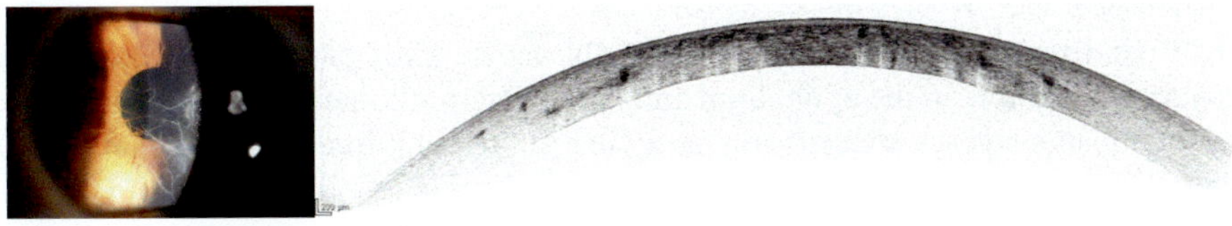

Fig. 11 Lattice Corneal Dystrophy. Lattice Corneal Dystrophy in slit-lamp photography and OCT. The grid lines are clearly visible in cross section as hyperreflective condensations in the anterior to mid-depth stroma. In addition, they protrude into the subepithelial area. The epithelium may also be irregular. In advanced stages, the grids may extend to the Descemet's membrane

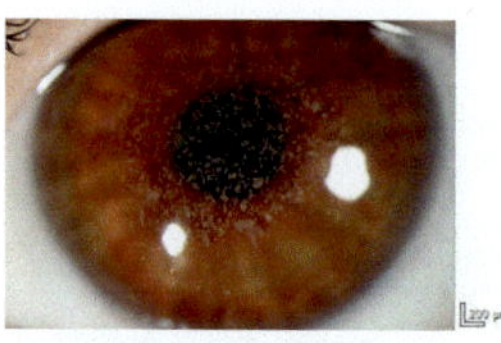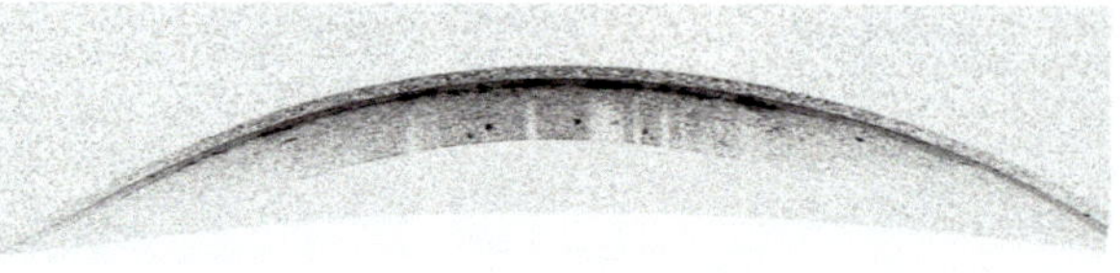

Fig. 12 Granular Corneal Dystrophy Type 1. Granular Corneal Dystrophy Type 1 as early form in slit-lamp photography and OCT. Hyperreflective deposits in the anterior stroma are visible by OCT. These cause streaky shadows towards the deeper stroma. The epithelium is partially thickened and the Bowman's layer seems to be irregular and interrupted. It is noticeable that the limbus is not affected

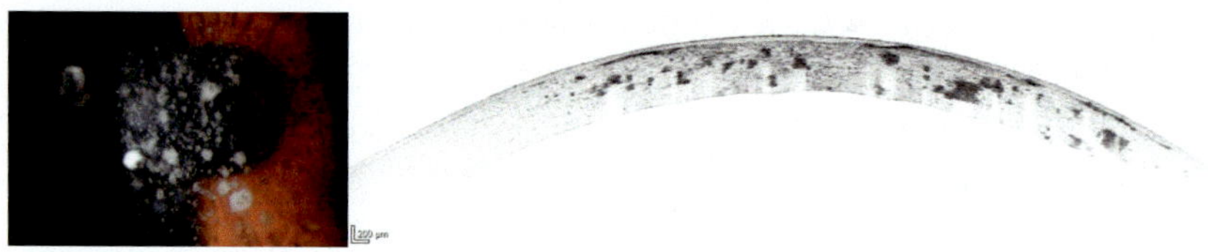

Fig. 13 Granular Corneal Dystrophy Type 1. Late form of Granular Corneal Dystrophy Type 1. In the OCT findings the deposits extend into the deep corneal stroma. Parts of the Descemet's membrane appear irregularly configured. It is also noticeable that the spaces between the deposits are clear

the cornea are excluded. Depending on the age of the patient, the granules extend into the deep corneal stroma (Møller 2016).

OCT findings: In imaging by OCT the deposits are visible as delimitable hyperreflective material. This extends from the epithelium, over the Bowman's layer, through the anterior to the deep corneal stroma. Epithelium and Bowman's layer are often interrupted and clearly irregular (Mori et al. 2009) (Figs. 12, 13).

(5) Granular Corneal Dystrophy Type 2 (GCD2)

In slit-lamp biomicroscopy, Granular Corneal Dystrophy Type 2 is characterized by superficial deposits in the anterior corneal stroma, which have small, thorn-like extensions. In addition, punctiform deposits, round spots and even grid-like lines are noticeable (Holland et al. 1992).

OCT findings: By means of OCT, partly lattice-like, partly dense, confluent deposits are visible in the epithelium and in the anterior corneal stroma. In addition, the Bowman's layer is affected and partly interrupted or raised (Holland et al. 1992) (Fig. 14).

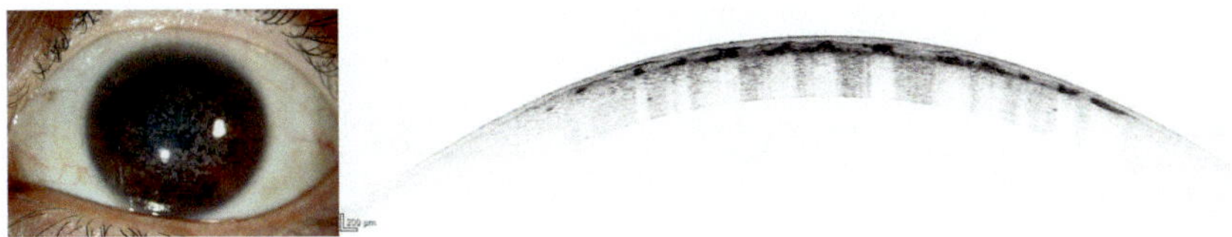

Fig. 14 Granular Corneal Dystrophy Type 2. slit-lamp image and OCT image of Granular Corneal Dystrophy, Type 2. The slit-lamp image shows confluent, partly line-forming, circular deposits in the anterior corneal stroma. These can be easily detected in OCT. Very dense, hyperreflective areas as well as brighter areas are particularly noticeable. The deposits penetrate the Bowman's layer and protrude into the epithelium

2 Stromal Corneal Dystrophies

(1) Macular Corneal Dystrophy (MCD)

In Macular Corneal Dystrophy (MCD), white and roundish, even spot-like opacities of the cornea are visible at the slit lamp. These are initially located in the anterior stroma, but later extend to the deep corneal stroma. The Descemet's membrane may also be involved. Also, the deposits extend to the limbus, which is important for the differential diagnosis to GCD1 and 2. Often the Macular Corneal Dystrophy is associated with a thinning of the cornea (Klintworth and Vogel 1964).

OCT findings: In OCT imaging, disseminated, hyperreflective deposits are initially noticeable, which usually affect the entire cornea. In addition, the overall reflectivity of the corneal collagen fibrils is increased (Nowinska et al. 2015) (Fig. 15).

(2) Schnyder Corneal Dystrophy (SCD)

The Schnyder Corneal Dystrophy (SCD) impresses at the slit lamp mostly by central and rather roundish opacities. These are mostly associated with subepithelial crystalline deposits. In older patients the deposits extend into the stroma and the middle corneal periphery. It can be observed that only about 50% of patients have crystalline deposits (McCarthy et al. 1994).

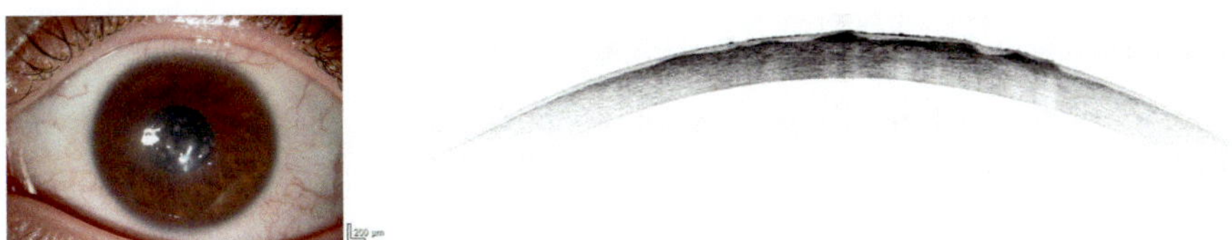

Fig. 15 Macular Corneal Dystrophy. In Macular Corneal Dystrophy the deposits extend to the limbus over the entire cornea. The interstitial spaces are not clear. This is also reflected in the OCT imaging. The deposits protrude into the epithelium. The epithelium itself is very irregular and partly thinned. Similar to the Granular Corneal Dystrophies, shadows are visible posterior to the deposits

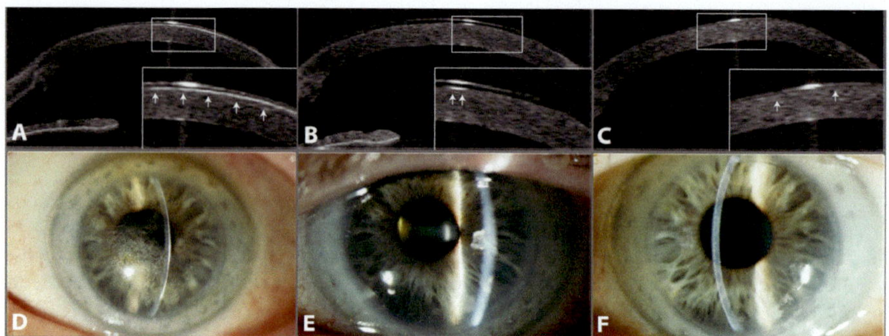

Fig. 16 Schnyder Corneal Dystrophy. Clinical images before and after phototherapeutic keratectomy in recurrence of Schnyder corneal dystrophy. **A + D** Show the clinical findings before PTK. The OCT image clearly shows the deposits in the anterior stroma. **B + E** Clinical image and OCT imaging directly after PTK. The deposits are completely removed and the cornea is clear. The therapeutic contact lens is also visible. **C + F** Findings after 4 weeks. The cornea is still clear

OCT findings: In OCT imaging especially central and subepithelial hyperreflective deposits are visible. These usually exclude the actual epithelium and the Bowman's layer (Jing and Wang 2009) (Fig. 16).

(3) Congenital Stromal Corneal Dystrophy (CSCD)

Congenital Stromal Corneal Dystrophy (CSCD) is a slit-lamp disease characterized by bilateral white–gray clouding of the corneal stroma. The clouding covers the entire cornea. In most cases, the cornea is thicker than normal (Pearce et al. 1969).

OCT findings: With the help of OCT, hyperreflective deposits diffusely distributed throughout the corneal stroma are visible. These are strictly distributed over the stroma so that Bowman's layer, epithelium and Descemet's membrane are not affected (Jing et al. 2014) (Fig. 17).

(4) Fleck Corneal Dystrophy (FCD)

To date, no studies with image data from optical coherence tomography on Fleck Corneal Dystrophy are known.

(5) Amorphous Posterior Corneal Dystrophy (PACD)

So far, no studies with image data on Amorphous Posterior Corneal Dystrophy are known.

(6) Central Cloudy Dystrophy of Francois (CCDF)

The Central Cloudy Dystrophy of Francois (CCDF) is characterized by polygonal opacities in the corneal stroma, which are restricted to the center of the cornea. This dystrophy can only be insufficiently distinguished from an often-visible crocodile chargrin.

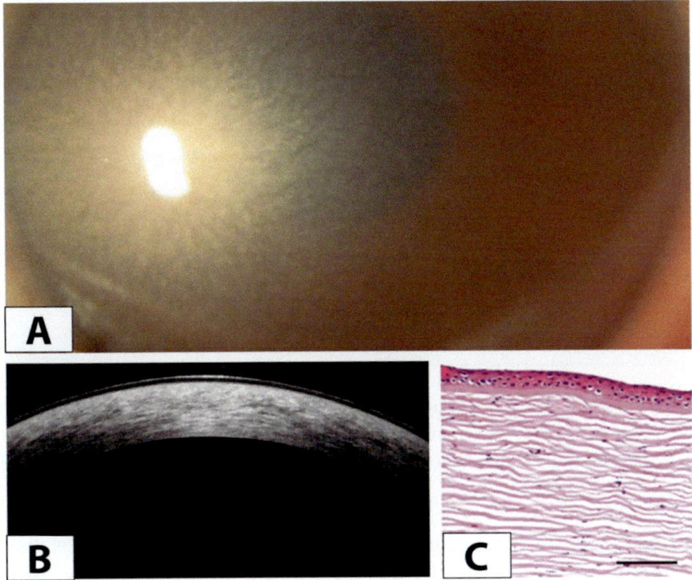

Fig. 17 Congenital Stromal Corneal Dystrophy. Clinical findings (**A**), OCT imaging (**B**) and histological findings (**C**) in Congenital Stromal Corneal Dystrophy. In the OCT image hyperreflective deposits are distributed throughout the corneal stroma. These are restricted to the corneal stroma and the epithelium and Bowman's layer as well as the Descemet membrane are unobtrusive. **C** Histologically (H&E) abnormal collagen fibrils are visible in the corneal stroma. From (Jing et al. 2014)

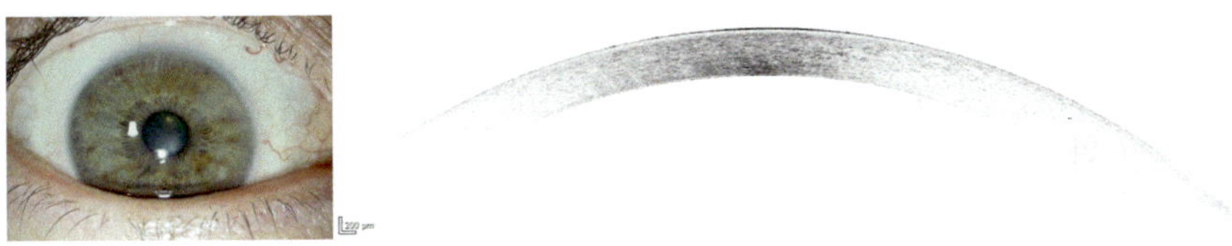

Fig. 18 Central Cloudy Dystrophy of Francois. Clinical findings and OCT in Central Cloudy Corneal Dystrophy. In OCT a stromal clouding of the cornea is clearly visible, which is especially limited to the center

OCT findings: OCT imaging clearly shows a clouding of the cornea, which is restricted to the central area of the cornea, especially in the posterior stroma. The Descemet's membrane is not affected (Fig. 18).

(7) Pre-Descemet Corneal Dystrophy (PDCD)

Pre-Descemet Corneal Dystrophy (PDCD) in the slit lamp usually does not show uniform findings. Rather focal, polymorphic as well as grayish opacities are striking, which extend to the deep corneal stroma near the Descemet's membrane. The epithelium or higher structures are not affected (Grayson and Wilbrandt 1967).

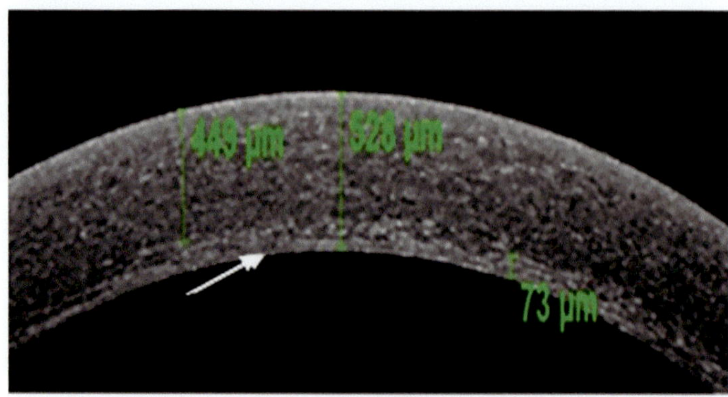

Fig. 19 Pre-Descemet Corneal Dystrophy. OCT findings in Pre-Descemet Corneal Dystrophy. Here, homogeneous bands can be seen directly in front of the Descemet's membrane in the entire corneal area, which partially extend into the posterior stroma. From (Malhotra et al. 2012)

OCT findings: Using OCT imaging, hyperreflective, homogeneous bands in the area immediately in front of the Descemet's membrane can usually be visualized. The posterior stroma is also partially affected (Malhotra et al. 2015) (Fig. 19).

3 Endothelial Corneal Dystrophies

(1) Fuchs Endothelial Corneal Dystrophy (FECD)

In Fuchs Endothelial Corneal Dystrophy (FECD), endothelial lesions resembling hammered copper are visible at the slit lamp. In addition, there are pigmented lesions, a thickened Descemet's membrane and in advanced stages subepithelial fibrosis (Adamis et al. 1993).

OCT findings: In anterior segment OCT imaging, a thickening of the Descemet's membrane and isolated nodular thickenings of endothelial cells are visible. In addition, epithelial changes can be detected, such as subepithelial fibrosis, epithelial edema and epithelial bullae in case of bullous keratopathy (Siebelmann et al. 2018b) (Figs. 20, 21 and 22).

(2) Posterior Polymorphous Corneal Dystrophy (PPCD)

Posterior Polymorphous Corneal Dystrophy (PPCD) is a slit-lamp disease characterized by helical track-like or bubble-shaped deposits on the Descemet's membrane. Sometimes fusiform or spindle-shaped figures are also visible (Grupcheva et al. 2001).

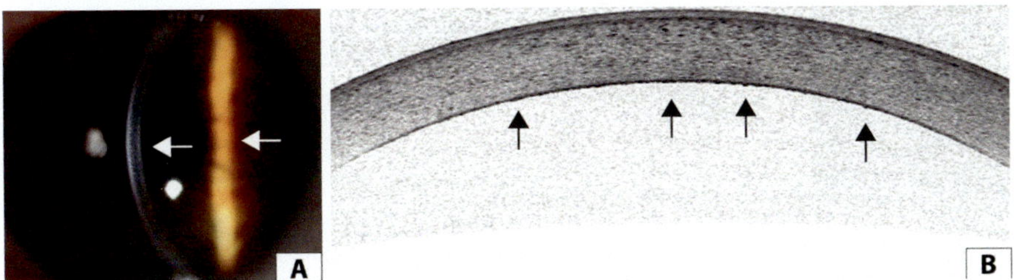

Fig. 20 Fuchs Endothelial Corneal Dystrophy. Clinical finding with typical corneal guttae in Fuchs Endothelial Corneal Dystrophy (**A**). The OCT image (**B**) shows a generally thickened cornea and the typical wart shaped thickenings (guttae) in the area of the Descemet's membrane, see arrows (from Siebelmann et al. 2018b)

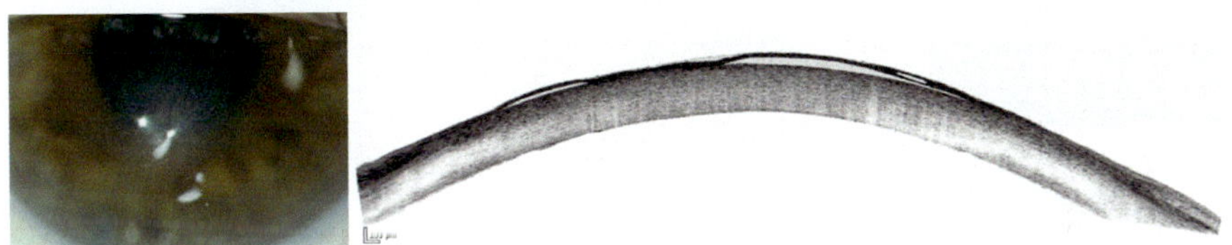

Fig. 21 Fuchs Endothelial Corneal Dystrophy. Advanced stage of Fuchs Endothelial Corneal Dystrophy with pronounced bullae and subepithelial fibrosis. Imaging by OCT clearly shows the blistered detached epithelial layer, as well as an underlying compression of the tissue. Also, a subtle hyperreflective fluid is visible in the bullae

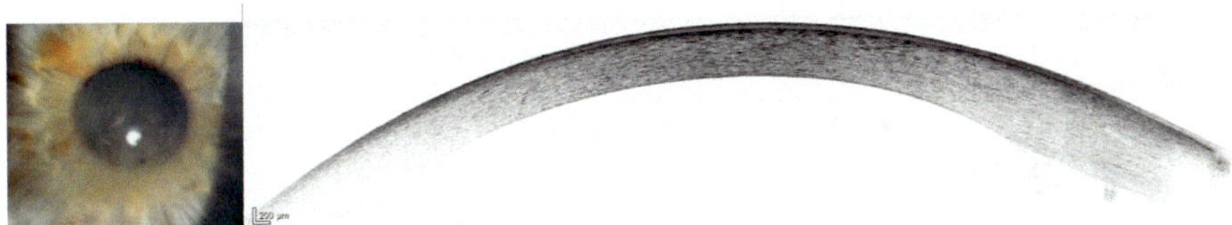

Fig. 22 Fuchs Endothelial Corneal Dystrophy. The slit-lamp photo also shows a clearly advanced stage of a Fuchs endothelial dystrophy treated with DMEK. OCT imaging shows a dense, subepithelial fibrosis. The patient requires an excimer laser PTK

OCT findings: OCT imaging reveals a generally thickened Descemet's membrane with partially amorphous deposits. These are hyperreflective and partially protrude into the lumen of the anterior chamber (Grupcheva et al. 2001) (Fig. 23).

(3) Congenital Hereditary Endothelial Dystrophy (CHED)

At the slit lamp, or often also during anesthesia, diffuse or focal opacities, which can look like spots or areas, are usually noticeable in Congenital Hereditary Endothelial Dystrophy (CHED). The cornea is generally thickened and there is diffuse corneal edema (Keates and Cvintal 1965).

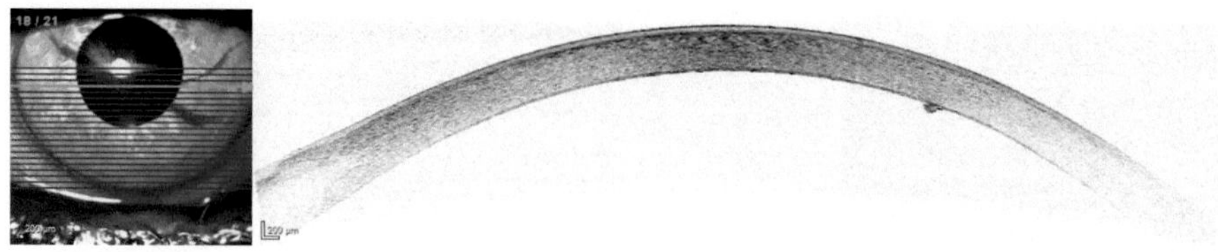

Fig. 23 Posterior Polymorphous Corneal Dystrophy. OCT imaging in Posterior Polymorphous Corneal Dystrophy. In OCT, the typical growths of the Descemet's membrane, which are impressive as snail traces on the slit lamp, are visible. These protrude into the lumen of the anterior chamber

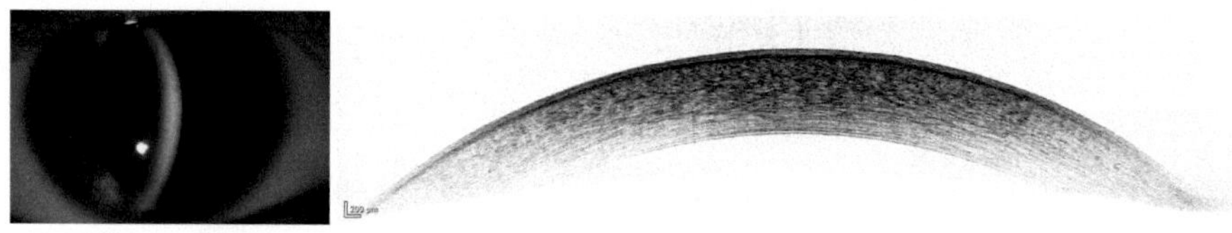

OCT findings: Congenital Hereditary Endothelial Dystrophy. OCT reveals diffuse corneal edema, a thickened Descemet's membrane and partly hyperreflective diffuse opacities. The Bowman's layer may also be irregular or partially degenerated (Mittal et al. 2011).

(4) X-chromosomal Endothelial Corneal Dystrophy (XECD)

There are no studies on the XECD that describe imaging by OCT.

4 Conclusion

Imaging by means of high-resolution anterior segment OCT in corneal dystrophies enables high-resolution cross-sectional imaging, which supplements important diagnostic information on the pure slit-lamp findings. This is particularly important if the cornea is very cloudy and no details or structures are visible in regressive light. All morphological changes that occur in the context of corneal dystrophies can be visualized in terms of localization and depth within the cornea as well as in terms of the affected corneal layers (Siebelmann et al. 2017). In this context, intraoperative OCT can provide particular added value, as it allows for an exact differentiation of the affected tissue parts, even in newborns and infants with cloudy corneas, as well as an imaging of the anterior chamber of the eye and thus, for example, a differentiation from dysgenesis of the anterior segment of the eye (Siebelmann et al. 2015a). However, the examination with a slit lamp is superior to imaging with OCT when it comes to recognizing certain patterns, as is necessary, for example, in Lattice Corneal Dystrophy. Nevertheless, anterior segment OCT provides important information regarding the depth and extent of corneal opacities, particularly for therapy planning (Hong et al. 2010) For example, the imaging data can be used to decide whether the deposits in the cornea can still be removed by superficial laser procedures, by anterior lamellar keratoplasty, or whether a penetrating procedure is necessary (Hong et al. 2010). In the future, this could play a role especially in image guided surgery, be it intraoperative microscope-integrated OCT or OCT integrated into femtosecond lasers or excimer laser devices. Initial studies have already shown that OCT-controlled ablation of corneal lesions using intraoperative OCT is possible and allows conclusions to be drawn about the remaining residual opacities (Siebelmann et al. 2018c).

In conclusion, it can be stated that OCT will certainly not replace slit-lamp examination in the diagnosis of corneal dystrophies, but it will add important information such as the exact depth and extent of the findings.

References

Adamis AP, Filatov V, Tripathi BJ. Fuchs' endothelial dystrophy of the cornea. Surv Ophthalmol. 1993;38(2):149–68.

Alvarez-Fischer M, de Toledo JA, Barraquer RI. Lisch corneal dystrophy. Cornea. 2005;24 (4):494–5.

Diez-Feijóo E, Durán JA. Optical coherence tomography findings in recurrent corneal erosion syndrome. Cornea. 2015;34(3):290–5.

Geerling G, Müller M, Winter C, et al. Intraoperative 2-dimensional optical coherence tomography as a new tool for anterior segment surgery. Arch Ophthalmol. 2005;123(2):253–7.

Ghouali W, Grieve K, Bellefqih S, et al. Full-field optical coherence tomography of human donor and pathological corneas. Curr Eye Res. 2015;40(5):526–34.

Goldman J, Dohlman C, Kravitt B. The basement membrane of the human cornea in recurrent epithelial erosion syndrome. Trans Am Acad Ophthalmol Otolaryngol. 1969;73(3):471.

Grayson M, Wilbrandt H. Pre-descemet dystrophy. Am J Ophthalmol. 1967;64(2):276–82.

Grupcheva CN, Chew GS, Edwards M, Craig JP, McGhee CN. Imaging posterior polymorphous corneal dystrophy by in vivo confocal microscopy. Clin Exper Ophthalmol. 2001;29(4):256–9.

Holland EJ, Daya SM, Stone EM, et al. Avellino corneal dystrophy: clinical manifestations and natural history. Ophthalmology. 1992;99(10):1564–8.

Hong JP, Ha BJ, Stulting RD, Kim EK. Determination of treatment strategies for granular corneal dystrophy type 2 using Fourier-domain optical coherence tomography. Br J Ophthalmol. 2010;94(3):341–5.

Jing Y, Wang L. Morphological evaluation of Schnyder's crystalline corneal dystrophy by laser scanning confocal microscopy and Fourier-domain optical coherence tomography. Clin Exper Ophthalmol. 2009;37(3):308–12.

Jing Y, Kumar PR, Zhu L, et al. Novel decorin mutation in a Chinese family with congenital stromal corneal dystrophy. Cornea. 2014;33(3):288–93.

Keates RH, Cvintal T. Congenital hereditary corneal dystrophy. Am J Ophthalmol. 1965;60 (5):892–4.

Klintworth GK, Vogel FS. Macular corneal dystrophy: an inherited acid mucopolysaccharide storage disease of the corneal fibroblast. Am J Pathol. 1964;45(4):565.

Kobayashi A, Sugiyama K. In vivo laser confocal microscopy findings for Bowman's layer dystrophies (Thiel–Behnke and Reis-Bücklers corneal dystrophies. Ophthalmology. 2007;114 (1):69–75.

Kobayashi A, Sakurai M, Shirao Y, Sugiyama K, Ohta T, Amaya-Ohkura Y. In vivo confocal microscopy and genotyping of a family with Thiel-Behnke (honeycomb) corneal dystrophy. Arch Ophthalmol. 2003;121(10):1498–9.

Lanier JD, Fine M, Brigitta T. Lattice corneal dystrophy. Arch Ophthalmol. 1976;94(6):921–4.

Liang Q, Pan Z, Sun X, Baudouin C, Labbé A. Reis-Bücklers corneal dystrophy: a reappraisal using in vivo and ex vivo imaging techniques. Ophthalmic Res. 2014;51(4):187–95.

Lisch W, Steuhl K-P, Lisch C, et al. A new, band-shaped and whorled microcystic dystrophy of the corneal epithelium. Am J Ophthalmol. 1992;114(1):35–44.

Magalhães OdA, Rymer S, Marinho DR, Kwitko S, Cardoso IH, Kliemann L. Optical coherence tomography image in gelatinous drop-like corneal dystrophy: case report. Arquivos brasileiros de oftalmologia. 2012;75(5):356–357.

Malhotra C, Rohit Shetty D, Kumar RS, Veluri H, Nagaraj H. In vivo imaging of riboflavin penetration during collagen cross-linking with hand-held spectral domain optical coherence tomography. J Refract Surg. 2012;28(11):776.

Malhotra C, Jain AK, Dwivedi S, Chakma P, Rohilla V, Sachdeva K. Characteristics of pre-Descemet membrane corneal dystrophy by three different imaging modalities—in vivo confocal microscopy, anterior segment optical coherence tomography, and Scheimpflug corneal densitometry analysis. Cornea. 2015;34(7):829–32.

McCarthy M, Innis S, Dubord P, White V. Panstromal Schnyder corneal dystrophy: a clinical pathologic report with quantitative analysis of corneal lipid composition. Ophthalmology. 1994;101(5):895–901.

Mittal V, Mittal R, Sangwan VS. Successful Descemet stripping endothelial keratoplasty in congenital hereditary endothelial dystrophy. Cornea. 2011;30(3):354–6.

Møller H. Granular corneal dystrophy Groenouw type I. Clinical and genetic aspects. Acta Ophthalmol Suppl. 1991(198):1.

Mori H, Miura M, Iwasaki T, et al. Three-dimensional optical coherence tomography-guided phototherapeutic keratectomy for granular corneal dystrophy. Cornea. 2009;28(8):944–7.

Nowinska AK, Teper SJ, Janiszewska DA, et al. Comparative study of anterior eye segment measurements with spectral swept-source and time-domain optical coherence tomography in eyes with corneal dystrophies. BioMed Res Int. 2015;2015.

Patel DV, Grupcheva CN, McGhee CN. Imaging the microstructural abnormalities of meesmann corneal dystrophy by in vivo confocal microscopy. Cornea. 2005;24(6):669–73.

Pearce W, Tripathi RC, Morgan G. Congenital endothelial corneal dystrophy. Clinical, pathological, and genetic study. Br J Ophthalmol. 1969;53(9):577.

Rodrigues MM, Fine BS, Laibson PR, Zimmerman LE. Disorders of the corneal epithelium: a clinicopathologic study of dot, geographic, and fingerprint patterns. Arch Ophthalmol. 1974;92(6):475–82.

Siebelmann S, Steven P, Cursiefen C. Intraoperative optical coherence tomography: ocular surgery on a higher level or just nice pictures? JAMA Ophthalmol. 2015b;133(10):1133–4.

Siebelmann S, Bachmann B, Matthaei M, et al. Mikroskopintegrierte intraoperative optische Kohärenztomographie bei der Narkoseuntersuchung von pädiatrischen Patienten. Ophthalmologe. 2018a;115(9):785–92.

Siebelmann S, Scholz P, Sonnenschein S, et al. Anterior segment optical coherence tomography for the diagnosis of corneal dystrophies according to the IC3D classification. Surv Ophthalmol. 2018b;63(3):365–80.

Siebelmann S, Horstmann J, Scholz P, et al. Intraoperative changes in corneal structure during excimer laser phototherapeutic keratectomy (PTK) assessed by intraoperative optical coherence tomography. Graefes Arch Clin Exp Ophthalmol. 2018c;256(3):575–81.

Siebelmann S, Hermann M, Dietlein T, Bachmann B, Steven P, Cursiefen C. Intraoperative optical coherence tomography in children with anterior segment anomalies. Ophthalmology. 2015a.

Siebelmann S, Scholz P, Sonnenschein S, et al. Anterior segment optical coherence tomography for the diagnosis of corneal dystrophies according to the IC3D classification. Surv Ophthalmol. 2017.

Siebelmann S, Bachmann B, Lappas A, et al. Intraoperative Optische Kohärenztomographie bei Hornhaut- und Glaukom-chirurgischen Eingriffen. Der Ophthalmologe: Zeitschrift der Deutschen Ophthalmologischen Gesellschaft. 2016(in print).

Tsujikawa M. Gelatinous drop-like corneal dystrophy. Cornea. 2012;31:S37–40.

Vajzovic LM, Karp CL, Haft P, et al. Ultra high-resolution anterior segment optical coherence tomography in the evaluation of anterior corneal dystrophies and degenerations. Ophthalmology. 2011;118(7):1291–6.

Weiss JS, Møller HU, Aldave AJ, et al. IC3D classification of corneal dystrophies—edition 2. Cornea. 2015;34(2):117–59.

Wu P, Cortes D, Li J, Chen M, Mannis M. Epithelial basement membrane dystrophy: a study with in vivo confocal microscopy and high-resolution anterior segment optical coherence tomography. Invest Ophthalmol vis Sci. 2013;54(15):564–564.

Refractive and Therapeutic Corneal Surgery

Stephan J. Linke and Johannes Steinberg

Laser systems used in refractive and therapeutic corneal surgery

The idea of "having laser surgery" in order to subsequently no longer need visual aids such as glasses or contact lenses for sharp vision is one of the most fascinating chapters of modern medicine for many people with ammetropia (and for some ophthalmologists). The first descriptions of corneal surgery using laser systems date back to Stephen Trockel in 1983 (Trokel et al. 1983).

The first applications of these "excimer" laser systems on humans were performed in Berlin as photorefractive keratectomy (PRK) by Theo Seiler in 1987 (Seiler et al. 1987).

In the context of modern therapeutic and refractive corneal surgery, two physically different laser systems are currently used to model the cornea: Excimer and femtosecond laser systems.

The controlled application of excimer-generated UV light of wavelength 193 nm in therapeutic and refractive corneal surgery allows very precise modulation of corneal tissue (Linke et al. 2013; Wilson et al. 2017). Today's excimer lasers emit UV light at a frequency of 500–1000 Hz. By means of a single pulse, a tissue ablation of approx. 0.25 µm in depth and of 0.6 mm^2 occurs. They are therefore used for surface treatment of the cornea, primarily either to change its shape (refractive treatment of hyperopia/myopia/astigmatism) or therapeutically to remove scars and/or regularize the corneal surface.

Femtosecond laser systems emit light in the infrared wave light range (>1000 nm) and therefore do not ablate corneal tissue at the surface, but perform intrastromal "cuts" by photodisruption with high precision and freely configurable

S. J. Linke (✉) · J. Steinberg
Department of Ophthalmology, University Eye Hospital Hamburg-Eppendorf
(Universitätsklinikum Hamburg-Eppendorf UKE), Martinistr. 52, 20246 Hamburg, Germany
e-mail: slinke@uke.de

S. J. Linke · J. Steinberg
Hamburg Vision Clinic, Martinistr. 64, 20251 Hamburg, Germany

cutting (spot size: 2 μm; pulse frequency: kilohertz (kHz) to megahertz (MHz) range; energy/pulse: nanojoule (nj) to microjule (μj) range—"low versus high energy Femtolaser"). In terms of classical therapeutic treatments, they are therefore used in the context of lamellar and perforating transplantations. In refractive surgery, they are mainly used for flap (LASIK) and lenticule (SMILE) preparation, but also to generate intrastromal "pockets" for implants.

Possible applications of optical coherence tomography (OCT) in the field of corneal refractive surgery

While placido and Scheimpflug techniques are still the goldstandard in the preoperative diagnosis and planning of refractive surgery, the diagnostic domain of optical coherence tomography (OCT) today is primarily in postoperative complication management and the assessment of (unclear) postoperative changes. Due to its highly accurate imaging of corneal tissue, it has become an indispensable "tool" in the armamentarium of modern, therapeutic corneal surgery.

In the context of corneal refractive surgery, OCT also allows precise in vivo visualization of the epithelium and corneal stroma in addition to visualization and assessment of the flap in LASIK (Fig. 1) and the interface after lenticule removal in the SMILE procedure (Fig. 2).

In the postoperative OCT image, the LASIK flap/interface can be identified by the white delicate line in the anterior stroma (continuous arrows). Furthermore, since the epithelium (dashed arrows) is well differentiated from the underlying stroma, a flap thickness of approximately 100 microns (twice the epithelial thickness) can be concluded.

OCT cross-sectional image with fine interface line/image at the level of the transition from the anterior to the middle third of the cornea. Due to the regular findings (i.e. absence of inflammatory processes, fluid deposition or lenticular remnants) the interface (continuous arrows) is hardly visible. Again, the border between epithelium and Bowman's lamella/anterior stroma is well visualized (dashed arrows).

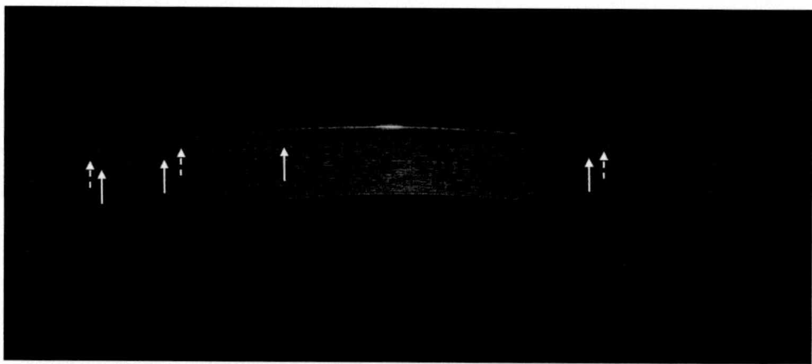

Fig. 1 Visualization of a cornea after LASIK (regular findings) with optical coherence tomography

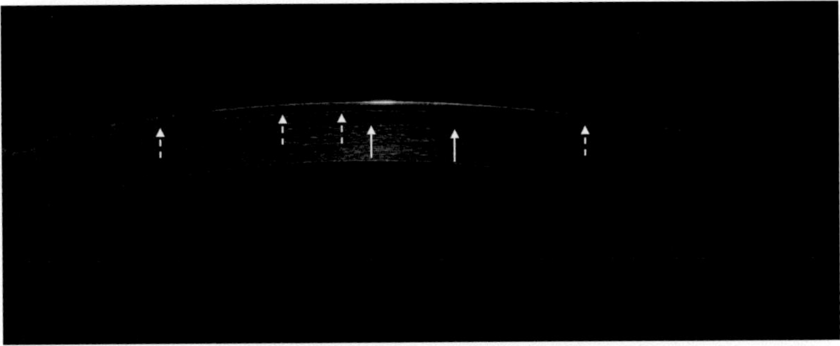

Fig. 2 Visualization of a cornea after SMILE (regular findings) using OCT

In the course of various intraoperative or postoperative complications, significant changes in morphology can sometimes occur. These can be detected by OCT.

In the following, selected examples are given in which OCT can be used advantageously in the context of postoperative complication management in refractive surgery:

Epithelial ingrowth after LASIK/SMILE:

During LASIK, an approximately 100 m thick corneal flap consisting of epithelium and anterior corneal stroma is generated. This flap is connected to the rest of the corneal stroma by a bridge structure ("hinge") about 0.5 mm wide and is "folded" out of the treatment area via the hinge before the subsequent excimer laser ablation. After excimer laser ablation of the corneal stroma, the flap is returned to its original position and the connection of the open corneal stroma to the ocular surface is thus reduced to a line-shaped incision in the transition area of the flap to the surrounding corneal tissue. This procedure leads to a very fast postoperative rehabilitation of the patient (symptom-free findings with visual acuity $\geq$ 0.7 already possible a few hours post-op). Epithelial ingrowth (EIG) is a rare postoperative complication after LASIK. Corneal epithelial cells enter the interface under the flap. The cause is either adhesion ("sealing") disorders in the flap margin area or epithelial cells introduced intraoperatively into the interface. In these cases, slit-lamp biomicroscopy and OCT can be used to visualize either individual epithelial "islands" (intraoperatively dispersed epithelial cells) or epithelial "roads" (epithelial cell accumulation moving from the flap margin to the center in the case of flap margin adhesion disorders). Whether EIG leads to a surgical indication in the form of a flap lift with mechanical removal of epithelial cells from the interface area is based on the localization (inside or outside the optic zone) and the risk assessment regarding possible flap melting above the EIG. Since epithelial cells can proliferate in principle or atrophy/regress spontaneously, morphological control of the findings is crucial. With OCT the extension of the EIG can be detected very well in the width (risk of progressive growth into the optical axis) as well as in the height (risk of flap melting and/or change of the corneal surface curvature which both potentially leading to an irregular astigmatism).

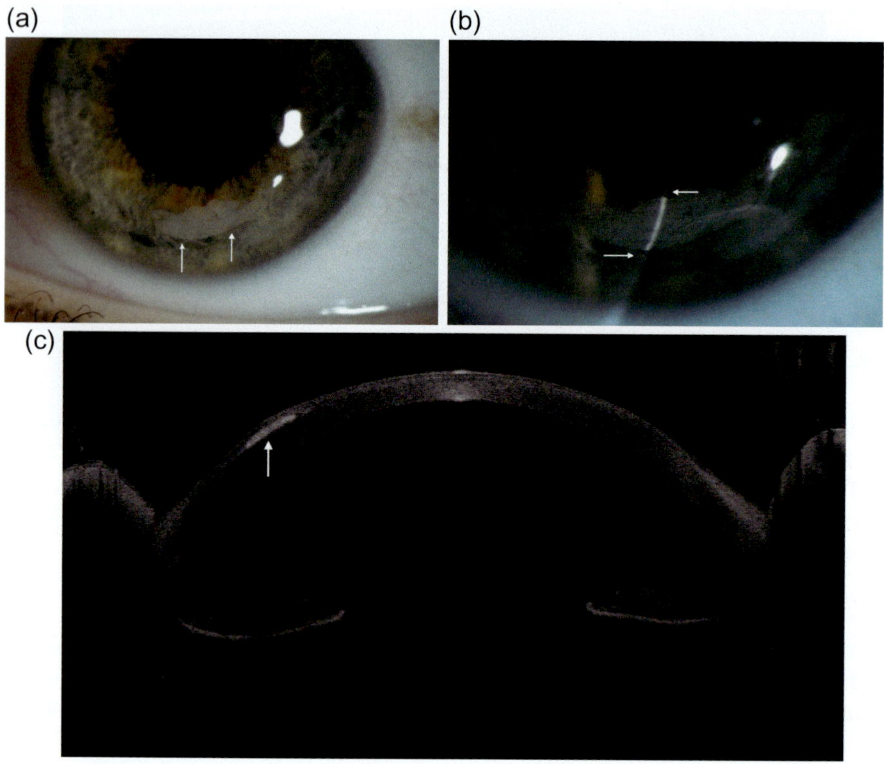

Fig. 3 Epithelial ingrowth (EIG) under the flap after LASIK (**A+B**: slit lamp biomicroscopy, **C**: imaging by OCT)

Biomicroscopic slit-lamp images A + B show the accumulation of whitish epithelial cells in the peripheral cornea (white arrow). The slit image (B) shows a superficial localization of the cells and suggests an elevation of the overlying flap. The OCT image (C) allows a precise localization and documentation of the epithelial cells in the interface area. Melting/thinning of the overlying stromal flap tissue is not visible.

Based on the width of the affected area and amount of accumulated cells as shown in Fig. 3, a flap lift with surgical removal of the epithelium (careful removal of the epithelium from the undersurface of the flap and the stromal interface using a field hockey knife) is indicated.

Although much rarer, EIG and the associated need for postoperative follow-up evaluation, possibly renewed surgical intervention, can also occur after SMILE (small incision lenticule extraction) (Wang et al. 2019). Again, there is a risk of intraoperative epithelial cells scattered into the corneal pocket or insufficient closure of the corneal manipulation tunnels through which superficial corneal epithelial cells may grow into the preformed intrastromal "space" (interface) (Fig. 4).

(a)

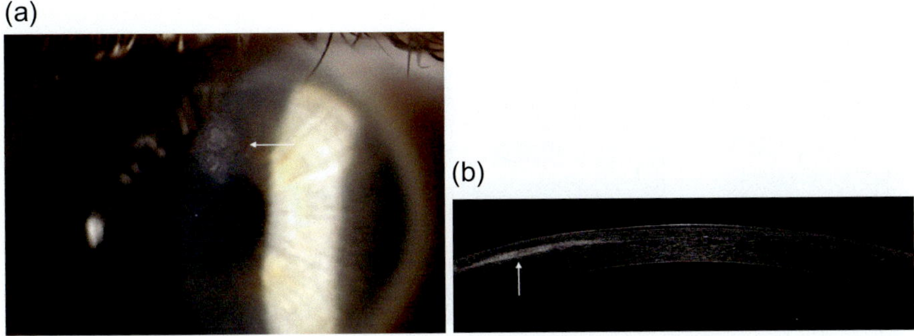

(b)

Fig. 4 EIG after SMILE, a) slit lamp b) OCT

Dislocated flap:

More so than in the case of striae, a completely dislocated flap after LASIK can lead to visual acuity and visual quality reduction. Dislocation can be difficult to diagnose by slit lamp biomicroscopy if it has been present for months due to partial melting of the flap. OCT allows a clear diagnosis even in the case of a dislocated, possibly partially melted flap due to a precise visualization of the flap morphology.

Keratitis/Haze:

Sterile as well as infectious keratitis may occur after corneal refractive surgery. Complication management includes intensive topical application of eye drops and/ or irrigation of the interface depending on severity. Topical therapy is administered based on the temporal evolution of the extent/density of the opacities.

In particular, sterile superficial stromal processes (haze) after surface ablation may require months of topical therapy and may require therapeutic excimer treatments (PTK). In addition to the indispensable slit lamp examination, OCT can contribute important, objectively quantifiable information to treatment planning by providing precise information on the depths and areal extent of the haze(s) (Fig. 5).

In the slit-lamp images A + B, the two-dimensional, honeycomb-shaped corneal scarring resembling pronounced haze after hyperopic excimer treatment in the paracentral/midperipheral corneal stroma is clearly visible (continuous arrows). The simultaneously present brownish iron deposition lines (dashed arrows) indicate an altered tear film due to prolonged corneal healing response. On the basis of slit-lamp images C + D, the superficial, subepithelial localization of the haze can be seen (white arrows). OCT images E and F allow precise localization in terms of area (proximity to optically relevant zone) and depth extent of post-inflammatory change (white arrows).

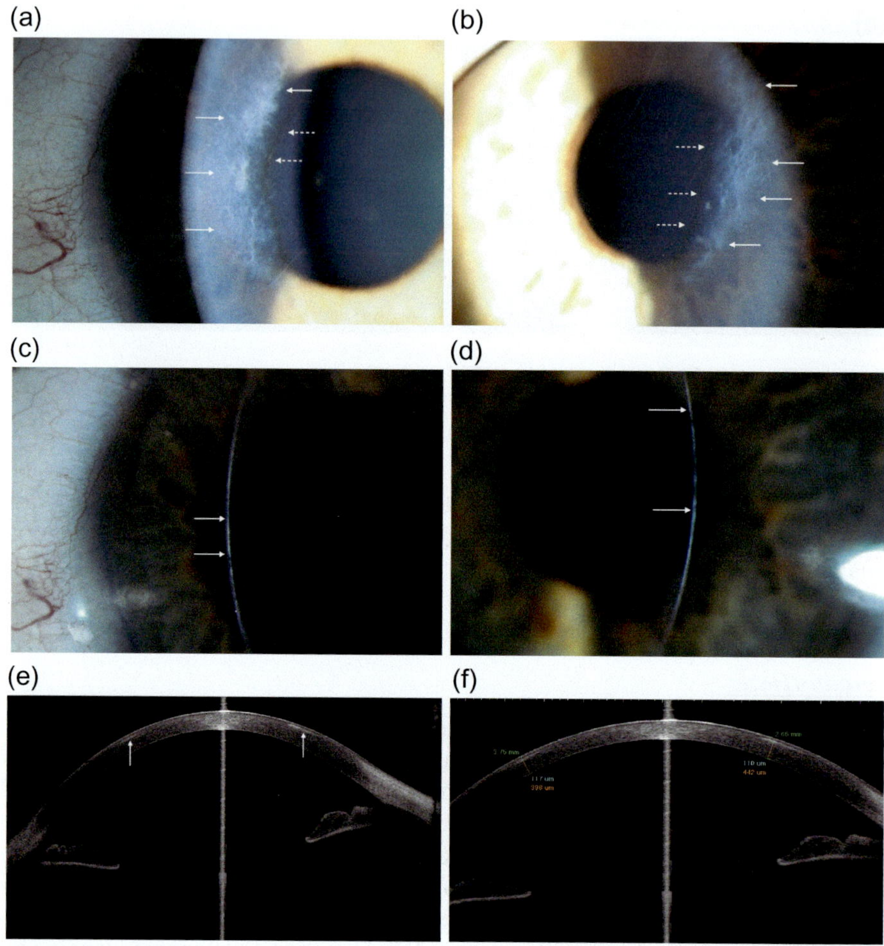

Fig. 5 Haze after hyperopic PRK (slit lamp [**a–d**] + OCT without [**e**] and with [**f**] depth of change)

An increased sterile inflammatory reaction with sometimes long-lasting, deep-stromal haze formation can also occur after corneal crosslinking (corneal crosslinking, CXL) (Fig. 6). Fortunately, haze formation after CXL shows a good response to high-frequency topical steroid administration.

The slit lamp photo shows the "cloudy" haze formation (continuous arrows) and the accompanying iron deposition (dashed arrows) due to the additionally present epithelial changes. By means of OCT, the extent of the post-inflammatory change is visible both in the area and in depth (white arrows) (Fig. 7).

The slit lamp images A + B show the diffuse, "speckled" distribution of the sterile infiltrates/inflammatory foci in the context of a DLK (white arrows). In the OCT image, the changes can be clearly assigned to the interface with regard to their depth localization (white arrows).

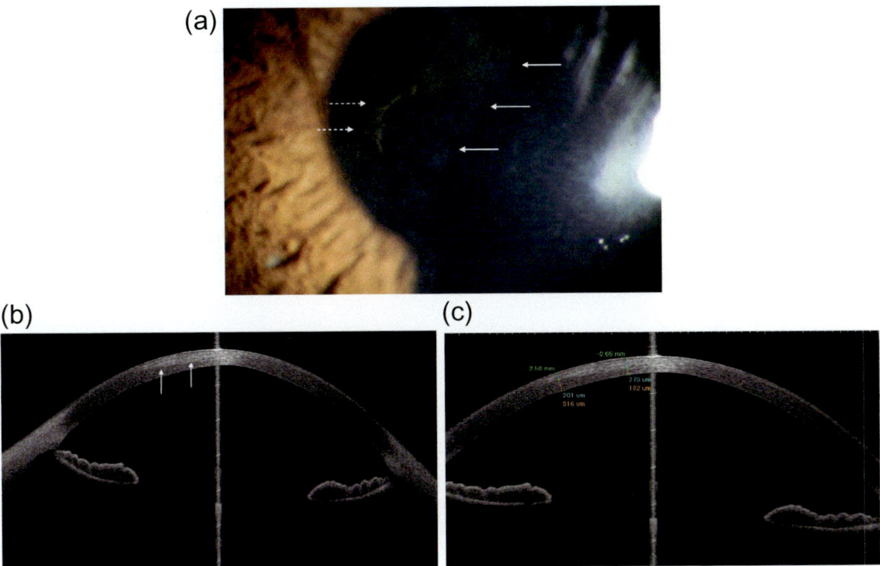

Fig. 6 Haze after corneal crosslinking (slit lamp image including superficial iron deposits [**A**] + OCT image without [**B**] and with [**C**] measurement of the depth of change)

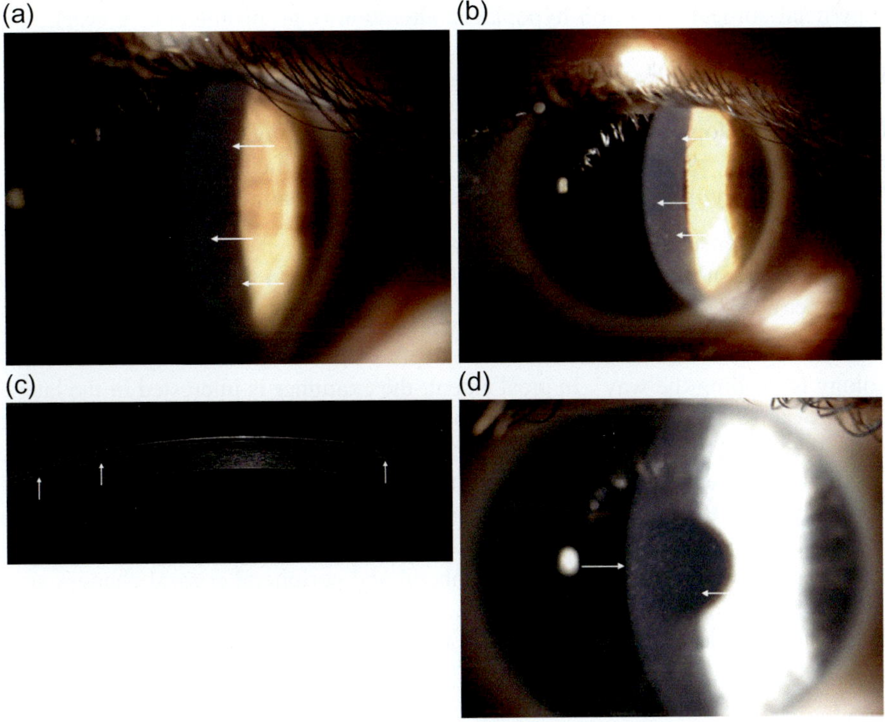

Fig. 7 Diffuse lamellar keratits (DLK) after SMILE (slit lamp [**A**, **B**] + OCT imaging [**C**]) and after LASIK (slit lamp [**D**])

The slit-lamp image of a DLK after LASIK (C) shows a typical configuration of the infiltrate according to stage II–III after Fantes with visually relevant, central cell aggregates (white arrows).

Therapeutic laser-assisted corneal surgery

Nowadays, it is impossible to imagine the therapeutic armamentarium without the excimer laser and in many cases it is **the** therapy of first choice. In the almost 30-year history of development of phototherapeutic keratectomy (PTK), three main indication areas have emerged. These are:

- epithelial adhesion problems
- corneal opacities and degenerations
- surface irregularities

Often different indications exist simultaneously or merge into each other. Decisive for the success of PTK is not only the indication, but also a thorough surgical planning, which has become much more precise due to the modern anterior segment OCT technology (Li et al. 2017; Ventura et al. 2012). An exact preoperative determination of the depth of the pathology is essential for the indication and differentiation from alternative surgical procedures such as anterior lamellar and perforating corneal transplantation. It is also necessary to differentiate whether the pathologic affection is a hyperplastic alteration (e.g., Salzmann nodule, subepithelial scars in pronounced basement membrane dystrophies, prominent superficial corneal scar) or a hypoplastic alteration (e.g., postulcerative scar).

Indication

Until the development of optical coherence tomography, a careful history and biomicroscopic slit lamp examination had to be sufficient for the indication. Morphologically, the most important factors for the treatment planning are the

- surface extension of the change (area)
- depth extension of the change (especially in relation to the total thickness of the cornea)

With regard to the assessment of the depth of pathological changes OCT technology is 'leading the way'. In areal extent, the examiner is interested in the lateral extent of a pathological corneal alteration as well as its distance from the effective optical zone. Thereby, special attention is paid to the central 3–4 mm zone (Sekundo and Geerling 2006). Optical coherence tomography allows a preoperative 3D analysis of the cornea in almost histological resolution and especially quantification of pathological areas for precise planning of a PTK (Ventura et al. 2012).

The situation is different for midperipheral and peripheral corneal changes such as those frequently encountered in Salzmann degeneration. Here, OCT helps to differentiate typical Salzmann degeneration (Fig. 8) from atypical Salzmannoid

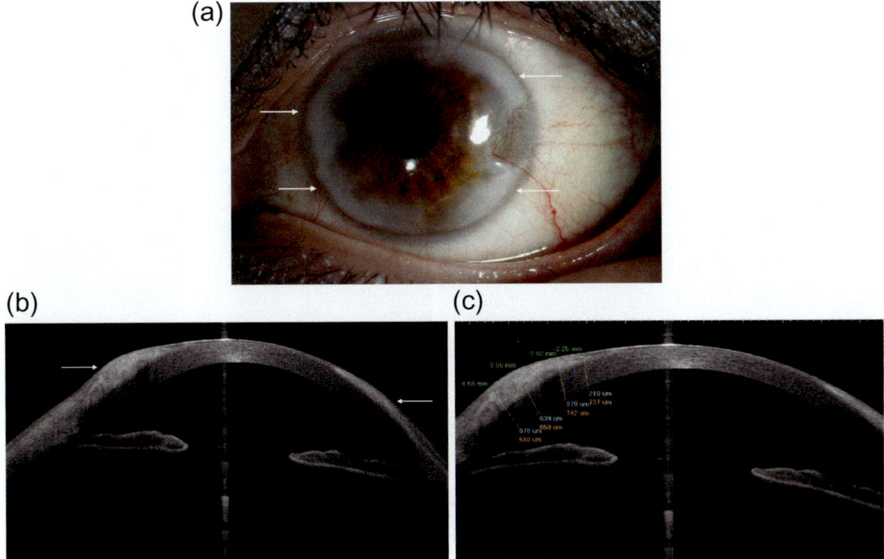

Fig. 8 Salzmann degeneration (slit lamp [A], OCT image [B+C])

changes and e.g. superficial corneal scars with migration through Bowman's membrane (Fig. 9A+B).

Slit lamp photography (A) clearly shows the practically circular whitish peripheral changes of the cornea in the present case (white arrows). OCT imaging (B) shows that this is a hyperplastic change that does not cross Bowman's membrane, but is located between Bowman's membrane and the epithelium (white arrows). As shown in Figure C, such changes can be measured well using appropriate software tools. Since in our case a software is used which automatically aligns the measurement path orthogonal to the corneal surface, especially in case of hyperplastic changes or pronounced tissue defects in the case of a deep ulcer, clear false measurements may occur (see the two right compared to the two left sections of measurement).

Intraoperatively, the Bowman membrane serves as a "guiding layer" when removing the Salzmann nodules. A migration of the Bowman membrane through a highly reflective structure visible in OCT argues against the diagnosis of Salzmann degeneration and will complicate a manual keratectomy, respectively make a supplementary PTK necessary with high probability. The following Figs. 9 and 10 clearly demonstrate the difference between a scar crossing the Bowman membrane (Fig. 9A–C) and a hyperplastic Salzmann degeneration (Figs. 10A–C and 11).

Slit lamp image A shows the planar extent of the scar in the central optic zone (white arrow). The slit-lamp image (B) allows an estimation of the depth extension, the OCT reveals the invasive character of the scar with enforcement of Bowman's membrane and involvement of the anterior stroma (white arrows). Manual keratectomy using a field hockey knife is not appropriate in this case.

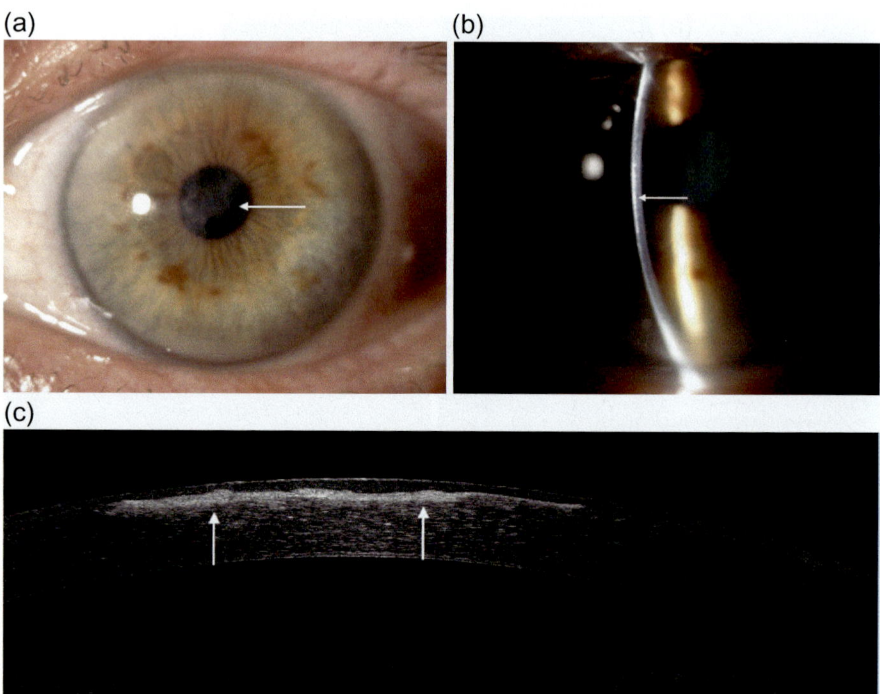

Fig. 9 Scar after herpes keratitis (**A+B** slit lamp, **C** OCT image)

Slit lamp photography (A) shows the typical arrangement of Salzmann degeneration-like changes of the cornea. In the diffuse illumination of slit-lamp biomicroscopy, the hyperplastic apposition of grayish/white tissue can be seen (white arrows). Since in focal illumination (slit) differentiation, such as depth extent "under the nodule" is difficult, OCT imaging should ideally be consulted. By means of the corresponding OCT image (B), the hyperplastic changes of the cornea respecting Bowman's membrane are well visible (white arrows). Manual removal using a hockey knife will most likely result in an opacity-free, clearly regularized corneal surface (Fig. 10B).

The whitish hyperplastic changes on Bowman's membrane are well visible. The manual removal of the visually relevant opacities by manual keratectomy is considered promising.

Here, the surgeon's focus is increasingly outside the central zone, since the paracentral hyperplastic processes can lead secondarily to visually relevant central changes in corneal curvature (hyperopia).

Treatment of hyperplastic changes is associated with a higher chance of success. Ultrasound pachymetry or ideally optical coherence tomography of the anterior segment or alternatively confocal microscopy is helpful in surgical planning. The advantage of OCT over confocal microscopy (HRT, Rostock Cornea Module,

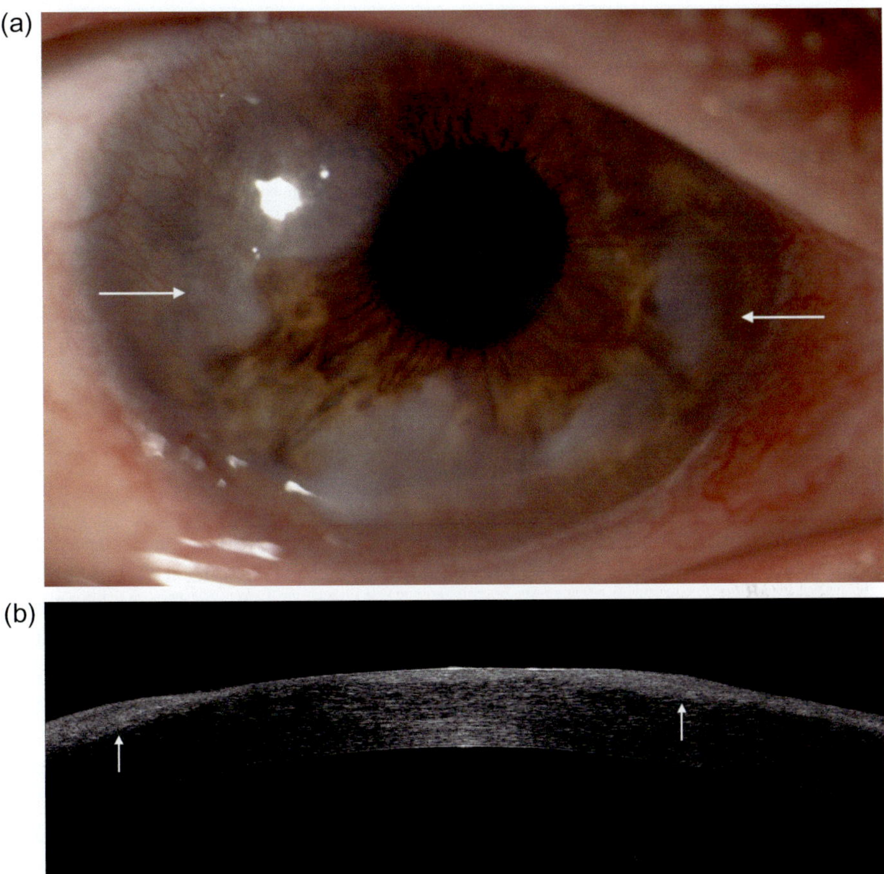

Fig. 10 Salzmann degeneration (**A** slit lamp, **B** OCT image)

Heidelberg Engineering, Heidelberg, Germany) is the better overview and the non-contact, much faster, more patient-friendly examination option.

Basics of phototherapeutic keratectomy (PTK)

If purely manual keratectomy of corneal pathology is not sufficient, phototherapeutic keratectomy (PTK) may be useful for (further) ablation of scar tissue. However, some basic principles have to be considered:

According to refractive surgery, the residual corneal stromal thickness should not fall below 250–300 μm to avoid postoperative corneal ectasia (Vinciguerra et al. 2005). In individual cases, the authors also consider a "deep" PTK of 120 up to 200 μm as a therapeutic option. Further attention is paid to concomitant pathologies. Depending on the ablation depth, PTK is often accompanied by a refractive shift in the form of myopia (Ginis et al. 2003). According to information

Fig. 11 OCT image of a recurrence of Salzmann degeneration on a corneal graft

from application specialists at Alcon (Erlangen, Germany), too much tissue tends to be ablated in the periphery with classic PTK, so that, for example, a myopic shift of up to 0.75 dpt should be expected with a tissue ablation of 50 μm in an optical zone (OZ) of 6.5 mm. Therefore, the refractive status of the partner eye should be considered in all unilateral changes to avoid postoperative high anisometropia as much as possible. Otherwise, the suffering of the patient due to the difference in refractive power may be greater than with unilateral opacification (Sekundo and Geerling 2006). In advance, therefore, the need for contact lens (CL) fitting should be discussed in detail with the patient in cases of deep ablation. A known CL intolerance is a relative contraindication to deep PTK. A coexisting cataract may be beneficial in such a case, as cataract surgery with target refraction emmetropia performed after refractive stability has been achieved may reduce anisometropia (Sekundo and Geerling 2006). In this context, PTK should be performed in most cases before a planned cataract surgery. Nevertheless, in case of deep ablation, irregularity of the cornea caused by this can be effectively corrected in many cases only with dimensionally stable contact lenses.

Re-epithelialization after PTK depends on various factors, especially on the status of the limbal stem cells. If the stem cells are clearly impaired (e.g. for example after chemical burn), PTK should not be performed, whereas PTK can still be considered if the limbus is only slightly involved (e.g. vascularization in one quadrant). In case of inflammatory diseases, e.g. after herpes keratitis, knowledge of the underlying disease, treatment in the inflammation-free interval and perioperative systemic aciclovir therapy are necessary to avoid recurrence.

Masking substances

Masking substances are liquids that are used to smooth the corneal surface during excimer laser treatment to achieve a flat and homogeneous ablation area.

In the case of an irregular contour of the corneal surface, laser treatment alone without masking substances would lead to a parallel displacement of this contour in depth (Fig. 12A). Only the filling of the "valleys" with a liquid leads to the selective ablation of the "hilltops", resulting in a "smoothed" surface at the end (Fig. 12B).

As schematically shown in figure A, a pure excimer laser treatment of an irregular corneal surface, no matter if with or without concomitant scarring, leads to an ablation of the anterior tissue (and thus to the removal/thinning of superficial opacities) but not to a regularization of the corneal surface. For this purpose, it is necessary to compensate the irregularities of the corneal surface with masking substances prior to the treatment to create a uniformly configured surface (B). The

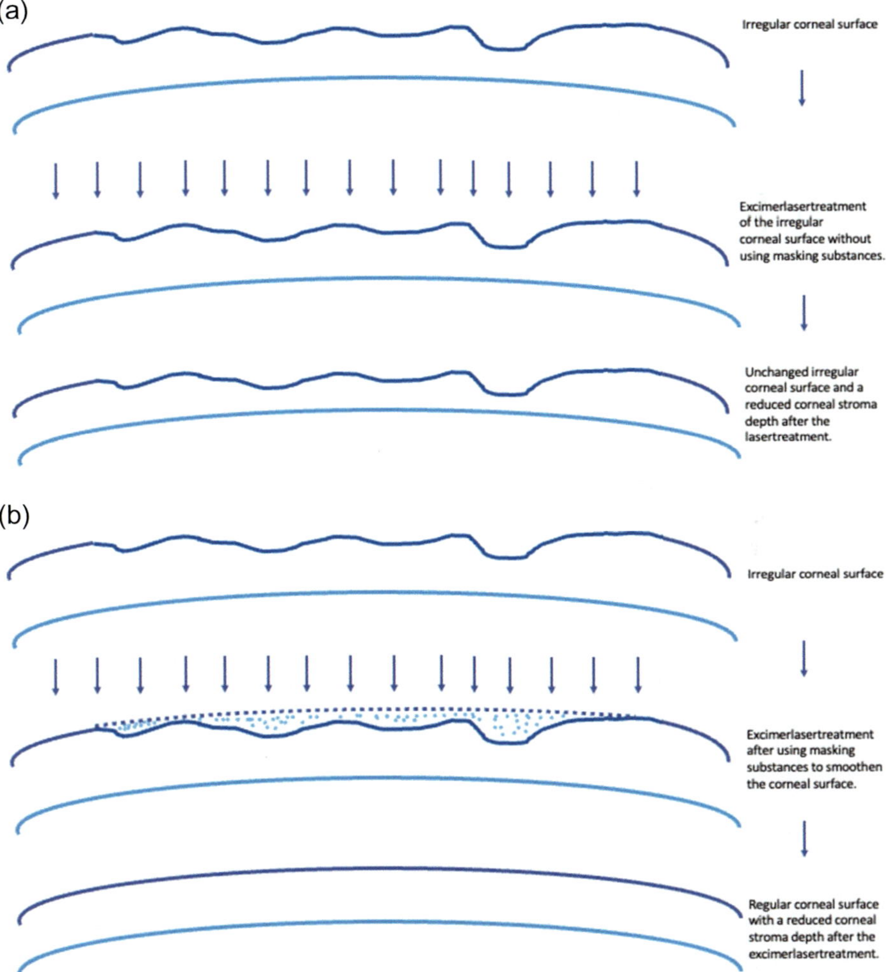

Fig. 12 Schematic representation of the modulation of an irregular corneal surface by the excimer laser without (**A**) and with the help of (**B**) a masking substance

subsequent excimer ablation leads to a regularization of the corneal surface, since both corneal tissue and masking substance are "ablated" uniformly.

Masking substances differ in their elastic properties (viscosity): they can be highly fluid (e.g. isotonic saline solution) or (thick) viscous (e.g. methyl cellulose). The ablation rate of a masking substance correlates with its viscosity. For example, the ablation rate of 0.25% sodium hyaluronate is comparable to the ablation rate of the cornea (Kornmehl et al. 1991). In many cases, a combination of viscous and low-viscosity substances can be useful: for example, in laser treatment of coarse-relief affections, which receive a "fine polish" under 0.9% NaCl after basic smoothing under 0.25% hyaluronate (Sekundo and Geerling 2006). However, the most effective masking "substance" is the corneal epithelium itself. For example, a recent study by Franco et al. indicates that in keratoconus, hypoplasia of the epithelium occurs around 20 μm at the cone apex and hyperplasia occurs around 30–40 μm at the cone base (Franco et al. 2020).

Due to these "remodeling" properties, irregularities of the corneal surface can already be compensated for naturally. To make the most of this effect, irregularities of the cornea should always be treated transepithelially, if necessary with additional application of masking substances (i.e. excimer laser ablation directly on the epithelium, not on the Bowman lamella after previous mechanical epithelial removal). Theoretically, if a large-area PTK is planned, the largest possible ablation diameter should be selected to minimize postoperative glare due to induction of higher-order aberrations in the area of the transition between ablated and nonablated tissue. At the same time, as described above, ablation-induced myopia increases as the ablation zone is enlarged. Modern excimer lasers offer ablation diameters up to 8 mm and above. When choosing the ablation diameter and effective optical zone, the transition zone should also be considered: since many laser platforms ablate tissue about 2 mm beyond the specified optical zone to the periphery, an extremely large zone can result in damage to the limbus. We therefore perform our standard PTK with the Wavelight® platform (WaveLight® GmbH, Erlangen, Germany) with an optical zone of 7 mm (total diameter including transition zone = 8.9 mm). It is important to know the characteristics of the excimer system used. For example, the Alcon EX-500 automatically reduces the ablation zone to a diameter of 5.0 mm at a ("refraction-neutral") PTK of > 50 μm in order to reduce the otherwise high myopic shift as much as possible. If a deeper ablation with a larger diameter is desired, ablation must be performed in several steps with a maximum of 50 μm.

Combination of PTK with manual abrasion in recurrent erosio corneae

Recurrent erosions of the cornea may develop due to trauma, spontaneously in the sense of recurrent corneal erosion syndrome, or on the ground of epithelial basement membrane dystrophy (EBMD) (Fagerholm 2003). According to current studies, about 50% of recurrent erosions are caused by trauma. In addition to the typical symptoms such as pain, foreign body sensation and epiphora, in our experience, initially unclear visual loss and refractive changes are often present as initial symptoms. With the help of VAA-OCT the diagnosis of EBMD can be verified.

As an example, we report on a patient who presented to our cornea consultation for co-evaluation due to unclear visual fluctuation, unstable refraction and visual acuity reduction (+0.25/−1.25/3° = 0.6) in the right eye. Biomicroscopically, the discreet changes in the sense of EBMD (formerly map-dot fingerprint dystrophy) shown in Fig. 13 were observed.

Slit-lamp biomicroscopy (A) clearly shows the partly line-shaped, partly diffuse opacity of the cornea (white arrows). OCT (A) allows a diagnosis to be confirmed by detecting epithelial duplications (small change within the epithelium, white arrow).

We performed manual abrasion corneae followed by 15 μm PTK on the right eye. Generally we recommend to initiate the abrasio without the use of alcohol in EBMD. If the diagnosis is correct, it is usually possible to remove the epithelium without alcohol with minimal mechanical manipulation due to the adhesion disorder to Bowman's membrane. Advantages of alcohol-less abrasio corneae are (a) minimization of corneal irritation due to shorter surgical time and omission of the inflammatory component due to alcohol application and (b) possibility of confirming the diagnosis. Half a year after treatment the corrected visual acuity had increased to 1.0 and the refraction (+1.75/−1.25/8°) was stable in the course with hyperopic shift.

The stabilization of the refraction, the regularization of topography and improvement of visual acuity usually achieved after PTK results in high satisfaction of the patient (Zalentein et al. 2007). From personal experience, the importance of informing the patient about a possible/probable refractive shift should also be pointed out, as otherwise, despite medically successful treatment, dissatisfaction could arise in the patient partly due to the slightly changed "spectacle values". Dry eye or chronic blepharitis should be ruled out by differential diagnosis before laser treatment, or if there are secondary findings, they should be treated consistently.

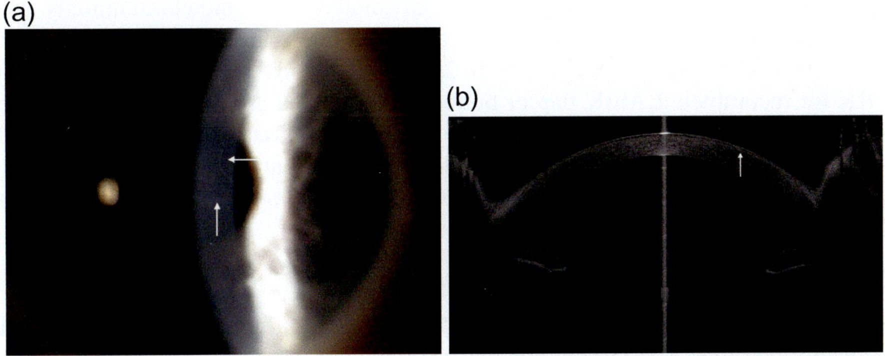

Fig. 13 Epithelial basement membrane dystrophy (EBMD); (**A** slit lamp, **B** OCT imaging)

In general, a differentiation is made between "intraepithelial" and "subepithelial" or "Bowman" PTK (Eschstruth and Sekundo 2006). Subepithelial PTK, i.e. PTK after manual removal of the epithelium, is performed most frequently and also appears to the authors as the logical and effective treatment strategy for recurrent erosions (see case study above).

A number of publications are available on this topic (Fagerholm 2003; Chow et al. 2005; Holzer et al. 2005; Baryla et al. 2006; Orndahl and Fagerholm 1998). Of particular note is Öhman and Fagerholm's (1998) published prospective and randomized study comparing long-term results of purely manual epithelial abrasion with combined (manual + 5 μm laser ablation of Bowman). Conclusion: 1. Additional laser treatment decreases the recurrence rate and 2. The majority of recurrences manifest within the first 4 months after surgery.

Combination of PTK with manual keratectomy

PTK can be combined with complementary or enhancing surgical procedures such as manual keratectomy. The prime example is the surgical treatment of Salzmann degeneration (see also Figs. 8 and 9B+C) (Linke et al. 2009; Khaireddin et al. 2011). Here, the hyperplastic, superficial and often midperipherally localized changes are preferentially "peeled off" with a hockey knife. Ideally, this allows the prominent Salzmann nodules to be removed in toto with the surrounding hyperplastic tissue— the Bowman membrane serves as the guiding layer. Since OCT shows that there is no sub-Bowman opacification of the cornea, subsequent PTK lasers with only a small ablation depth (10–15 μm) are used for "fine polishing" of any remaining degenerated tissue. Our standard treatment includes the subsequent application of Mitomycin C (0.02%) for 30 s with the aim of recurrence prophylaxis.

Combination of PTK with photorefractive keratectomy

As previously described, the epithelium exhibits compensatory hyperplasia in the area of the depressions when there are gross changes in the corneal surface (Sekundo and Geerling 2006). This is also the case after PRK and can lead to a temporary, "opposing false refraction" in the first months after laser treatment. In such pathological cases of coarse-relief changes, laser treatment through the epithelium (transepithelial) brings obvious advantages: The epithelium initially acts as the body's own "masking substance" as, for example, in the appearance of flap macrostriae after LASIK (Steinert et al. 2004). A second example is transepithelial PRK for incomplete LASIK flap or buttonhole (Kapadia and Wilson 1998). In the refractive stable interval (stable refraction > 6 months) laser treatment is performed as transepithelial PRK (TPRK). For follow-up treatment of flap-associated complications, the authors prefer TPRK due to mostly existing fine scarring and risk of flap distortion in case of ReLASIK with deep incision.

Subepithelial and stromal corneal dystrophies

In general, PTK is preferable to corneal transplantation (lamellar or perforating) if clinically possible. The reasons for this are obvious:

1. No donor material is needed 2. The intact endothelium is preserved 3. The surgery is less invasive 4. Because of the recurrent nature of corneal dystrophies, recurrence on the graft may also occur.

The recurrence rate of corneal dystrophies also enters into the treatment planning. Ideally, a distinction should be made between clinically significant and clinically non-significant recurrences (Orndahl and Fagerholm 1998; Dinh et al. 1999). Important information on the clinical picture, localization and recurrence frequency can be taken from the new classification of dystrophies (Seitz and Lisch 2011; Lisch and Seitz 2011).

The success or failure of PTK in corneal dystrophies is decisively influenced by the extension in depth of the deposits in the stroma and the targeted ablation. From our own experience, refractive changes/irregularities of the cornea after superficial ablation (up to approx. 50 µm from Bowman's membrane; i.e. approx. 100 µm from epithelium) can often still be sufficiently corrected by optimized spectacle coordination. Especially in these cases, PTK is an ideal treatment option.

Granular corneal dystrophy, type 1 (classic) (GCD1) seems to be particularly well suited for PTK (Das et al. 2005). The changes are usually localized within the central 7-mm zone and can often be successfully treated again even in recurrences (Fig. 14).

By means of biomicroscopic imaging well recognizable central opacites in the sense of granular corneal dystrophy, type 1 (GCD1) (A). The slit image (B) shows the superficial localization of the opacities, well recognizable by the shadowing (dashed arrows) caused by the opacities (continuous arrows), OCT allows an objective, quantifiable/"measurable" representation of the pathological change (continuous arrows) (C).

The frequently recurrent character of the dystrophy must be considered and conveyed in particular in the educational discussion. Depending on the localization of the pathology, early (epithelial) or delayed (stromal) recurrence is to be expected (Seitz and Lisch 2011; Hafner et al. 2005). Due to a strong tendency to recurrence, or exacerbation, PTK seems to be relatively contraindicated in lattice/macular corneal dystrophy (Orndahl and Fagerholm 1998; Das et al. 2005). In individual cases, however, good results can also be obtained.

Degeneration and scarring

Calcifications in band keratopathy were among the early indications for PTK (Dighiero et al. 2000; O'Brart et al. 1993). From our point of view, in the case of band keratopathy and intact Bowman's lamella, EDTA abrasio alone is often sufficient and is therefore our preferred primary therapy. However, often the Bowman is eroded, so that a combined EDTA-abrasio/PTK with masking fluid leaves a much smoother surface (Stewart and Morrell 2003). In the case of degenerative-hyperplastic changes such as extensive epithelial scarring on a corneal graft, it may be helpful to perform the entire ablation using an excimer laser. This should always be considered when the changes are primarily intraepithelial and subepithelial and a regular corneal surface is present. If ablation of the epithelium were to be performed primarily with a sharp instrument (e.g., field hockey knife) in

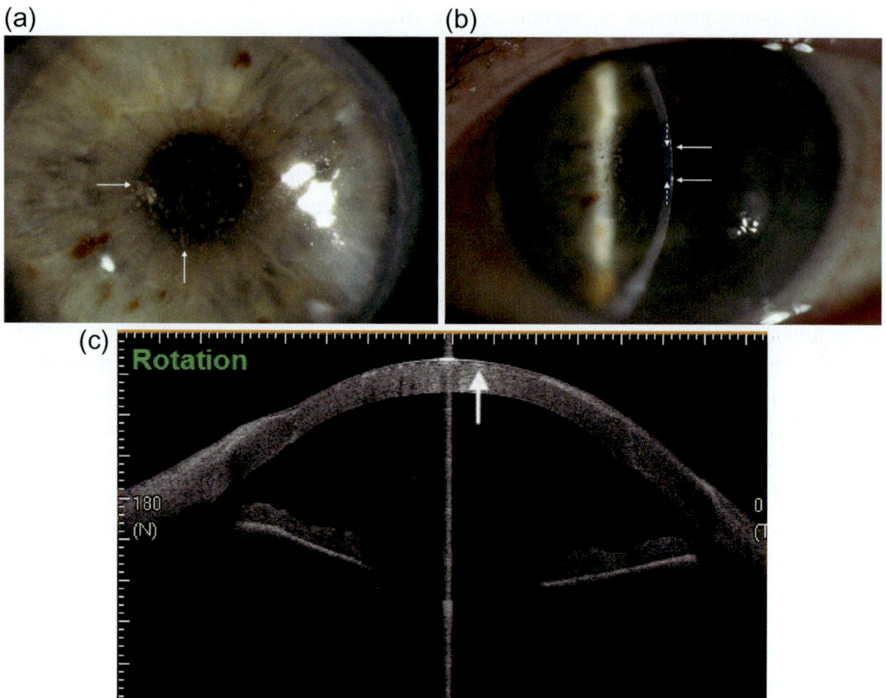

Fig. 14 Granular corneal dystrophy (GCD1) (recurrence on graft; slit lamp [**A+B**] and OCT image [**C**])

this case, there is a risk that this would result in an irregular surface configuration due to scarring and partial destruction of the Bowman's lamella. Although this can be compensated for using masking agents prior to excimer laser application, it carries a higher risk of postoperative irregularities than primary ablation using excimer laser. Shows such a case of superficial scarring of a 20-year-old corneal graft extending to a depth of approximately 110 μm including epithelial parts. After multistage ablation of the superficial 115 μm under biomicroscopic control (50 μm + 40 μm + 20 μm), topical 0.02% mitomycin was applied for 30 s as recurrence prophylaxis. According to our explanations before (section "masking substances"), in case the Bowman lamella/epithelium is affected, we recommend to use the excimer laser transepithelially to regularize the cornea and benefit from the masking effect (Fig. 15).

Central, subepithelial scar on a corneal transplant that can be well visualized by different OCT devices (A+B Tomey Casia®, C+D Topcon Maestro 2® OCT, Topcon Deutschland Medical GmbH, Willich, Germany). The companies inherent software and resolution, as well as the necessity to manually mark the changes, sometimes lead to slight deviations of the measurement results (compare pachymetry data image B + D).

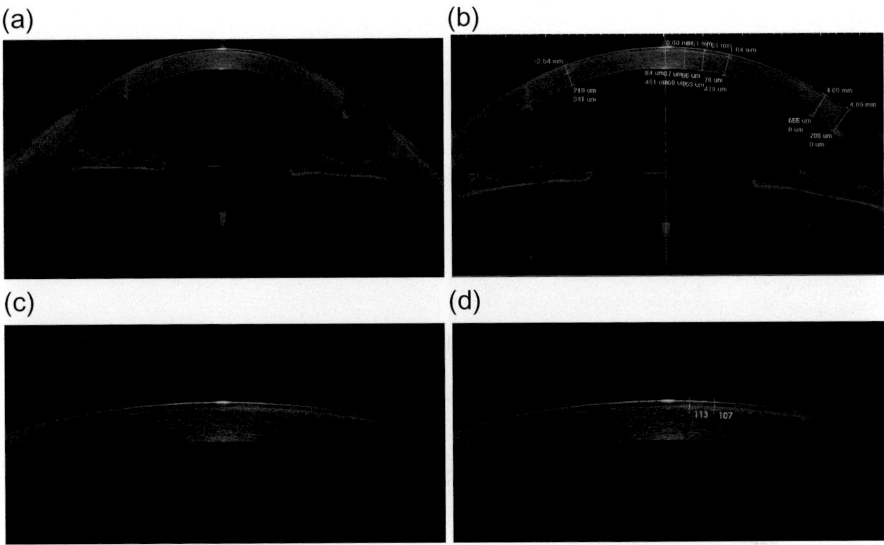

Fig. 15 Scars on a corneal graft (**A+B** Tomey Casia OCT; **C + D** Topcon Maestro 2 OCT each with manual pachymetry)

For deep-located changes, the indication must be well considered. In our experience, haze-free laser treatment with corneal ablation up to 150–180 μm can be performed using antimetabolites such as mitomycin C (MMC).

According to the recommendations from the literature, the authors apply 0.02% MMC for up to 60 s in almost every PTK, except the treatment of EBMD, despite off-label status (Wilson et al. 2017; Arranz-Marquez et al. 2019).

However, one should remain cautious applying MMC in all diseases with possible wound healing disorders/delays such as diabetes mellitus, pronounced keratoconjunctivitis sicca, rheumatic diseases, limbal insufficiencies (see above), but also per (post-)herpetic scars.

Regardless of the effective keratitis suppression by MMC, in our opinion a maximum relative ablation of 30% should not be exceeded because of the resulting biomechanical destabilization of the corneal tissue and inherent risk of keratectasia development. However, hyperopia of 6 dpt and above is not uncommon with such high ablation. Close cooperation with an optometrist for contact lens fitting is therefore essential for the success of treatment in deep PTK.

For larger substance defects and scars (e.g., after a corneal ulcer, see Figs. 16 and 17), lamellar or penetrating keratoplasty often offers a visually more attractive alternative.

Shown is a large central deep shield-like ulcer (A) with fluorescein-positive epithelial defect (B) and thinning of the corneal stroma, well assessable in terms of depth extent by OCT (white arrows) (C).

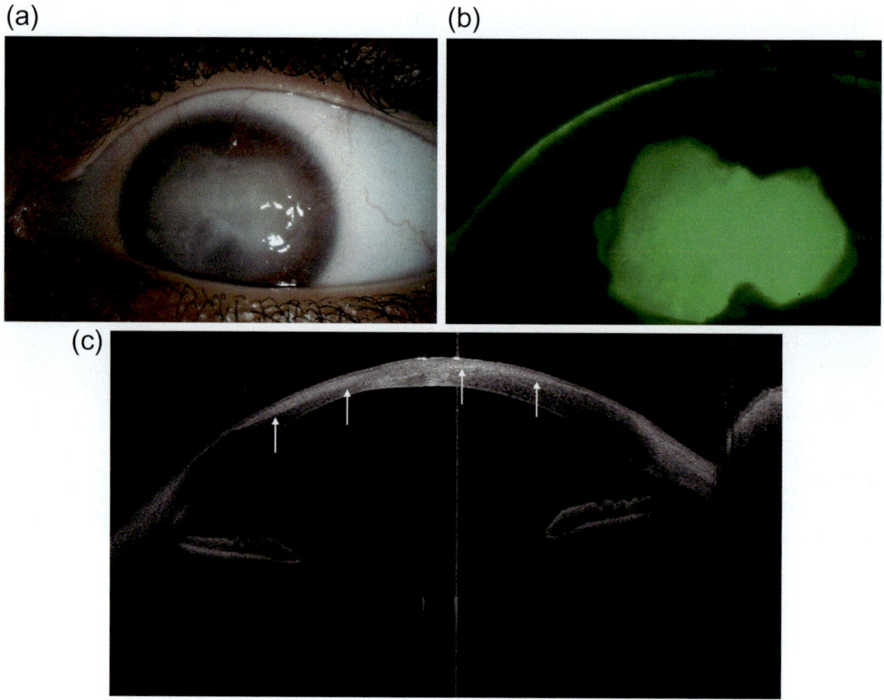

Fig. 16 Deep shield-ulcer in keratitis vernalis (slit lamp [**A**], fluorescein slit lamp [**B**], and OCT imaging [**C**])

Shown is a corneal scar (A) involving the optical zone. Involvement of at least the anterior stromal third can already be seen by slit imaging with biomicroscopy. By OCT (C) the stromal defect, the stromal scar and the hyperplastic epithelium "compensating" the defect can be well differentiated. Because the opacity extends too deep into the stroma, PTK is not indicated. In this case, lamellar grafting would be discussed as a reasonable therapeutic option.

Another example of a useful combination of manual keratectomy and, if necessary, subsequent PTK treatment of residual scar tissue is the pterygium. It is not uncommon for superficial and even paracentral scar areas to remain after pterygium excision. These can be minimized with the aid of PTK. However, the success is often limited by a strong irregularity of the scar, which is difficult to regularize even with masking substances (Fig. 18) (Fagerholm et al. 1993).

By slit lamp biomicroscopy (A) and OCT (B) well recognizable hyperplastic tissue proliferation in the sense of a pterygium spreading to the cornea. By OCT the "riding" of the pterygium on the Bowmann membrane, similar to Salzmann degeneration, is well visible (white arrow).

After PTK in the setting of pterygium treatment, activation of keratocytes in the ablation area and surrounding scar areas has been observed, which may lead to dense and persistent scarring/haze (Fagerholm 2003; Fagerholm et al. 1993).

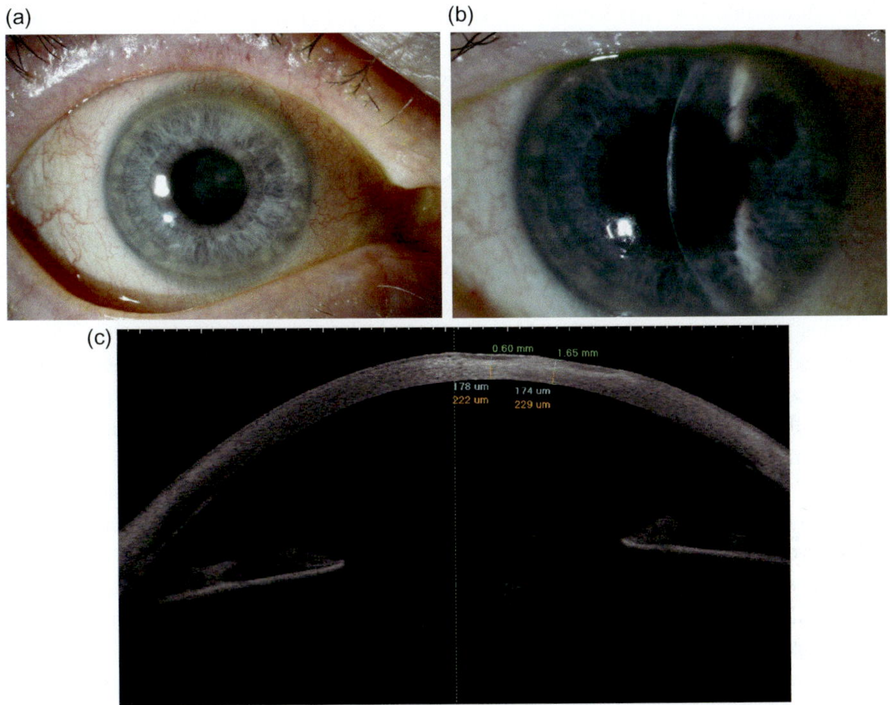

Fig. 17 Central corneal scar after foreign body—associated keratitis (slit lamps [**A**], [**B**] and OCT image [**C**])

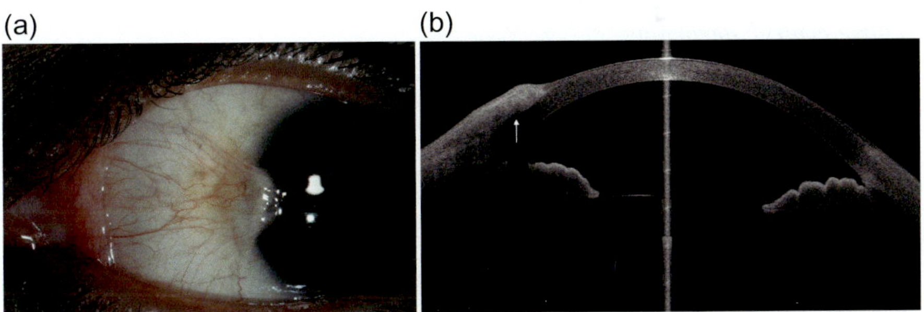

Fig. 18 Pterygium (slit lamp [**A**]—and OCT image [**B**])

Overall, there is only a small number of publications and also own experiences show a rather moderate success of PTK in post pterygium scars despite application of MMC (Hahn et al. 1993; Maloney et al. 1996; Rapuano 1997). The strong tendency of surrounding keratocytes to transform into activated keratocytes and transdifferentiate into myofibroblasts seems to be partly responsible for the reduced predictability of PTK in this situation.

Topography-guided PTK

Nowadays, topography-guided PTK/PRK laser treatment is increasingly used (Seitz et al. 1998; Pasquali and Krueger 2012; Knorz and Jendritza 2000; Lin et al. 2012). This treatment aims to regularize irregular areas and is thus a highly individualized form of treatment. Compared to wavefront-guided laser treatment, topography-guided laser treatment offers the advantage of more robust and reliable data collection, especially in the case of very irregular corneas and/or media opacities such as corneal scars or lens opacities (Lin et al. 2008; Krueger 2006).

Nowadays, different systems (Placido versus Scheimpflug based) are available for the collection of curvature data. Due to the underlying physical principles, Scheimpflug based methods seem to be more robust and reliable for the analysis of central irregularities (Cummings and Mascharka 2010). This is caused by a "central scotoma" due to the central camera position in Placido-based topography. This results in a necessary extrapolation of the central corneal data. The application field of topography-guided PTK/PRK range from the treatment of irregular astigmatisms after corneal transplantation (Lin et al. 2012; Ohno 2011) (Fig. 19), via post excimer laser irregularities (Toda et al. 2007), to CL intolerant keratoconus patients (Kanellopoulos and Binder 2007, 2011).

Topographic image of an irregular corneal surface after corneal transplanta-tion (A). Excimer laser treatment profile created by topographic data (B) and post-operative topography (C). The aim of the treatment was to regularize the optical zone by ablation in the area of the paracentral-nasal steep cornea and ablation of peripheral corneal areas superiorly and temporally. The peripheral ablation led via biomechanical weakening in the ablation area to a planned con-secutive central steepening.

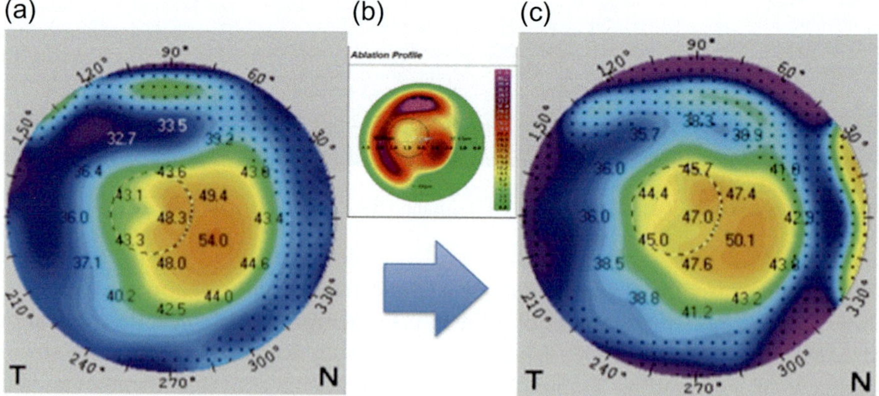

Fig. 19 PTK in irregular astigmatism after corneal transplantation

Such regularization by topography-guided PTK is potentially also a useful therapeutic strategy in the treatment of visual deterioration in patients with keratoconus. However, since topography-guided laser treatment potentially induces progression of keratoconus due to tissue ablation, the safety and efficacy of PTK in combination with corneal cross-linking is the subject of current studies (Kanellopoulos and Binder 2007, 2011). The authors use PTK combined with directly subsequent corneal cross-linking according to the Athens protocol (max. ablation 50 μm) to regularize the cornea in progressive keratoconus (Kanellopoulos 2019). A case treated by the authors is shown by means of Figs. 20 (topographies before/after PTK/CXL incl. difference plot) and 28 (applied treatment profile of the excimer laser). The central optical zone of the patient with progressive keratoconus was regularized, and the findings were stabilized with CXL treatment immediately following. The patient demonstrated stable morphologic as well as functional findings 10 months after treatment, at the time of this article. Despite a clear morphologic regularization of the corneal surface, the corrected visual acuity, with a clear cornea, could not be increased (refraction + decimal visual acuity before post-op: +2.5/−4.75/95° = 0.6; −1.5/−3.0/77° = 0.6). However, the reduction of refractive astigmatism as well as the postoperative myopia due to the steepening of the central optical zone made it possible to compensate the remaining refractive error again by means of glasses. In addition, subjectively perceived halos decreased

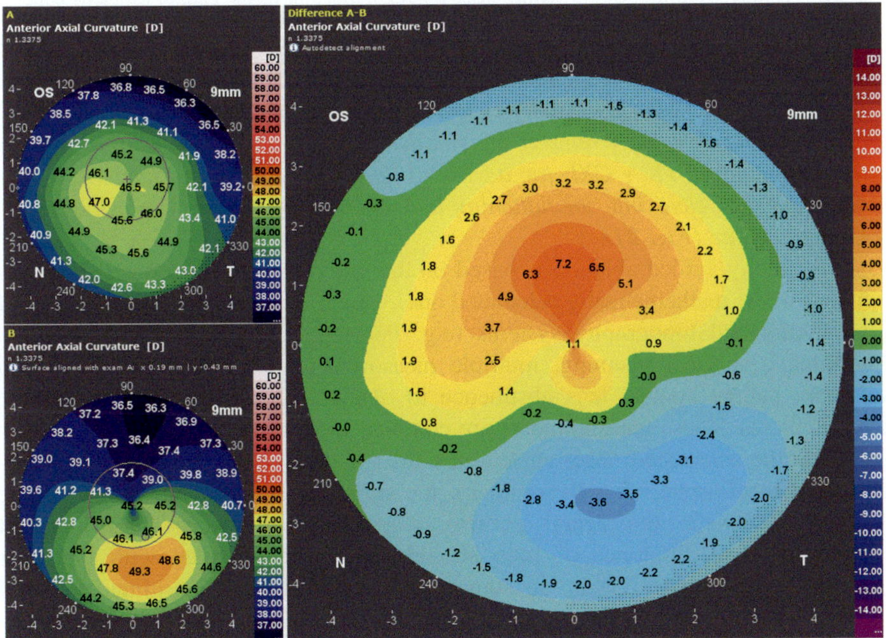

Fig. 20 Topography of a keratoconus patient before and after treatment using topography-guided PTK with the aim of regularizing the cornea

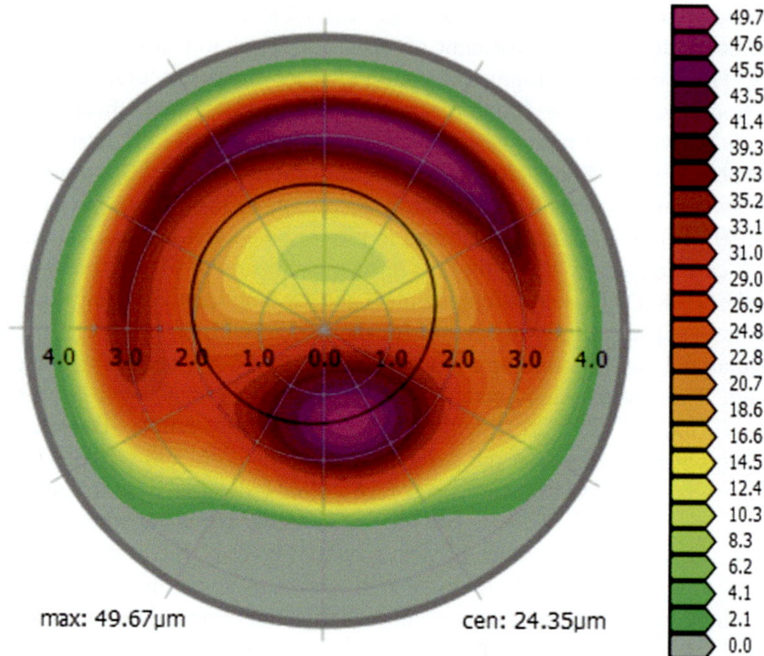

Fig. 21 Treatment profile of the excimer laser for regularization of the central (optical) zone

and image quality/contrast increased. The regularized cornea also leads to a better fitting with contact lenses in many cases according to our own experience.

Topography showing irregular astigmatism before (lower left) and 10 months after (upper left) PTK + CXL for advanced keratoconus. Right: Differential representation with clear inferior flattening and superior steepening according to the treatment profile (Fig. 21).

Topography-guided ablation is based on the individual "real" corneal shape (as opposed to the mathematically calculated one), which is determined with the help of tomography and topography systems (e.g. Pentacam®/Topolyzer®; Orbscan®). For reliable surgical planning, multiple measurements are often necessary with sufficient patient contact lens abstinence to obtain meaningful and reproducible measurements. These measurements are combined with refraction and pachymetry data, and the subsequent laser algorithm aims to "remove the peaks" while maintaining corneal asphericity. In summary, the software analyzes and calculates the difference between the actual corneal shape (curvature data) and a target asphericity. The difference of both should ideally be removed with the laser (Pasquali and Krueger 2012). In some cases, the software algorithms not only "flatten" the abnormally steep areas, but also steepening individual areas by peripheral ablation to achieve a central optical zone that is as homogeneous as possible (see Figs. 19 and 20). One challenge of topography-guided laser treatment is the refractive predictability: Each stromal modulation of the cornea induces a refractive change—but since it is an individual ablation, no nomograms exist (yet) (Lin et al. 2012). Despite interesting study data on sequential PTK/PRK (PTK for correction of opacities followed directly by PRK for additive refractive correction) (Nakamura et al. 2018) the authors therefore prefer a two-stage procedure for the treatment of irregular corneal surfaces as a result of superficial scars or post-keratoplasty: first, topography-guided treatment is performed with the aim of regularizing the corneal surface and improving the corrected visual acuity. In the refractive stable interval, refractive surface laser treatment (if desired) can then be planned if corneal thickness is sufficient.

Rare indications based on selected examples

The extent to which topography-guided laser treatment of e.g. irregular cornea after transplantation still falls under the term PTK can be controversially discussed. However, the therapeutic use of the laser in these cases is undisputed.11 Persistent and visual acuity-reducing haze after PRK can be reduced with the help of PTK (Fig. 22).

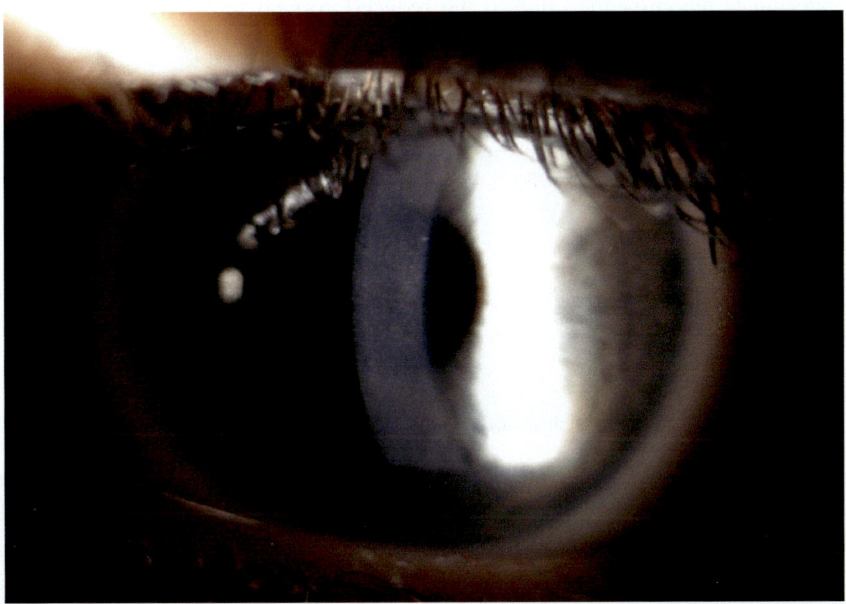

Fig. 22 Haze after PRK

However, based on current studies, MMC should be applied intraoperatively and not postoperatively in the form of eye drops (Shalaby et al. 2009). For haze prophylaxis after refractive surface ablation, many surgeons already use MMC during a primary procedure and can thereby minimize the occurrence of clinically significant haze (Shalaby et al. 2009; Raviv et al. 2000; Majmudar et al. 2000; Shah and Wilson 2010). The authors also apply MMC as standard for all primary refractive surface ablations (PRK/transepithelial PRK/LASEK/EpiLASIK) between 15 and 45 s depending on preoperative refraction.

Scars after viral keratitis

Herpes simplex, herpes zoster and keratoconjunctivitis epidemica can lead to superficial corneal scars, which can be subjected to PTK in the low-stimulus interval. Postherpetic scars are often associated with stromal thinning—this must be estimated/recorded preoperatively on the slit lamp or ideally using tomographic techniques. The more advanced the stromal thinning, the lower the chances of success of PTK treatment (Fagerholm et al. 1993; Campos et al. 1993). Critically, UV exposure has been described as a trigger for a flare-up of herpetic keratitis. Prophylactically, a preoperative systemic antiviral therapy should be planned to reduce the probability of recurrence (Fagerholm et al. 1993). Close postoperative monitoring is recommended due to the reduced corneal sensitivity caused by the herpes infection and the laser treatment itself (Figs. 23 and 24).

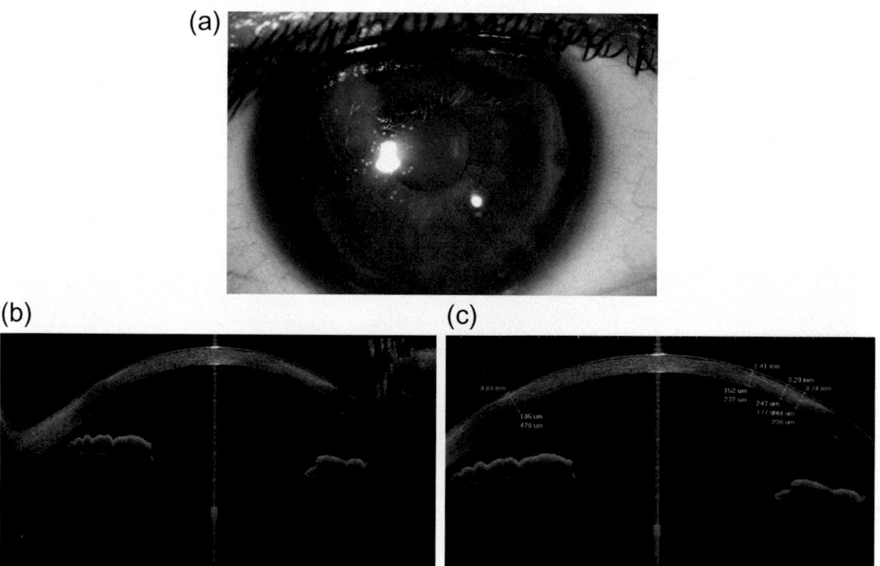

Fig. 23 Corneal scar after herpes keratitis (slit lamp [A] and OCT image [B, C])

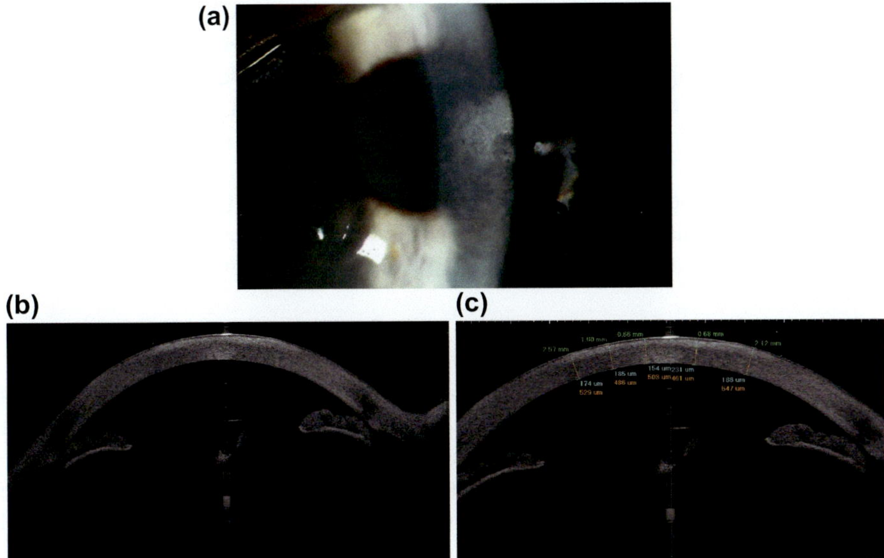

Fig. 24 Central corneal scar after herpes keratitis (slit lamp [**A**] and OCT image [**B, C**])

In slit lamp biomicroscopy well recognizable almost circular, peripheral corneal scar with clear areal extension into paracentral areas at 10 o'clock. By OCT (B, C) a precise measurement of the depth extension of the changes is well possible.

Central, dense corneal scar well visible in slit lamp biomicroscopy. By OCT (B, C) a precise measurement of the depth extension of the changes is well possible. Transepithelial PTK is a potential therapeutic option.

Visual acuity—relevant nummuli after keratoconjunctivitis epidemica should initially be treated with CsA 2% 4x/d on a trial basis if there is no improvement and only be treated with PTK as ultima ratio (>8 months after keratitis) (Binder et al. 1994; Quentin et al. 1999).

Mitomycin C application in combination with therapeutic corneal laser applications.

As can be seen from the individual case presentations above, an important new development in recent years has been the introduction of intraoperative application of mitomycin C 0.02% (MMC) in laser surgery of the cornea.

MMC leads to a reduction of keratocytes in the application area and thus effectively suppresses scar formation (Majmudar et al. 2000; Hashemi et al. 2004; Schipper et al. 1997). As mentioned above, adjuvant MMC allows a depth of ablation of up to 150 μm without significant haze development. Reduction of the keratocyte population also has advantages in the treatment of stromal dystrophies.

Early reports suggest that recurrence rates decrease with MMC use (Kim et al. 2006; Miller et al. 2004). Due to potential side effects, responsible use of this chemotherapeutic agent is necessary (Geerling and Sekundo 2006). In addition, patients should be educated about off-label treatment. With the exception of the treatment of recurrent erosions, the authors use MMC in the majority of therapeutic laser treatments with the goal of haze prevention and recurrence prophylaxis. Exceptions are secondary diseases associated with delayed epithelial wound healing such as keratoconjunctivitis sicca, blepharitis, or limbal stem cell insufficiency. However, these secondary diseases are often themselves a contraindication to laser treatment.

Summary

In parallel to continuous innovations in the field of refractive excimer surgery and phototherapeutic keratectomy, anterior segment OCT is gaining more importance and provides new sophisticated applications.

PTK is nowadays an effective treatment method for diseases especially of the corneal surface. Main indications are epithelial adhesion problems, superficial opacities and irregularities. Particularly successful is the treatment of recurrent erosio corneae and corneal dystrophies and degenerations in the anterior stromal third.

The very reliable histopathologic in vivo correlation by anterior segment OCT allows precise planning and targeted, tissue-saving use of the surgical modalities available today.

Diseases associated with hyperplastic changes, such as Salzmann degeneration, have a higher chance of success than diseases leading to stromal melting, such as deep postulcerative scars. For the indication and individual surgical planning, factors such as depth and areal extend of the pathologic findings in addition to the refractive status of both eyes play as important a role as the knowledge of the underlying disease and the limbal stem cell status. Regarding the preoperative 3D measurement of the cornea, VAA-OCT has proven to be indispensable.

In contrast to refractive surgery, phototherapeutic keratectomy and topography-guided laser treatment is not an automated or standardized surgical technique, but rather a customized procedure.

Conflict of Interest There are no financial, political or economical conflicts of interests of the authors in regard to this work.

References

Arranz-Marquez E, Katsanos A, Kozobolis VP, Konstas AGP, Teus MA. A critical overview of the biological effects of mitomycin C application on the cornea following refractive surgery. Adv Ther. 2019;36(4):786–97.

Baryla J, Pan YI, Hodge WG. Long-term efficacy of phototherapeutic keratectomy on recurrent corneal erosion syndrome. Cornea. 2006;25(10):1150–2.

Binder PS, Anderson JA, Rock ME, Vrabec MP. Human excimer laser keratectomy. Clinical and histopathologic correlations. Ophthalmology. 1994;101(6):979–89.

Campos M, Nielsen S, Szerenyi K, Garbus JJ, McDonnell PJ. Clinical follow-up of phototherapeutic keratectomy for treatment of corneal opacities. Am J Ophthalmol. 1993;115(4):433–40.

Chow AM, Yiu EP, Hui MK, Ho CK. Shallow ablations in phototherapeutic keratectomy: long-term follow-up. J Cataract Refract Surg. 2005;31(11):2133–6.

Cummings AB, Mascharka N. Outcomes after topography-based LASIK and LASEK with the wavelight oculyzer and topolyzer platforms. J Refract Surg. 2010;26(7):478–85.

Das S, Langenbucher A, Seitz B. Excimer laser phototherapeutic keratectomy for granular and lattice corneal dystrophy: a comparative study. J Refract Surg. 2005;21(6):727–31.

Dighiero P, Boudraa R, Ellies P, Saragoussi JJ, Legeais JM, Renard G. Therapeutic photokeratectomy for the treatment of band keratopathy. J Fr Ophtalmol. 2000;23(4):345–9.

Dinh R, Rapuano CJ, Cohen EJ, Laibson PR. Recurrence of corneal dystrophy after excimer laser phototherapeutic keratectomy. Ophthalmology. 1999;106(8):1490–7.

Eschstruth P, Sekundo W. [Recurrent corneal erosion. Different treatment options with the excimer laser with emphasis on aggressive PTK]. Ophthalmologe. 2006;103(7):570–5.

Fagerholm P. Phototherapeutic keratectomy: 12 years of experience. Acta Ophthalmol Scand. 2003;81(1):19–32.

Fagerholm P, Fitzsimmons TD, Orndahl M, Ohman L, Tengroth B. Phototherapeutic keratectomy: long-term results in 166 eyes. Refract Corneal Surg. 1993;9(2 Suppl):S76-81.

Fagerholm P, Ohman L, Orndahl M. Phototherapeutic keratectomy in herpes simplex keratitis. Clinical results in 20 patients. Acta Ophthalmol (Copenh). 1994;72(4):457–60.

Franco J, White CA, Kruh JN. Analysis of compensatory corneal epithelial thickness changes in keratoconus using corneal tomography. Cornea. 2020;39(3):298–302.

Galvis V, Tello A, Revelo ML, Valarezo P. LASIK interface complications: what is the appropriate term for PISK? J Refract Surg. 2013;29(2):81.

Geerling G, Sekundo W. [Phototherapeutic keratectomy. Undesirable effects, complications, and preventive strategies]. Ophthalmologe. 2006;103(7):576–82.

Ginis HS, Katsanevaki VJ, Pallikaris IG. Influence of ablation parameters on refractive changes after phototherapeutic keratectomy. J Refract Surg. 2003;19(4):443–8.

Hafner A, Langenbucher A, Seitz B. Long-term results of phototherapeutic keratectomy with 193-nm excimer laser for macular corneal dystrophy. Am J Ophthalmol. 2005;140(3):392–6.

Hahn TW, Sah WJ, Kim JH. Phototherapeutic keratectomy in nine eyes with superficial corneal diseases. Refract Corneal Surg. 1993;9(2 Suppl):S115–8.

Hashemi H, Taheri SM, Fotouhi A, Kheiltash A. Evaluation of the prophylactic use of mitomycin-C to inhibit haze formation after photorefractive keratectomy in high myopia: a prospective clinical study. BMC Ophthalmol. 2004;4:12.

Holzer MP, Auffarth GU, Specht H, Kruse FE. Combination of transepithelial phototherapeutic keratectomy and autologous serum eyedrops for treatment of recurrent corneal erosions. J Cataract Refract Surg. 2005;31(8):1603–6.

Kanellopoulos AJ. Ten-Year Outcomes of Progressive Keratoconus Management With the Athens Protocol (Topography-Guided Partial-Refraction PRK Combined With CXL). J Refract Surg. 2019;35(8):478–83.

Kanellopoulos AJ, Binder PS. Collagen cross-linking (CCL) with sequential topography-guided PRK: a temporizing alternative for keratoconus to penetrating keratoplasty. Cornea. 2007;26 (7):891–5.

Kanellopoulos AJ, Binder PS. Management of corneal ectasia after LASIK with combined, same-day, topography-guided partial transepithelial PRK and collagen cross-linking: the athens protocol. J Refract Surg. 2011;27(5):323–31.

Kapadia MS, Wilson SE. Transepithelial photorefractive keratectomy for treatment of thin flaps or caps after complicated laser in situ keratomileusis. Am J Ophthalmol. 1998;126(6):827–9.

Khaireddin R, Katz T, Baile RB, Richard G, Linke SJ. Superficial keratectomy, PTK, and mitomycin C as a combined treatment option for Salzmann's nodular degeneration: a follow-up of eight eyes. Graefes Arch Clin Exp Ophthalmol. 2011;249(8):1211–5.

Kim TI, Pak JH, Chae JB, Kim EK, Tchah H. Mitomycin C inhibits recurrent Avellino dystrophy after phototherapeutic keratectomy. Cornea. 2006;25(2):220–3.

Knorz MC, Jendritza B. Topographically-guided laser in situ keratomileusis to treat corneal irregularities. Ophthalmology. 2000;107(6):1138–43.

Kornmehl EW, Steinert RF, Puliafito CA. A comparative study of masking fluids for excimer laser phototherapeutic keratectomy. Arch Ophthalmol. 1991;109(6):860–3.

Krueger RR. Corneal topography vs ocular wavefront sensing in the retreatment of highly aberrated post surgical eyes. J Refract Surg. 2006;22(4):328–30.

Li Y, Yokogawa H, Tang M, Chamberlain W, Zhang X, Huang D. Guiding flying-spot laser transepithelial phototherapeutic keratectomy with optical coherence tomography. J Cataract Refract Surg. 2017;43(4):525–36.

Lin DT, Holland SR, Rocha KM, Krueger RR. Method for optimizing topography-guided ablation of highly aberrated eyes with the ALLEGRETTO WAVE excimer laser. J Refract Surg. 2008;24(4):S439–45.

Lin DT, Holland S, Tan JC, Moloney G. Clinical results of topography-based customized ablations in highly aberrated eyes and keratoconus/ectasia with cross-linking. J Refract Surg. 2012;28(11):S841–8.

Linke S, Kugu C, Richard G, Katz T. An in vivo confocal microscopic analysis of Salzmann's nodular degeneration: pre- and post-surgical intervention. Acta Ophthalmol. 2009;87(2):233–4.

Linke SJ, Steinberg J, Katz T. Therapeutic excimer laser treatment of the cornea. Klin Monbl Augenheilkd. 2013;230(6):595–603.

Lisch W, Seitz B. [New international classification of corneal dystrophies (CD)]. Ophthalmologe. 2011;108(9):883–96; quiz 97.

Majmudar PA, Forstot SL, Dennis RF, et al. Topical mitomycin-C for subepithelial fibrosis after refractive corneal surgery. Ophthalmology. 2000;107(1):89–94.

Maloney RK, Thompson V, Ghiselli G, Durrie D, Waring GO, 3rd, O'Connell M. A prospective multicenter trial of excimer laser phototherapeutic keratectomy for corneal vision loss. The Summit Phototherapeutic Keratectomy Study Group. Am J Ophthalmol. 1996;122(2):149–60.

Miller A, Solomon R, Bloom A, Palmer C, Perry HD, Donnenfeld ED. Prevention of recurrent Reis-Bucklers dystrophy following excimer laser phototherapeutic keratectomy with topical mitomycin C. Cornea. 2004;23(7):732–5.

Nakamura T, Kataoka T, Kojima T, Yoshida Y, Sugiyama Y. Refractive outcomes after phototherapeutic refractive keratectomy for granular corneal dystrophy. Cornea. 2018;37(5):548–53.

O'Brart DP, Gartry DS, Lohmann CP, Patmore AL, Kerr Muir MG, Marshall J. Treatment of band keratopathy by excimer laser phototherapeutic keratectomy: surgical techniques and long term follow up. Br J Ophthalmol. 1993;77(11):702–8.

Ohman L, Fagerholm P. The influence of excimer laser ablation on recurrent corneal erosions: a prospective randomized study. Cornea. 1998;17(4):349–52.

Ohno K. Customized photorefractive keratectomy for the correction of regular and irregular astigmatism after penetrating keratoplasty. Cornea. 2011;30(Suppl 1):S41–4.

Orndahl MJ, Fagerholm PP. Treatment of corneal dystrophies with phototherapeutic keratectomy. J Refract Surg. 1998;14(2):129–35.

Orndahl MJ, Fagerholm PP. Phototherapeutic keratectomy for map-dot-fingerprint corneal dystrophy. Cornea. 1998;17(6):595–9.

Pasquali T, Krueger R. Topography-guided laser refractive surgery. Curr Opin Ophthalmol. 2012;23(4):264–8.

Quentin CD, Tondrow M, Vogel M. Phototherapeutic keratectomy (PTK) after epidemic keratoconjunctivitis. Ophthalmologe. 1999;96(2):92–6.

Rapuano CJ. Excimer laser phototherapeutic keratectomy: long-term results and practical considerations. Cornea. 1997;16(2):151–7.

Raviv T, Majmudar PA, Dennis RF, Epstein RJ. Mytomycin-C for post-PRK corneal haze. J Cataract Refract Surg. 2000;26(8):1105–6.

Schipper I, Suppelt C, Gebbers JO. Mitomycin C reduces scar formation after excimer laser (193 nm) photorefractive keratectomy in rabbits. Eye (London). 1997;11(Pt 5):649–55.

Seiler T, Bende T, Wollensak J. Correction of astigmatism with the Excimer laser. Klin Monbl Augenheilkd. 1987;191(3):179–83.

Seitz B, Lisch W. Stage-related therapy of corneal dystrophies. Dev Ophthalmol. 2011;48:116–53.

Seitz B, Langenbucher A, Kus MM, Harrer M. Experimental correction of irregular corneal astigmatism using topography-based flying-spot-mode excimer laser photoablation. Am J Ophthalmol. 1998;125(2):252–6.

Sekundo W, Geerling G. [Phototherapeutic keratectomy. Basic principles, techniques and indications]. Ophthalmologe. 2006;103(7):563–9.

Shah RA, Wilson SE. Use of mitomycin-C for phototherapeutic keratectomy and photorefractive keratectomy surgery. Curr Opin Ophthalmol. 2010;21(4):269–73.

Shalaby A, Kaye GB, Gimbel HV. Mitomycin C in photorefractive keratectomy. J Refract Surg. 2009;25(1 Suppl):S93–7.

Steinert RF, Ashrafzadeh A, Hersh PS. Results of phototherapeutic keratectomy in the management of flap striae after LASIK. Ophthalmology. 2004;111(4):740–6.

Stewart OG, Morrell AJ. Management of band keratopathy with excimer phototherapeutic keratectomy: visual, refractive, and symptomatic outcome. Eye (London). 2003;17(2):233–7.

Tello A, Galvis V, Mendoza BF. LASIK interface complications: Pressure-Induced Stromal Keratitis (PISK), Interface Fluid Syndrome (IFS) and Post-LASIK Edema-induced Keratopathy (PLEK). Int Ophthalmol Clin. 2016;56(3):185–7.

Toda I, Yamamoto T, Ito M, Hori-Komai Y, Tsubota K. Topography-guided ablation for treatment of patients with irregular astigmatism. J Refract Surg. 2007;23(2):118–25.

Tourtas T, Kopsachilis N, Meiller R, Kruse FE, Cursiefen C. Pressure-induced interlamellar stromal keratitis after laser in situ keratomileusis. Cornea. 2011;30(8):920–3.

Trokel SL, Srinivasan R, Braren B. Excimer laser surgery of the cornea. Am J Ophthalmol. 1983;96(6):710–5.

Ventura BV, Moraes HV Jr, Kara-Junior N, Santhiago MR. Role of optical coherence tomography on corneal surface laser ablation. J Ophthalmol. 2012;2012: 676740.

Vinciguerra P, Munoz MI, Camesasca FI, Grizzi F, Roberts C. Long-term follow-up of ultrathin corneas after surface retreatment with phototherapeutic keratectomy. J Cataract Refract Surg. 2005;31(1):82–7.

Wang Y, Ma J, Zhang L, et al. Postoperative corneal complications in small incision lenticule extraction: long-term study. J Refract Surg. 2019;35(3):146–52.

Wilson SE, Marino GK, Medeiros CS, Santhiago MR. Phototherapeutic keratectomy: science and art. J Refract Surg. 2017;33(3):203–10.

Zalentein WN, Holopainen JM, Tervo TM. Phototherapeutic keratectomy for epithelial irregular astigmatism: an emphasis on map-dot-fingerprint degeneration. J Refract Surg. 2007;23 (1):50–7.

Optical Coherence Tomography of the Anterior Segment of the Eye in Corneal Transplantation

Takahiko Hayashi, Alexander Händel, Mario Matthaei, Claus Cursiefen, and Sebastian Siebelmann

1 Introduction

Corneal transplantation has been the most common and successful type of tissue transplantation worldwide in the last century (Zirm 1906; Coster and Williams 2005). In recent years, however, a technological revolution in corneal transplantation has emerged, as lamellar corneal transplants have been introduced in addition to the previous gold standard of penetrating keratoplasty, which still achieves excellent results (Flockerzi et al. 2018). Despite the increasing number of lamellar surgeries such as deep anterior lamellar keratoplasty (DALK), endothelial kerato-plasties (EK) such as Descemet's stripping-automated endothelial keratoplasty (DSAEK) and Descemet's membrane endothelial keratoplasty (DMEK), approximately half of all keratoplasties performed worldwide continue to be penetrating keratoplasties (PK) (Flockerzi et al. 2018; Hos et al. 2019). Nevertheless, the trend toward lamellar procedures is strongly increasing.

Compared to lamellar keratoplasties, there are disadvantages of penetrating keratoplasty, such as suture-associated problems (e.g. astigmatism, infections), graft rejection, slower recovery of postoperative visual acuity, but also the risk of traumatic postoperative ruptures (Stechschulte and Azar 2000). Despite this risk profile, PK can significantly improve vision in patients with severe corneal disease or damage (Yokogawa et al. 2018). Nevertheless, lamellar keratoplasties are superior to PK in many indications. These include, in particular, indications in which only a part of the cornea is opacified.

T. Hayashi (✉)
Division of Ophthalmology, Department of Visual Sciences, Nihon University School of Medicine, Itabashi, Tokyo, Japan
e-mail: Takamed@gmail.com

A. Händel · M. Matthaei · C. Cursiefen · S. Siebelmann
Department of Ophthalmology, University Hospital of Cologne, Cologne, Germany

© The Author(s), under exclusive license to Springer Nature Switzerland AG 2022
L. M. Heindl and S. Siebelmann (eds.), *Optical Coherence Tomography of the Anterior Segment*, https://doi.org/10.1007/978-3-031-07730-2_10

175

Simple anterior stromal opacities can be treated with DALK, corneal edema caused by endothelial dysfunction with endothelial keratoplasty like DMEK or DSAEK (Reinhart et al. 2011; Ple-Plakon and Shtein 2014). However, most corneal pathologies requiring PKP are complex, and patients may have a history of corneal injury, infection, or severe corneal dystrophy. Thus, deciding which keratoplasty is right for an individual patient is often challenging. In addition, in many cases of superficial corneal changes such as epithelial-stromal corneal dystrophies, phototherapeutic keratectomy with an excimer laser can provide good visual rehabilitation without the need for corneal transplantation (Seitz et al. 2004). The axial as well as the lateral extension of the corneal opacities or their absolute localization and depth in the cornea is decisive (Seitz et al. 2004). In addition to slit lamp microscopy, this can be detected and assessed with near histologic resolution using optical coherence tomography. In addition to the purely volumetric information about how much corneal tissue is opacified, OCT also provides important information about the location of the corneal tissue that is opacified (Siebelmann et al. 2018a). If this is the case, for example, in the upper third of the cornea, an excimer laser PTK can usually be chosen as the treatment method (Seitz et al. 2004). If the opacity is deeper, deep anterior lamellar keratoplasty (DALK) or penetrating keratoplasty (PK) is usually necessary. In contrast, for purely endothelial disease, DMEK or DSAEK can be chosen without damaging the integrity of the anterior portion of the cornea (Anshu et al. 2012).

OCT can be helpful in this context for corneal assessment for indication, but also for postoperative follow-up for all types of keratoplasty, both in terms of corneal topography and in terms of corneal cross-sectional imaging.

For example, to assess postoperative corneal astigmatism after keratoplasty, the analysis of topo- and tomographic maps obtained either by OCT or Scheimpflug imaging is very important. In addition, it is important to assess the corneal status after grafting, especially to evaluate graft adherence or detachment .

In this context, modern AS-OCT devices automatically acquire images of the anterior segment of the eye. The devices then analyze the image data and provide a variety of information such as topographic data on the elevation of the anterior and posterior surface of the cornea, maps showing the curvature of the cornea as well as thickness maps. OCT has been shown to be superior to current Scheimpflug systems in certain areas, providing accurate information on higher order corneal aberrations and higher resolution in the presence of pronounced corneal opacities (Antonios et al. 2016; Lu et al. 2019).

In the following chapter, examples of the opportunities and limitations of anterior segment OCT in indication, preoperative, intraoperative, and postoperative corneal evaluation of various keratoplasties are given.

2 Optical Coherence Tomography in Deep Anterior Lamellar Keratoplasty (DALK)

In Deep Anterior Lamellar Keratoplasty (DALK), after trephination and preparation of the anterior corneal stroma, Descemet's membrane or the posterior corneal complex consisting of Dua's layer, Descemet's membrane and endothelium is prepared. (Reinhart et al. 2011). Thus, all corneal stromal opacities are removed and the remaining recipient cornea is prepared for corneal transplantation. Subsequently, a graft consisting of the anterior corneal portions is transferred and sutured in place (Reinhart et al. 2011). OCT of the anterior segment of the eye can be very helpful in DALK, both in surgical planning and in postoperative follow-up (see the "Intraoperative OCT" infobox for information obtained intraoperatively) (Lim et al. 2008). First, important information such as the general corneal thickness and, crucially, the depth and extent of corneal scar tissue can be obtained preoperatively (Fig. 1) (Siebelmann et al. 2016a; Scorcia et al. 2020). In addition, statements can be made about the configuration of the posterior corneal surface. This may include scar tissue, which also affects the posterior corneal complex, but also a particularly bulging Descemet's membrane, as in keratoconus, due to which DALK may also be difficult (Scorcia et al. 2020).

In the postoperative course, both the posterior interface between the recipient bed and the donor cornea and the border between the graft margins and the trephination surface can be assessed (Figs. 2 and 3) (Lyall et al. 2012). Special attention is paid to the postoperative formation of a second anterior chamber, i.e., fluid located in the interface between the posterior corneal complex and the donor

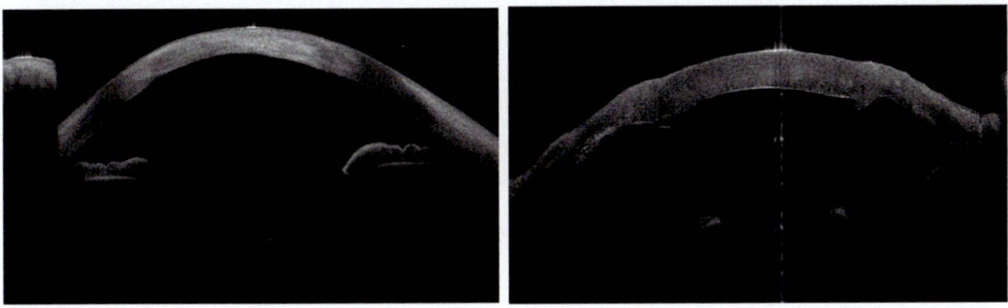

Fig. 1 **A** Preoperative findings of a cornea with central scars before DALK. OCT clearly shows the opacities in the corneal stroma. **B** OCT findings one week after DALK. The opacities are removed, the graft is completely attached

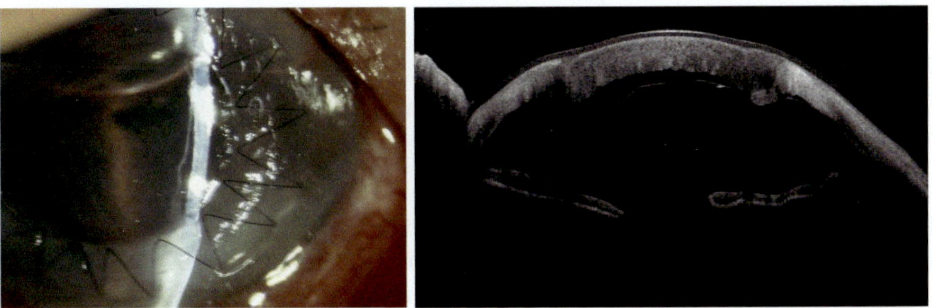

Fig. 2 Graft detachment after DALK. A second anterior chamber is visible during slit lamp examination. This is confirmed by OCT

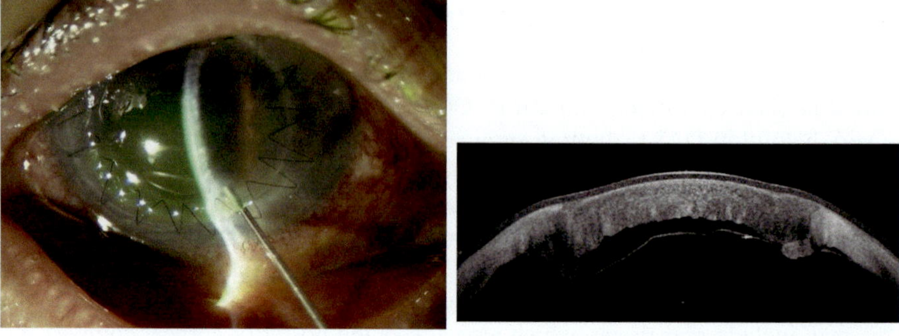

Fig. 3 Due to a big bubble technique using a ophthalmic viscoelastic device (OVD) to separate the Descemet's Membrane, residual OVD may cause delayed reattachment of the Descemet's Membrane to the graft. Flushing of the interface may be helpful in this case

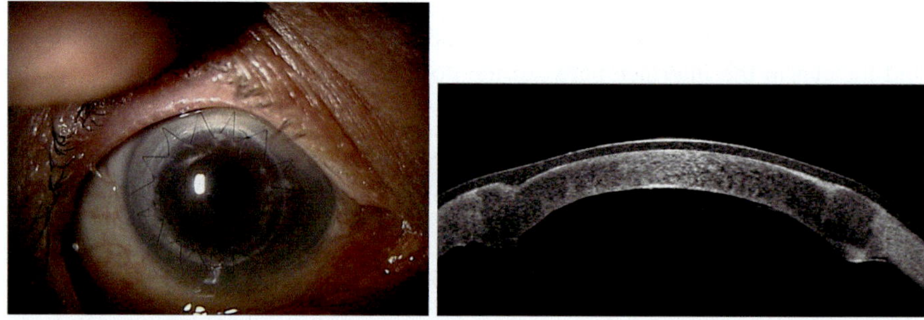

Fig. 4 Complete reattachment of Descemet's membrane to the graft after interface flushing

cornea (Figs. 4, 5, 6 and 7) (Myerscough et al. 2019). In addition, however, correct placement of the trephination margins can also be assessed. This information can be particularly helpful if the graft is not yet completely epithelialized or edematous. In addition, complications such as acute graft rejection or epithelial ingrowth into the interface can be monitored by OCT (Fig. 8).

3 Anterior Segment OCT in Posterior Lamellar Keratoplasties

In Descemet's Membrane Endothelial Keratoplasty, the surgeon's greatest challenge is usually the correct diagnosis and intervention planning in the face of advanced corneal edema and reduced anterior chamber visibility. The view into the anterior chamber of the eye may be reduced, for example, in diseases of the endothelium, such as Fuchs' endothelial corneal dystrophy (FECD), posterior

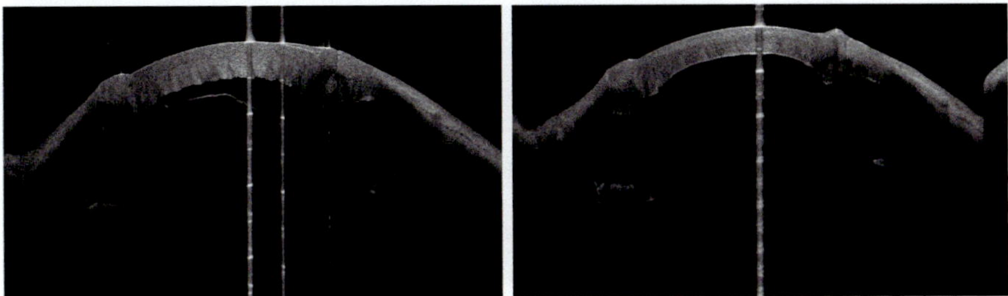

Fig. 5 DALK is often still possible after small perforation of the Descemet's Membrane during preparation. Nevertheless, it should be considered that the risk of formation of a second anterior chamber or detachment of Descemet's membrane from the graft is rather higher. Therefore, the anterior chamber should be filled with gas. In the graft detachment shown here, the anterior chamber was completely filled with gas for 2 h postoperatively. Subsequently, half of the gas was drained again. OCT showed complete graft apposition. Especially in inferior perforations, the anterior chamber should be filled almost completely with gas

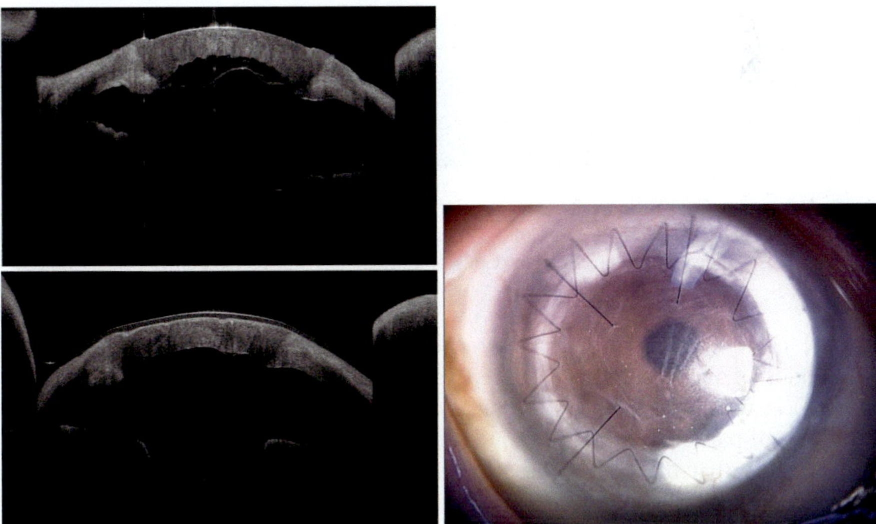

Fig. 6 If reattachment of the Descemet's membrane does not occur despite multiple reinjections of gas into the anterior chamber (**A**, **B**), placement of pre-Descemet's sutures may be necessary. These sutures can be removed after 1–2 months after complete reattachment of the graft as shown here. OCT can be used to verify complete graft attachment (**C**)

polymorphous corneal dystrophy (PPCD), but also in glaucomatous endothelial decompensation after acute eye pressure decompensation or after complicated cataract surgery (Figs. 9 and 10). (Corneal edema after cataract surgery: incidence and etiology 2002). All signs of corneal decompensation are visible on OCT. The cornea may be edematous on OCT imaging, epithelial bullae may be visualized,

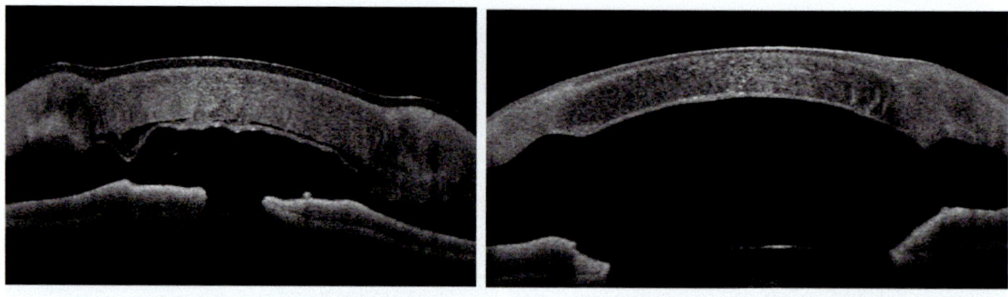

Fig. 7 In case of a not or only incompletely successful Big Bubble, a manual preparation of the corneal stroma as close as possible to the Descemet's membrane is necessary (layer-by-layer technique). Here, specially designed instruments such as the Hayashi DALK hook can be helpful. Likewise, intraoperative OCT can provide information about the remaining residual stroma during surgery. In the eye shown here, a large part of the anterior corneal stroma was removed. Nevertheless, some residual stroma remained. Immediately after surgery, a complete graft attachement is visible

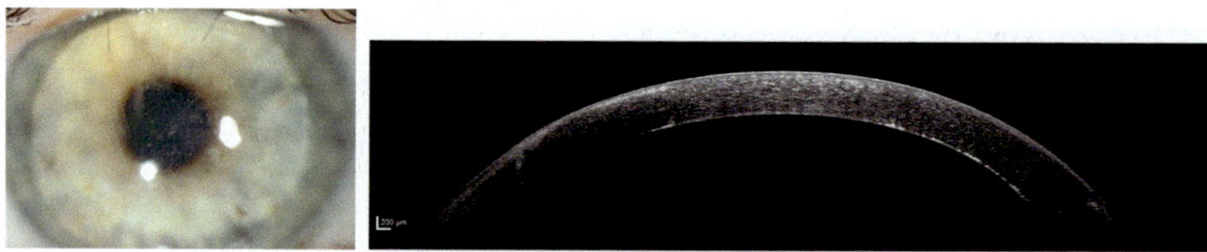

Fig. 8 Ingrowth of epithelium after Deep Anterior Lamellar Keratoplasty (DALK). The clinical picture shows clearly opacified areas of epithelial conglomerates. Using spectral domain OCT, these can be localized as hyperreflective deposits immediately above Descemet's membrane

and the posterior curvature is wavy and irregular (Figs. 9, 10 and 11). Other pathologies of the posterior corneal surface (e.g., Haab striae, other corneal dystrophies) in which DMEK is a reasonable option can also be visualized by OCT.

OCT is of particular importance in DMEK for postoperative follow-up (Fig. 12). It is possible that the transplanted Descemet's membrane is not yet completely adherent and that it is therefore not possible to completely assess the position and morphology of the graft using a slit lamp due to epithelial and stromal edema. Here, OCT can contribute significant information on graft position and its adherence (Figs. 13, 14 and 15). Previous studies have shown that spectral domain OCT (SD-OCT) has a higher resolution and is thus particularly suitable for imaging central graft detachments, whereas time domain OCT (TD-OCT) nevertheless detects more graft detachments overall (Siebelmann et al. 2016b). This can be explained by the fact that TD-OCT allows better visualization and, above all, a better overview of the entire anterior chamber due to the higher penetration depth, thus making it possible to analyze the complete graft. In addition, the vast majority of graft detachments occur in the lower periphery of the cornea (Siebelmann et al. 2016b). Furthermore, it is noted that when carefully and manually examined by

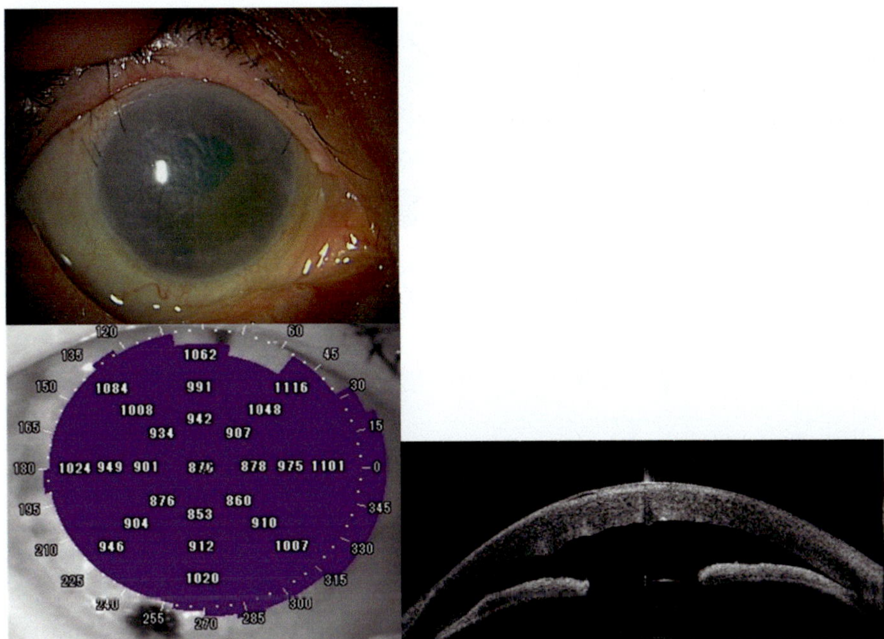

Fig. 9 This patient suffers from bullous keratopathy caused by complex cataract surgery. There is a significant increase in corneal thickness. An irregular posterior corneal surface is also visible by OCT. In addition, general swelling of the cornea and epithelial detachment are evident

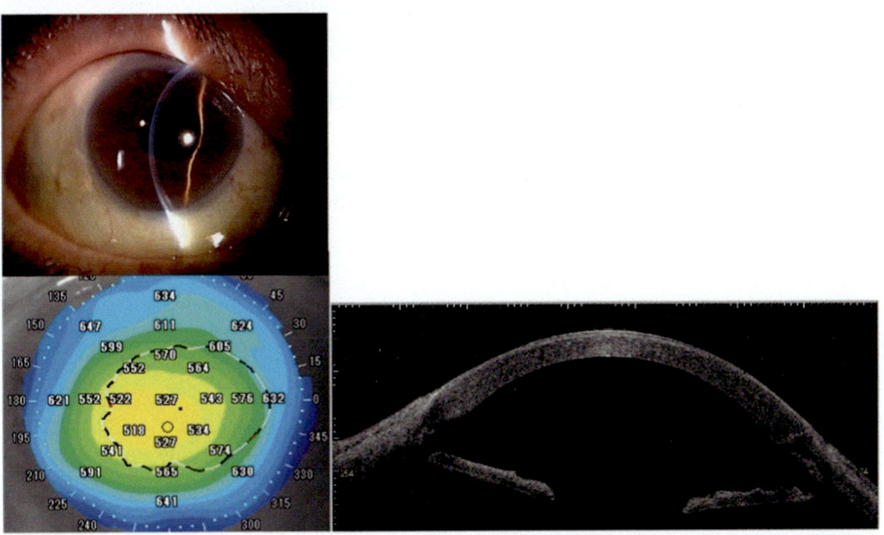

Fig. 10 Clinical findings after successfully performed DMEK, corneal thickness decreased significantly after DMEK and undulation of the posterior corneal surface is no longer visible

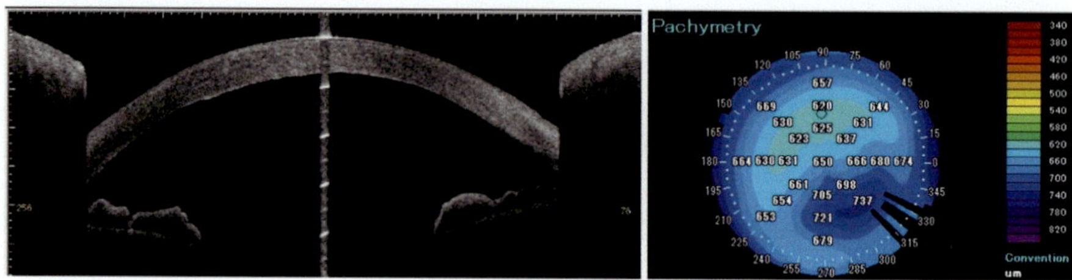

Fig. 11 This patient suffers from Fuchs endothelial corneal dystrophy. OCT shows corneal edema and irregular posterior curvature of the cornea. OCT pachymetry confirms these findings

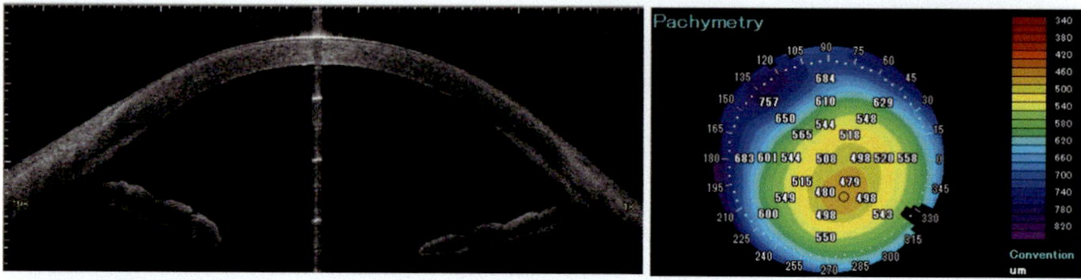

Fig. 12 After successful DMEK, the cornea is much thinner and the posterior surface is smooth. The corneal thickness has decreased significantly

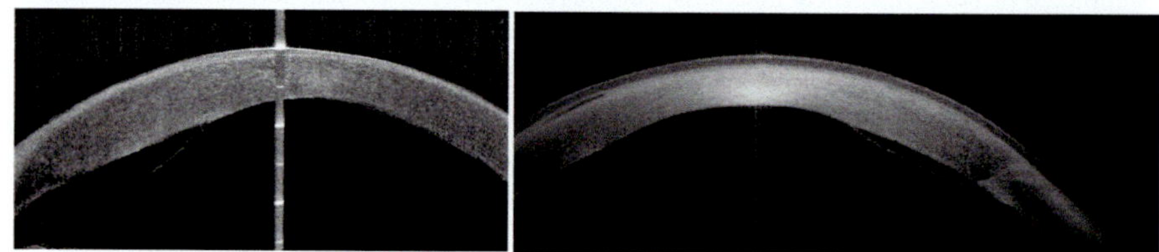

Fig. 13 OCT shows two peripheral graft detachments 4 days after DMEK was performed. Since the detachment is peripheral, it was decided against rebubbling. In most cases, spontaneous reattachment occurs here. Very peripheral, remaining detachments are also usually not relevant for visual acuity

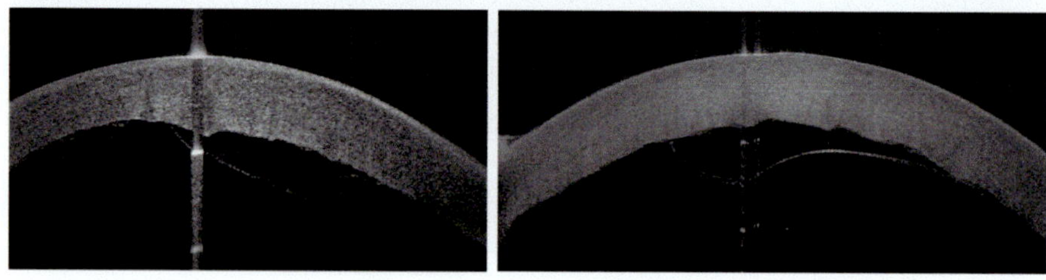

Fig. 14 Special attention should be paid to central graft detachments, as they usually do not spontaneously reattach. Therefore, they should be rebubbled as soon as possible

Fig. 15 Large graft detachment in an eye that had previously undergone vitrectomy. Due to the flexible iris-lens diaphragm, the counterpressure by the endotamponade was probably missing in places and the graft detached

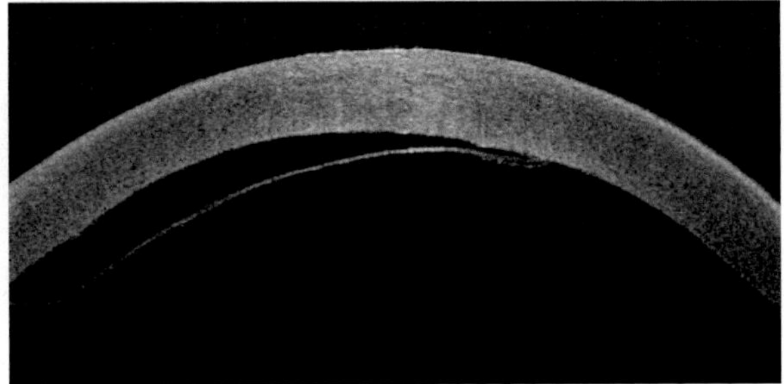

OCT, single areas of graft detachments can be detected in almost all patients. (Siebelmann et al. 2016b). This leads to the crucial question, at which characteristics of a graft detachment a rebubbling, respectively a reinjection of air or gas into the anterior chamber of the eye should be performed. A large study from the University of Cologne, Cologne, Germany could show on the basis of 624 rebubblings, by measuring with OCT, that the average lateral diameter of graft detachments that had to be rebubbled was about 4.5 mm (Siebelmann et al. 2020). In most cases, these detachments were of an axial depth of about 380 μm. Rebubbling occurred after approximately 7 days for anterior chamber endotamponade with air and after 13 days for SF6 gas (Siebelmann et al. 2020). In contrast to patients who were not rebubbled, who tended to show detachments in the lower periphery, the graft detachments in rebubbled patients were evenly distributed over the entire cornea, especially centrally and superior (Siebelmann et al. 2020).

A surprising finding of this study was that patients who previously had to be treated with rebubbling in the first eye also had a significantly increased risk of rebubbling in the second eye, even when the second eye was not operated on by the same surgeon.

A limitation of previous studies, however, is that the surgical indication for rebubbling is usually made at the slit lamp, considering the vertical detachment size of the graft. However, most OCT devices only perform horizontal measurements as part of volume scans, so this distance must be estimated from the OCT images usually on the entire volume scan. New scanning patterns optimized for the analysis of corneas after corneal transplantation could be advantageous here. As is already possible with some devices, these should include vertical or star scans in addition to horizontal scan grids in order to capture all areas of the graft and the entire morphology of the detachments. Automatic detection and volumetric recording of interface fluid would also be desirable in order to have an even more precise, absolute value for the indication of rebubbling.

It is generally true that graft detachment mostly occurs in the lower periphery of the graft, since a loss of backpressure of the early missing endotamponade presumably occurs at this site due to resorption of the gas. By using 20% sulfur hexafluoride gas (SF6) as an endotamponade after DMEK, it was shown by OCT that the number and size of graft detachments were significantly reduced due to almost twice the resorption time of gas in the anterior chamber (Siebelmann et al.

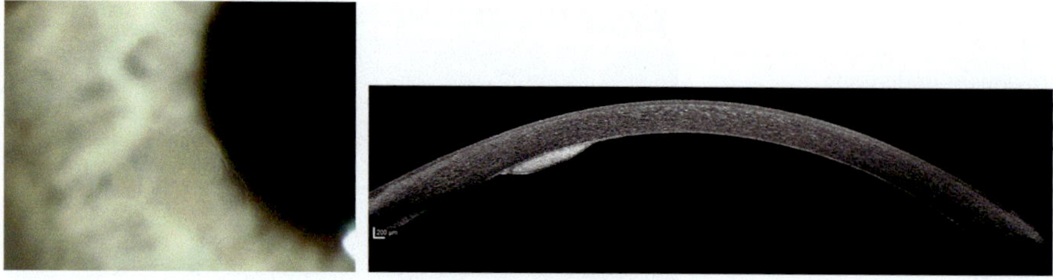

Fig. 16 Epithelial ingrowth on the graft after DMEK. The patient's visual acuity is not affected. OCT shows an adherent graft and the conglomerate of migrated epithelium on the posterior cornea

2018b). This was also reflected in the study cited here in a significantly reduced incidence of rebubbling when comparing room air and SF6 (Siebelmann et al. 2018b; Schaub et al. 2017). The influence of back pressure for the endotamponade in the sense of an intact iris lens diaphragm or the presence of the vitreous body to build up sufficient pressure for the graft is currently controversial (Siebelmann et al. 2018c). Thus, one study demonstrated that pseudophakic and aphakic patients had more graft detachments after DMEK and had to be rebubbled more often (Siebelmann et al. 2018c). Similar findings were observed for patients with post-vitrectomy conditions (Figs. 16, 17, 18 and 19).

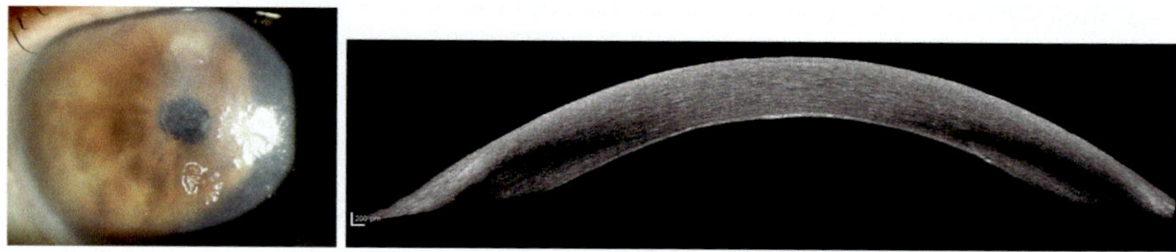

Fig. 17 Acute transplant rejection after DMEK. Clinically, corneal edema is visible. Spectral domain OCT shows hyperreflective endothelial deposits

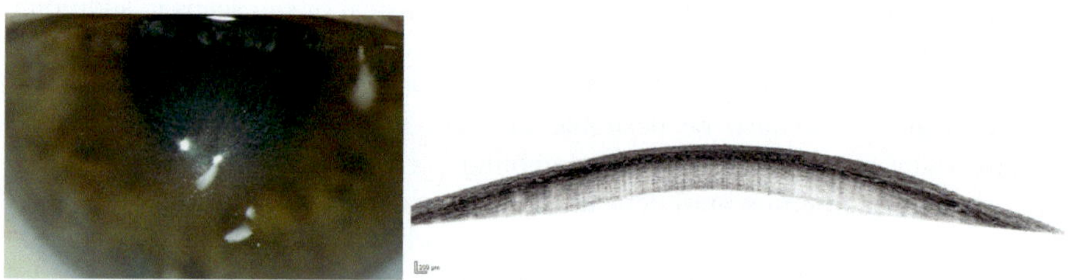

Fig. 18 Even after successful DMEK, subepithelial fibrosis may develop after longstanding corneal edema (left). In this case, excimer laser PTK can be an useful treatment option. OCT can be used to determine the depth of subepithelial opacification of the cornea and to plan PTK

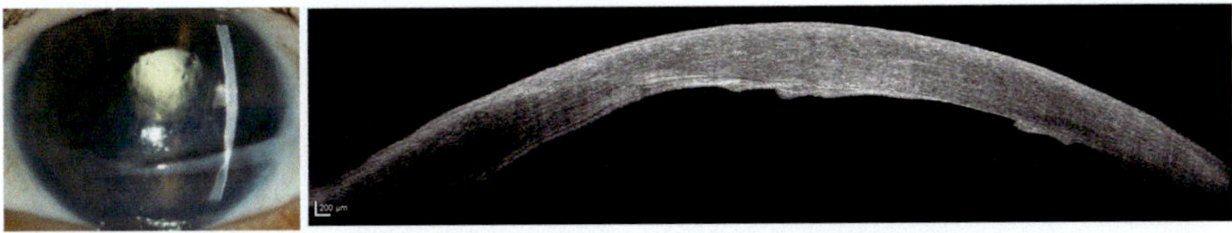

Fig. 19 Pronounced graft folds after DMEK. Clinically, a distinct folding of the graft can be seen in the inner corneal region after DMEK ("PVR-like DM folding"). OCT confirms this finding and shows a pronounced thickening of the graft

4 Intraoperative OCT in Corneal Transplantation

Microscope-integrated optical coherence tomography (MI-OCT) is particularly important in lamellar keratoplasty. MI-OCT devices are surgical microscopes in which an OCT device is integrated in such a way that cross-sectional imaging of the surgical area can be performed without interruption and in real time (Geerling et al. 2005). It could be worked out in the past that this technology is particularly advantageous when the view into the anterior chamber of the eye is reduced or when very thin and partly transparent structures are handled (Siebelmann et al. 2015). Since these two conditions apply in many cases to the lamellar keratoplasties such as DMEK, DALK or DSAEK, these procedures were one of the first published applications of MI-OCT in the anterior segment of the eye. It was shown that in posterior lamellar keratoplasties such as DMEK and DSAEK, all steps of the operations can be followed and monitored (Fig. 20) (Sharma et al. 2016). In addition, at the end of the operation it is possible to detect a correct graft placement and at the same time to exclude interface fluid (Steven et al. 2013, 2014). In DSAEK, the presence of interface fluid at the end of surgery was even associated with an increased risk of interface opacification on MI-OCT imaging (Hallahan et al. 2017; Juthani et al. 2014). In addition, the view into the anterior chamber is often significantly reduced due to endothelial diseases such as corneal dystrophies or pseudophakic bullous keratopathy. Again, MI-OCT has been shown to provide valuable information beyond what can be visualized using a surgical microscope alone. Similarly, this is true for anterior lamellar keratoplasties such as DALK (Liu et al. 2019; Benito-Llopis et al. 2014). Particularly critical surgical steps such as trephination of the recipient tissue at the beginning of the operation, placement of the cannula in front of the Descemet's membrane for injection of air or fluid to induce the Big Bubble, and preparation of the stroma down to the bare Descemet's membrane can also be shown here (Steven et al. 2014). Also, correct graft placement can be verified at the end of surgery. In recent years, lamellar corneal transplants revolutionized the surgical treatment of patients with corneal diseases. With regard to the indication, which lamellar transplantation procedure should be chosen, or whether even a pure laser ablation by means of excimer laser

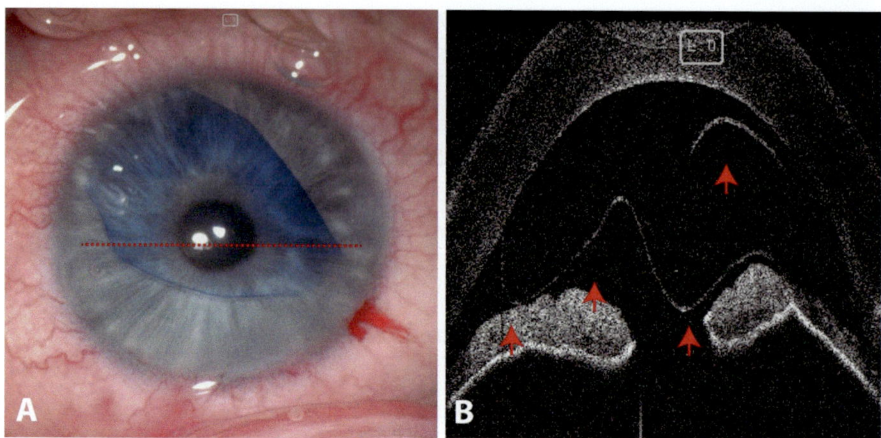

Fig. 20 Intraoperative imaging using MI-OCT in DMEK. **A** shows the position of the graft in the anterior chamber through the microscope. **B** shows imaging by intraoperative OCT in cross-section and the position of the graft (red arrows) (Siebelmann et al. 2018d)

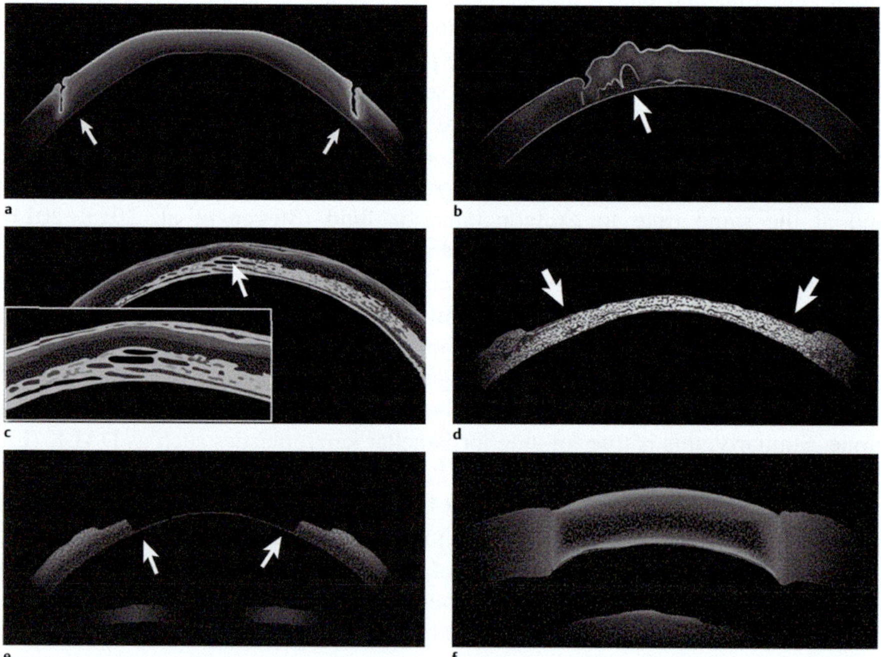

Fig. 21 Intraoperative imaging during DALK. Using MI-OCT, both the depth of trephination (**A**) and the position of the cannula (**B**) during air injection to generate a big bubble (**C**) can be tracked. During preparation, the remaining corneal stroma or posterior corneal complex can be visualized (**D**). **E** shows the further preparation of Descemet's membrane with subsequent bare Descemet's membrane. The correct adaptation of the graft with the Descemet's membrane in place can also be seen (**F**). (From Siebelmann et al. 2016c)

phototherapeutic keratectomy is sufficient for the removal of a corneal scar, OCT technology could thus become groundbreaking pre-, intra-, and postoperatively.

Intraoperative OCT can also be used in conventional penetrating keratoplasty to exclude iris incarcerations and to ensure correct positioning and adaptation of the graft to the recipient bed. This also applies to the Boston Keratoprosthesis. Here it could be shown that during implantation of a Boston keratoprosthesis not only the correct assembly could be checked and corrected, but also the correct position in the recipient bed could be confirmed after implantation (Fig. 22). Future prospective studies should investigate whether surgery with MI-OCT is really verifiably safer and possibly even better visual outcomes are achieved.

More abstract complications beyond graft detachment can also be detected by anterior segment OCT (Figs. 17, 18 and 19). These include, for example, upside-down implantation of the graft (Fig. 23), graft folds (Fig. 19) an epithelial ingrowth (Fig. 17), or down-growth, which is the migration of epithelium between the graft and the recipient cornea or onto the endothelium or Descemet's membrane of the graft. A not very rare complication is also the migration of gas, which was injected into the anterior chamber as an endotamponade, behind the iris, which then leads to an angle block by pushing the iris forward with consecutive closure of the chamber angle (Fig. 24). Here, a sufficiently large basal (YAG laser) iridotomy is of particular importance. Often, supine positioning simply causes gas to displace the iridotomy, which also leads to an angle block configuration. In this case, an initial attempt can be made to bring the patient into an upright sitting position so that the flow of aqueous humor is ensured again. Likewise, after the corneal edema has subsided following PTK, subepithelial fibrosis can be seen in individual cases, which can be treated with excimer laser PTK (Fig. 18). In conclusion, the observations made with DMEK can also be transferred almost without exception to DSAEK. Correct graft attachment as well as non-attachment, dislocations and complications can be visualized by OCT (Figs. 25 and 26) (Lim et al. 2008).

5 Optical Coherence Tomography in Penetrating Keratoplasty and Keratoprostheses

Due to the increasing indications for lamellar keratoplasty in terms of selective corneal replacement, OCT is also gaining importance for the indication of penetrating keratoplasty. In this context, preoperative OCT imaging can be used to determine on an almost histologic level which corneal layers are affected by opacities such as scars or deposits, e.g., due to corneal dystrophies. Due to the faster visual rehabilitation, the lower rejection rates and generally the fact that the integrity and stability of the eye is preserved in lamellar keratoplasties, penetrating keratoplasty should actually only be performed in cases of opacities completely affecting the cornea, where no selective corneal replacement can be performed.

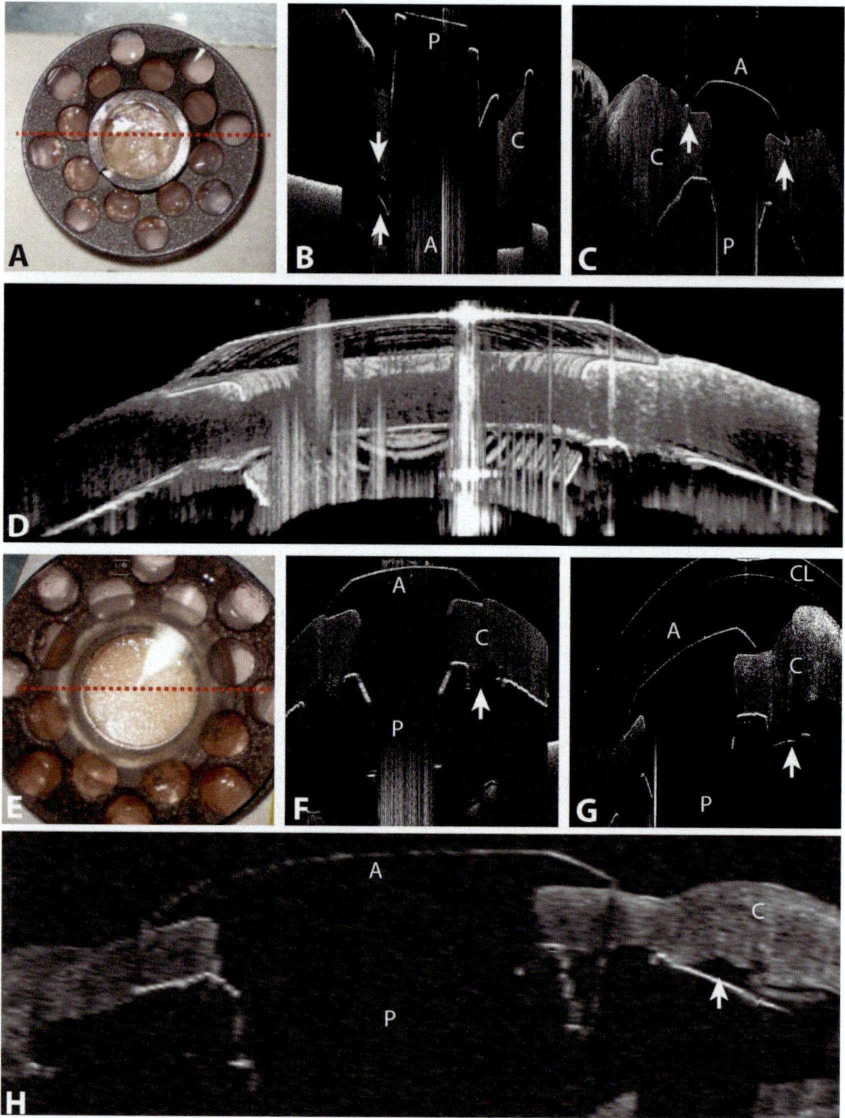

Fig. 22 **A** shows the titanium ring, the optic cylinder and a locking clip. Below the titanium ring, the donor cornea can be seen through the perforation. **B** A gap between the optic cylinder and the graft is visible by OCT. **C** After re-fixation of the locking ring, this gap has disappeared. **D** By means of MI-OCT, a three-dimensional view of the assembled scan sections is also possible. **E** View from the front. **F** OCT shows the correct assembly of the prosthesis. Gaps are also visible in the area of the holes in the titanium ring towards the graft. **G** After implantation of the prosthesis, individual gaps are also visible in this area. However, further fixation or even revision of this area is not necessary, as it is located inside the eye. **H** shows the same area postoperatively by time domain OCT. It can be seen that the depth of penetration and overview is significantly greater using TD-OCT. (From Siebelmann et al. 2016)

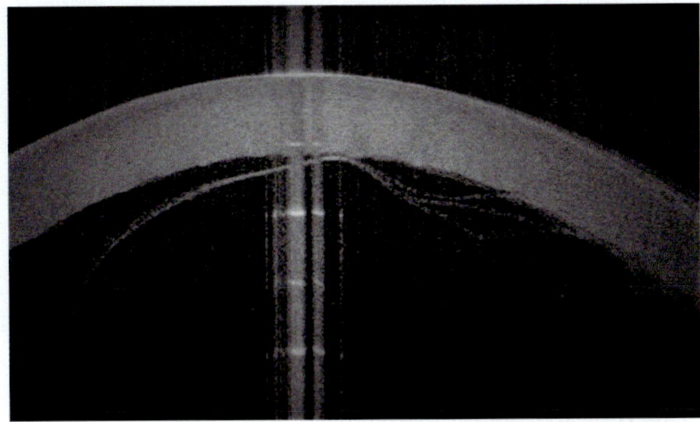

Fig. 23 The figure shows a graft in upside-down position. The multiple folded graft parts and the mispositioned graft margin are clearly visible

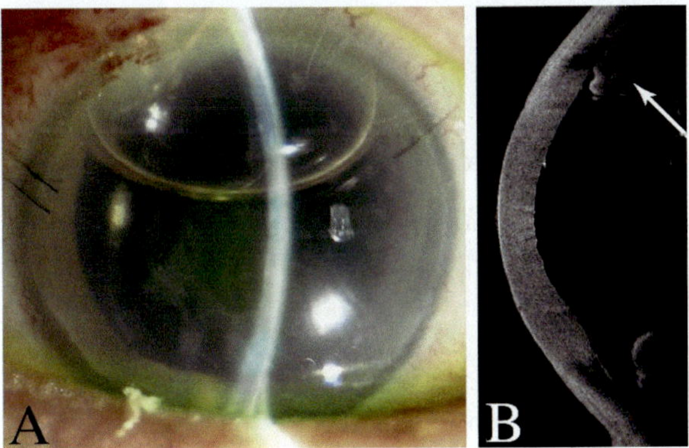

Fig. 24 **A** eye after DMEK with a partial gas filling of approx. 40%. The patient complained of severe postoperative pain. Slit lamp showed angle block and decompensation of intraocular pressure. **B** showed that gas was dislocated behind the iris, which exerted pressure on it and occluded the chamber angle. After application of topical mydriatics the block could be released and the eye pressure normalized

Furthermore, explicitly extended posterior opacities of the cornea, e.g. after herpetic endotheliitis or extended posterior stromal keratitis, can also be treated with penetrating keratoplasty (Keane et al. 2014). However, in addition to DMEK and DSAEK, further femtosecond laser-assisted procedures could be added in the future, which also allow the selective treatment of posterior corneal stromal opacities (Maier et al. 2010). In addition, Bowman membrane transplantation for keratoconus and various lenticule and stroma implantation procedures have recently been added to the list of stromal transplantation procedures, which could further limit the range of indications for penetrating keratoplasty (Dijk et al. 2015; Damgaard et al. 2018).

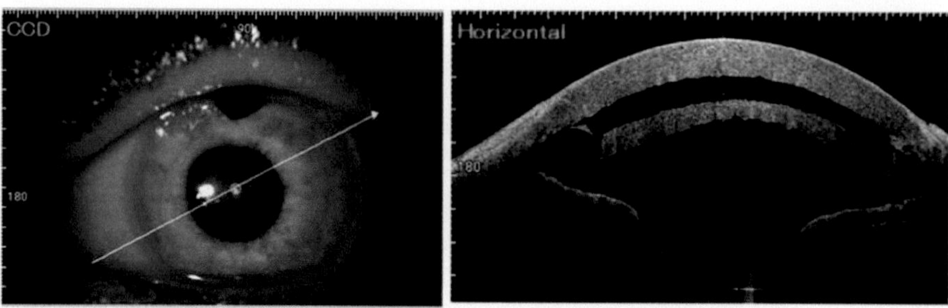

Fig. 25 Dislocation of a DSAEK graft. OCT imaging clearly shows the graft floating freely in the anterior chamber. This is clearly thicker than in DMEK

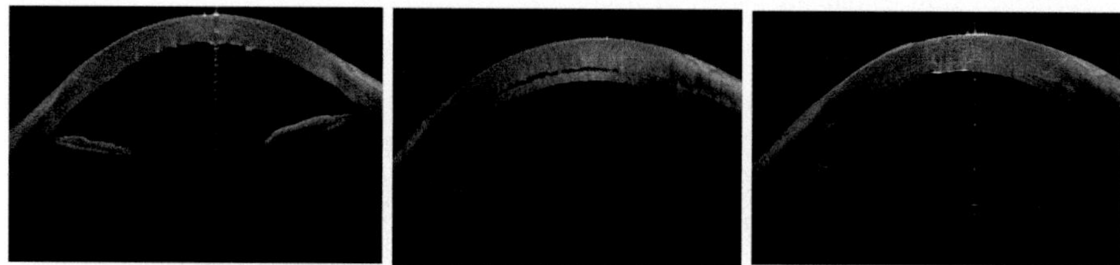

Fig. 26 The OCT images show the corneal findings before surgery and immediately after DSAEK. There is still interface fluid, so it was decided to do a rebubbling. Afterwards, a completely adherent graft was seen

In penetrating keratoplasty, OCT can also be used preoperatively to obtain a good overview of the entire anterior segment of the eye, especially if the cornea is opacified or even vascularized (Fig. 27). For example, in unclear initial situations, the anterior chamber depth, lens status, anterior or posterior synechiae, and glaucoma implants (e.g., Baerveldt or Ahmed Valve implant) can be visualized. This can provide the surgeon with important information for planning the surgical procedure. (For intraoperative imaging, see infobox "MI-OCT").

OCT can also be used for postoperative evaluation of corneal grafts (Fig. 28). Among other things, the correct fit of the graft and the suture tension can be assessed (Kaiserman et al. 2008; Jhanji et al. 2011). In this context, perforations or perforation sites can also be assessed by OCT after coverage (Figs. 29, 30 and 31).

Furthermore, the configuration of the anterior chamber can also be assessed after transplantation. Precipitates in acute corneal rejection can also be identified (e.g. Khodadoust line) (Fig. 32).

Another important indication of anterior segment OCT, is the evaluation before and after implantation of keratoprostheses, if penetrating keratoplasty is not possible or grafts have been rejected or vascularized more than once (Shapiro et al. 2013). In addition to the aforementioned advantages for preoperative assessment of the anterior chamber with reduced visibility due to an opacified cornea (e.g., anterior chamber depth, synechiae, glaucoma implants, lens status, etc.), OCT can

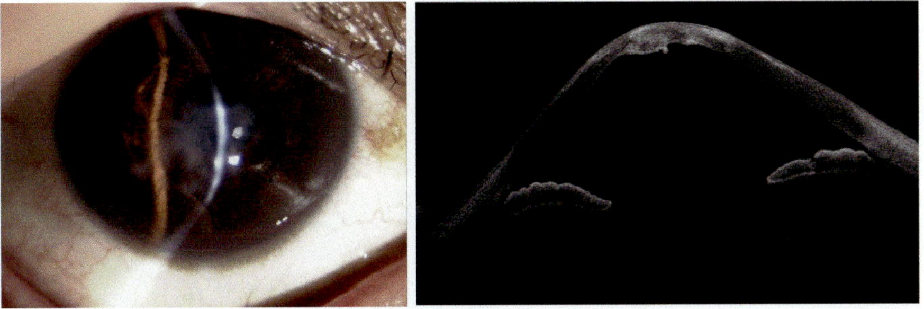

Fig. 27 The clinical photograph shows a cornea in a patient with keratoconus after acute corneal hydrops. OCT shows that Descemet's membrane is extensively ruptured in the optical axis. In addition, a scar encompassing the entire cornea is evident. Therefore a penetrating keratoplasty was performed

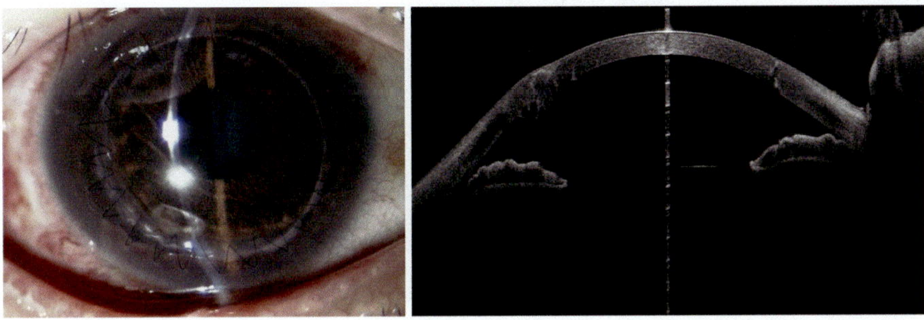

Fig. 28 Clinical image shows eye shown in Fig. 27 after PK has been performed. OCT imaging shows a well adapted, perfectly clear corneal graft

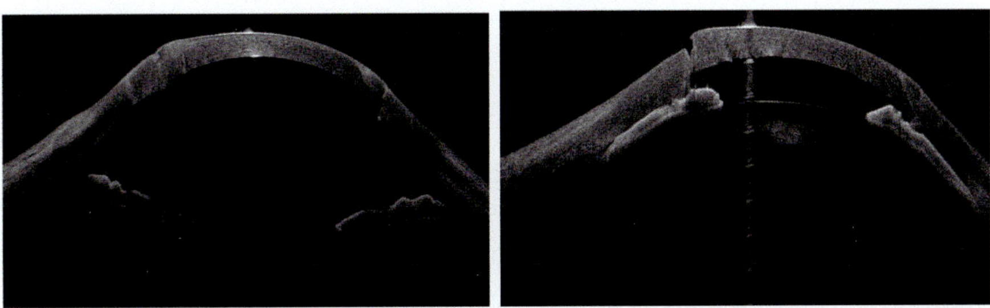

Fig. 29 The OCT image on the left shows a corneal graft that appears generally well adapted. The interface on the left is slightly thickened. After suture traction, the right image shows a partial dislocation of the graft. The anterior chamber is lifted and there is contact between iris and endothelium

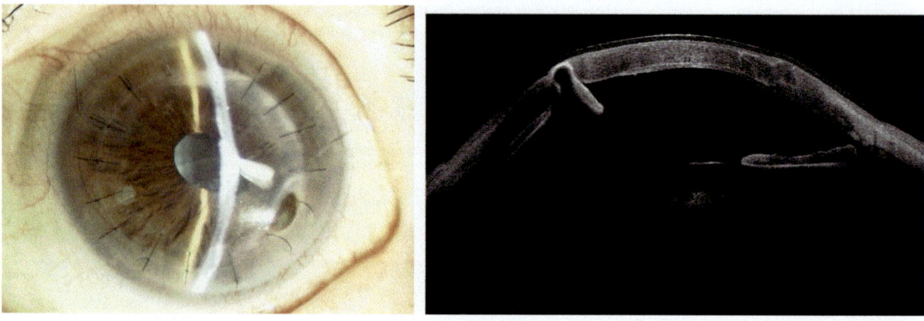

Fig. 30 Even small perforations can be detected and assessed by OCT. Left: A perforation in the graft interface can be seen in the clinical image. In addition, an iris prolapse is visible. The OCT image shows a standing anterior chamber, as well as the iris prolapse, which completely fills the perforation site. In addition, a nuclear cataract is indicated

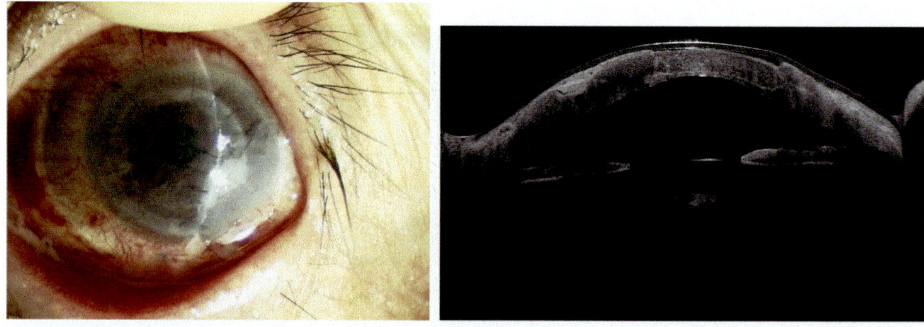

Fig. 31 The perforation site was covered by an amniotic patch and the iris prolapse was reduced. Despite the amniotic membrane, OCT shows that the iris is no longer adherent and the substance defect in the corneal stroma is completely covered

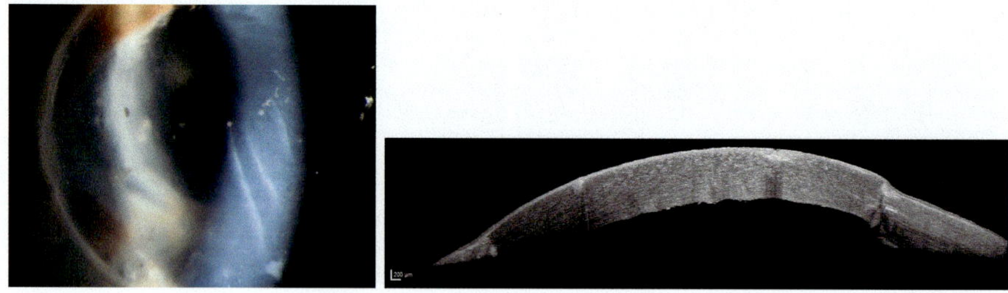

Fig. 32 Acute corneal rejection with Khodadoust line in slit lamp photo. OCT shows clear precipitates on the posterior surface of the cornea

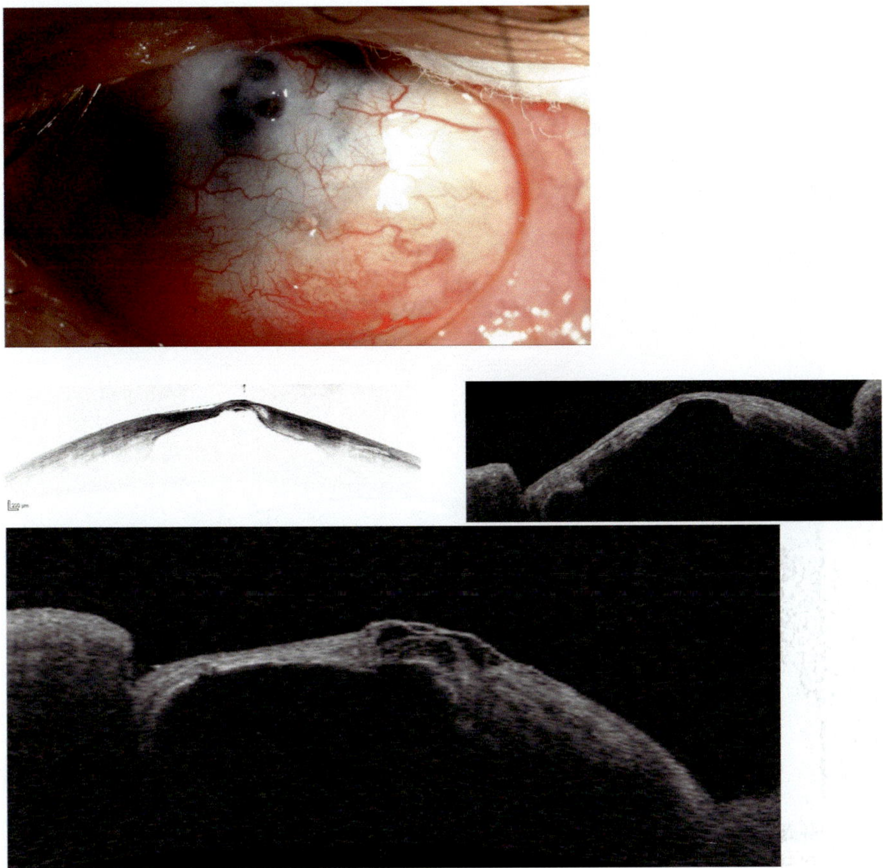

Fig. 33 Preoperative images before Boston keratoprosthesis after corneal burn. While the clinical image (**A**) allows almost no conclusions about the configuration of the anterior chamber, OCT provides much more information. The corneal thickness as well as a standing anterior chamber (**B** + **C**) are recognizable. In addition, the imaging differences between Spectral Domain (**B**) and Time Domain OCT (**C**) are clearly visible in corresponding images. **D** shows another area of the anterior segment with clear conjunctivalization of the cornea with cystic parts

also provide important information on the condition of the implant postoperatively (Fig. 33). In the following, this will be illustrated using the example of the Boston keratoprosthesis, one of the most frequently implanted keratoprostheses.

In Boston keratoprosthesis, a central optic cylinder is fixed in a donor cornea with a posteriorly located perforated titanium disc and then implanted (Fig. 34). In the postoperative course, the newly transplanted cornea can now vascularize and become opacified, as the central optic cylinder remains clear, allowing vision despite an opacified cornea (Chew et al. 2009). However, frequent postoperative complications are prosthesis loosening and melting of the graft, especially in the area of the optic cylinder, which partly overlaps the graft (Fig. 35) (Chew et al.

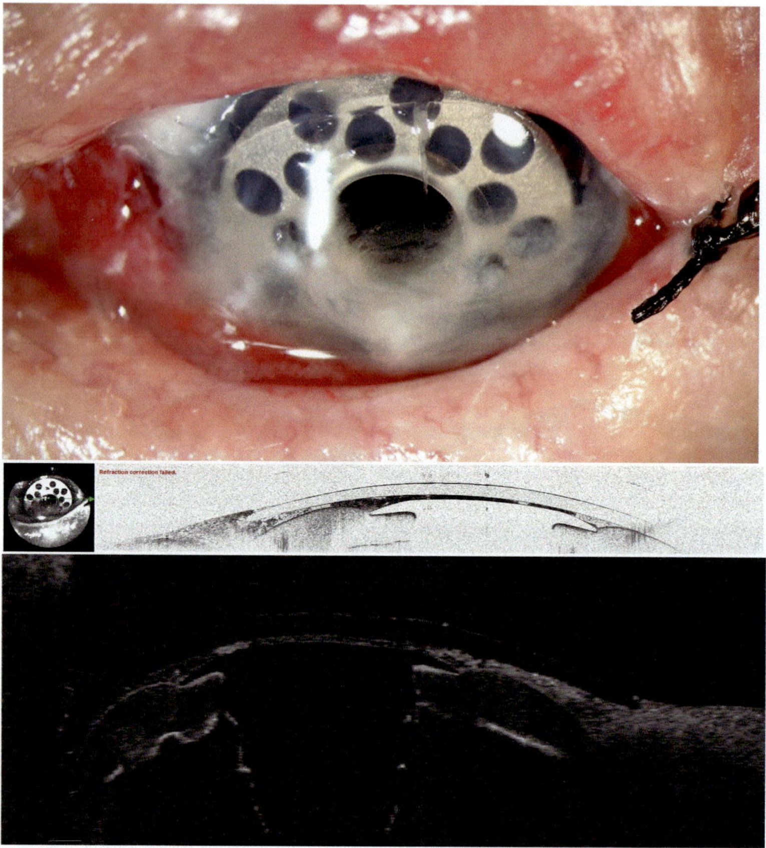

Fig. 34 Immediate postoperative findings (**A**). The freshly implanted Boston keratoprosthesis with therapeutic contact lens and suture material after tarsorrhaphy is shown. The OCT image (**B + C**) shows that due to the low penetration depth the parts of the keratoprosthesis can be visualized much better with Time Domain OCT (**C**) than with Spectral Domain OCT. In contrast, the epithelialization of the prosthesis as well as the status of the anterior part of the optic cylinder and its surface can be assessed in detail much better with Spectral Domain OCT

2009). These can often be detected better with OCT than with the slit lamp, since they are usually covered by the optic cylinder or the therapeutic bandage contact lens, that has to be worn permanently (Fig. 35) (Fernandez et al. 2012). Thus, therapy can be adjusted early on, or a surgical response can be made with an amniotic membrane patch, corneal crosslinking, or corneal partial grafting before infection or perforation of the graft occurs. OCT can also be used to check the degree of epithelialization after implantation of the keratoprosthesis (Kiang et al. 2012). Because some patients develop glaucoma after implantation, OCT can help detect early risk factors, such as a shallow anterior chamber or anterior synechiae,

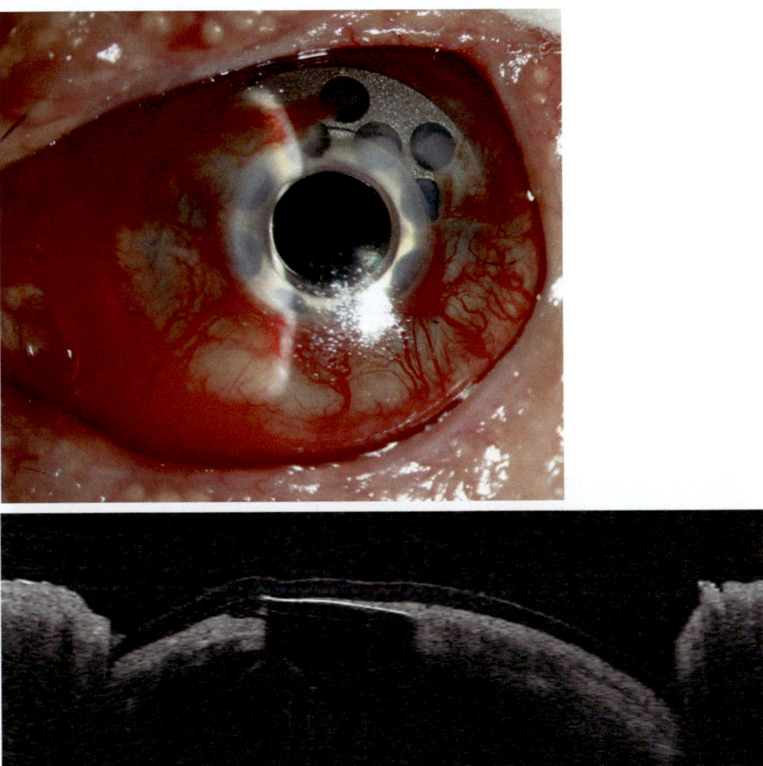

Fig. 35 Assessment of complications after implantation of a keratoprosthesis. The upper image shows the clinical findings of a Boston keratoprosthesis with a melting graft in the upper portion of the donor cornea (area without vascularization). The remaining graft portion is well vascularized but partially hyperemic. By OCT the extent of melting of the graft is visible. In addition, a fistula between the optic cylinder and donor cornea is evident. It was decided to revise the keratoprosthesis

before eye pressure increases, which are particularly difficult to detect after Boston keratoprosthesis. (Kang et al. 2013; Qian et al. 2015).

Finally, limitations of OCT imaging are mainly extremely dense opacities of the cornea, partly the sclera and especially strongly pigmented parts like iris tissue, optically dense elements e.g. of keratoprostheses or glaucoma implants or metallic particles as used e.g. for corneal tattoos. Thus, a complete shading of the anterior chamber can be seen after a corneal tattoo because the tattoo ink contains iron oxide particles (Fig. 36). In summary, it can be said that OCT is not only gaining importance in the planning, performance and postoperative assessment of all types of keratoplasty, but also makes certain procedures possible in the first place, and the indication for individual lamellar procedures can be made in a much more

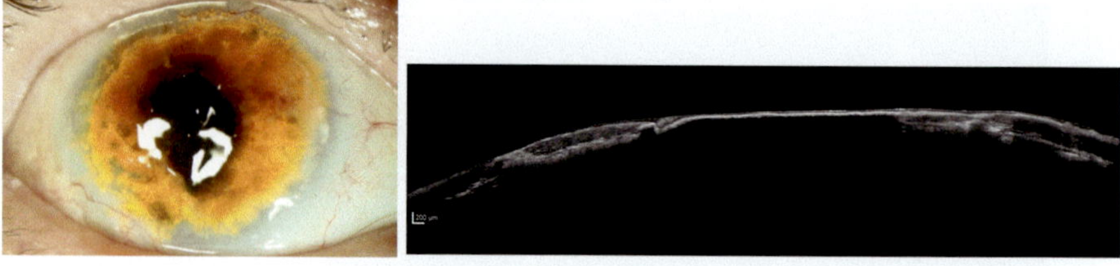

Fig. 36 Limitations of imaging due to a corneal tattoo. **A** Clinical findings of a corneal tattoo where two different tattoo inks were used. In OCT imaging, massive shadowing can be seen, especially due to the black ink, because the inks contain iron oxide particles that are not penetrable by the OCT laser

differentiated manner. In the future, the implementation of automatic image data analysis of OCT image data by artificial intelligence could lead to a further, significant improvement in the decision-making process for certain surgical procedures, but also in the postoperative assessment. For example, the first algorithms are already available that can predict the probability of a big bubble developing during DALK or the need for rebubbling after DMEK (Hayashi et al. 2020). It is questionable, however, whether these algorithms, which are often based on the assessment of surgical data from specific surgeons, can be readily applied to other surgeons.

References

Anshu A, Price MO, Tan DT, Price FW Jr. Endothelial keratoplasty: a revolution in evolution. Surv Ophthalmol. 2012;57(3):236–52.

Antonios R, Fattah MA, Maalouf F, Abiad B, Awwad ST. Central corneal thickness after cross-linking using high-definition optical coherence tomography, ultrasound, and dual Scheimpflug tomography: a comparative study over one year. Am J Ophthalmol. 2016;167:38–47.

De Benito-Llopis L, Mehta JS, Angunawela RI, Ang M, Tan DT. Intraoperative anterior segment optical coherence tomography: a novel assessment tool during deep anterior lamellar keratoplasty. Am J Ophthalmol. 2014;**157**(2):334–41. e3.

Chew HF, Ayres BD, Hammersmith KM, et al. Boston keratoprosthesis outcomes and complications. Cornea. 2009;28(9):989–96.

Corneal edema after cataract surgery: incidence and etiology. Seminars in ophthalmology; 2002. Taylor & Francis.

Coster DJ, Williams KA. The impact of corneal allograft rejection on the long-term outcome of corneal transplantation. Am J Ophthalmol. 2005;140(6):1112–22.

Damgaard IB, Ivarsen A, Hjortdal J. Biological lenticule implantation for correction of hyperopia: an ex vivo study in human corneas. J Refract Surg. 2018;34(4):245–52.

Fernandez AGA, Radcliffe NM, Sippel KC, et al. Boston type I keratoprosthesis-donor cornea interface evaluated by high-definition spectral-domain anterior segment optical coherence tomography. Clin Ophthalmol (Auckland, NZ). 2012;6:1355.

Flockerzi E, Maier P, Böhringer D, et al. Trends in corneal transplantation from 2001 to 2016 in Germany: a report of the DOG–section cornea and its keratoplasty registry. Am J Ophthalmol. 2018;188:91–8.

Geerling G, Müller M, Winter C, et al. Intraoperative 2-dimensional optical coherence tomography as a new tool for anterior segment surgery. Arch Ophthalmol. 2005;123(2):253–7.

Hallahan KM, Cost B, Goshe JM, Dupps WJ Jr, Srivastava SK, Ehlers JP. Intraoperative interface fluid dynamics and clinical outcomes for intraoperative optical coherence tomography–assisted Descemet stripping automated endothelial keratoplasty from the PIONEER study. Am J Ophthalmol. 2017;173:16–22.

Hayashi T, Tabuchi H, Masumoto H, et al. A deep learning approach in Rebubbling after Descemet's membrane endothelial keratoplasty. Eye Contact Lens. 2020;46(2):121–6.

Hos D, Matthaei M, Bock F, et al. Immune reactions after modern lamellar (DALK, DSAEK, DMEK) versus conventional penetrating corneal transplantation. Prog Retin Eye Res. 2019;73: 100768.

Jhanji V, Constantinou M, Beltz J, Vajpayee RB. Evaluation of posterior wound profile after penetrating keratoplasty using anterior segment optical coherence tomography. Cornea. 2011;30(3):277–80.

Juthani VV, Goshe JM, Srivastava SK, Ehlers JP. The association between transient interface fluid on intraoperative OCT and textural interface opacity following DSAEK surgery in the PIONEER study. Cornea. 2014;33(9):887.

Kaiserman I, Bahar I, Rootman D. Corneal wound malapposition after penetrating keratoplasty: an optical coherence tomography study. Br J Ophthalmol. 2008;92(8):1103–7.

Kang JJ, Allemann N, De La Cruz J, Cortina MS. Serial analysis of anterior chamber depth and angle status using anterior segment optical coherence tomography after Boston keratoprosthesis. Cornea. 2013;32(10):1369–74.

Keane M, Coster D, Ziaei M, Williams K. Deep anterior lamellar keratoplasty versus penetrating keratoplasty for treating keratoconus. Cochrane Database Syst Rev. 2014(7)

Kiang L, Rosenblatt MI, Sartaj R, et al. Surface epithelialization of the type I Boston keratoprosthesis front plate: immunohistochemical and high-definition optical coherence tomography characterization. Graefes Arch Clin Exp Ophthalmol. 2012;250(8):1195–9.

Lim LS, Aung HT, Aung T, Tan DT. Corneal imaging with anterior segment optical coherence tomography for lamellar keratoplasty procedures. Am J Ophthalmol. 2008;145(1):81–90.

Liu Y-C, Wittwer VV, Yusoff NZM, et al. Intraoperative optical coherence tomography-guided femtosecond laser-assisted deep anterior lamellar keratoplasty. Cornea. 2019;38(5):648–53.

Lu W, Li Y, Savini G, et al. Comparison of anterior segment measurements obtained using a swept-source optical coherence tomography biometer and a Scheimpflug-Placido tomographer. J Cataract Refract Surg. 2019;45(3):298–304.

Lyall DA, Tarafdar S, Gilhooly MJ, Roberts F, Ramaesh K. Long term visual outcomes, graft survival and complications of deep anterior lamellar keratoplasty in patients with herpes simplex related corneal scarring. Br J Ophthalmol. 2012;96(9):1200–3.

Maier P, Birnbaum F, Reinhard T. Therapeutic applications of the femtosecond laser in corneal surgery. Klin Monatsbl Augenheilkd. 2010;227(6):453.

Myerscough J, Bovone C, Mimouni M, Elkadim M, Rimondi E, Busin M. Factors predictive of double anterior chamber formation following deep anterior lamellar keratoplasty. Am J Ophthalmol. 2019;205:11–6.

Ple-Plakon PA, Shtein RM. Trends in corneal transplantation: indications and techniques. Curr Opin Ophthalmol. 2014;25(4):300–5.

Qian CX, Hassanaly S, Harissi-Dagher M. Anterior segment optical coherence tomography in the long-term follow-up and detection of glaucoma in Boston type I keratoprosthesis. Ophthalmology. 2015;122(2):317–25.

Reinhart WJ, Musch DC, Jacobs DS, Lee WB, Kaufman SC, Shtein RM. Deep anterior lamellar keratoplasty as an alternative to penetrating keratoplasty: a report by the American Academy of Ophthalmology. Ophthalmology. 2011;118(1):209–18.

Schaub F, Enders P, Snijders K, et al. One-year outcome after Descemet membrane endothelial keratoplasty (DMEK) comparing sulfur hexafluoride (SF6) 20% versus 100% air for anterior chamber tamponade. Br J Ophthalmol. 2017;101(7):902–8.

Scorcia V, Giannaccare G, Lucisano A, et al. Predictors of bubble formation and type obtained with pneumatic dissection during deep anterior lamellar keratoplasty in keratoconus. Am J Ophthalmol. 2020;212:127–33.

Seitz B, Behrens A, Fischer M, Langenbucher A, Naumann GO. Morphometric analysis of deposits in granular and lattice corneal dystrophy: histopathologic implications for phototherapeutic keratectomy. Cornea. 2004;23(4):380–5.

Shapiro BL, Cortés DE, Chin EK, et al. High-resolution spectral domain anterior segment optical coherence tomography in type 1 Boston keratoprosthesis. Cornea. 2013;32(7):951.

Sharma N, Aron N, Kakkar P, Titiyal JS. Continuous intraoperative OCT guided management of post-deep anterior lamellar keratoplasty descemet's membrane detachment. Saudi J Ophthalmol. 2016;30(2):133–6.

Siebelmann S, Steven P, Cursiefen C. Intraoperative optical coherence tomography: ocular surgery on a higher level or just nice pictures? JAMA Ophthalmol. 2015;133(10):1133–4.

Siebelmann S, Bachmann B, Lappas A, et al. Intraoperative optical coherence tomography in corneal and glaucoma surgical procedures. Der Ophthalmologe: Zeitschrift Der Deutschen Ophthalmologischen Gesellschaft. 2016a;113(8):646.

Siebelmann S, Steven P, Hos D, Hüttmann G, Lankenau E, Bachmann B, Cursiefen C. Advantages of microscope-integrated intraoperative online optical coherence tomography: usage in Boston keratoprosthesis type I surgery. J Biome Optics. 2016;21(1):016005.

Siebelmann S, Steven P, Cursiefen C. Intraoperative optische Kohärenztomografie bei der tiefen anterioren lamellären Keratoplastik. Klin Monbl Augenheilkd. 2016c;233(06):717–21.

Siebelmann S, Scholz P, Sonnenschein S, et al. Anterior segment optical coherence tomography for the diagnosis of corneal dystrophies according to the IC3D classification. Surv Ophthalmol. 2018a;63(3):365–80.

Siebelmann S, Ramos SL, Scholz P, et al. Graft detachment pattern after Descemet membrane endothelial keratoplasty comparing air versus 20% SF6 tamponade. Cornea. 2018b;37(7):834–9.

Siebelmann S, Ramos SL, Matthaei M, et al. Factors associated with early graft detachment in primary Descemet membrane endothelial keratoplasty. Am J Ophthalmol. 2018c;192:249–50.

Siebelmann S, Matthaei M, Heindl LM, Bachmann BO, Cursiefen C. Die Bedeutung der intraoperativen optischen Kohärenztomografie (MI-OCT) bei der Behandlung von Hornhautdystrophien. Klin Monbl Augenheilkd. 2018d;235(06):714–20.

Siebelmann S, Kolb K, Scholz P, et al. The Cologne rebubbling study: a reappraisal of 624 rebubblings after Descemet membrane endothelial keratoplasty. Br J Ophthalmol. 2020

Stechschulte SU, Azar DT. Complications after penetrating keratoplasty. Int Ophthalmol Clin. 2000;40(1):27–43.

Steven P, Le Blanc C, Velten K, et al. Optimizing descemet membrane endothelial keratoplasty using intraoperative optical coherence tomography. JAMA Ophthalmol. 2013;131(9):1135–42.

Steven P, Le Blanc C, Lankenau E, et al. Optimising deep anterior lamellar keratoplasty (DALK) using intraoperative online optical coherence tomography (iOCT). Br J Ophthalmol. 2014;98(7):900–4.

van Dijk K, Liarakos VS, Parker J, et al. Bowman layer transplantation to reduce and stabilize progressive, advanced keratoconus. Ophthalmology. 2015;122(5):909–17.

Yokogawa H, Kobayashi A, Okuda T, Mori N, Masaki T, Sugiyama K. Combined keratoplasty, pars plana vitrectomy, and flanged intrascleral intraocular lens fixation to restore vision in complex eyes with coexisting anterior and posterior segment problems. Cornea. 2018;37:S78–85.

Zirm E. Eine erfolgreiche totale Keratoplastik. Albrecht Von Graefes Archiv Für Ophthalmologie. 1906;64(3):580–93.

Optical Coherence Tomography of the Anterior Chamber and the Chamber Angle

Stefan J. Lang and Rafael S. Grajewski

1 Introduction

The anterior chamber of the eye is bounded anteriorly by the endothelium of the cornea and the anterior chamber angle, including the trabecular meshwork, and posteriorly by the iris and lens anterior surface in the region of the pupil.

The chamber angle is not directly visible on the slit lamp due to total reflection of the cornea. Visualization is possible by using a gonioscope. From anterior to posterior, the following structures can be distinguished in the chamber angle:

- Schwalbe's line
- Trabecular meshwork
- Scleral spur
- Ciliary body band

The chamber angle is usually narrowest in the superior quadrant and therefore should be assessed in each quadrant (superior, inferior, nasal, and temporal).

Although gonioscopy remains highly valued in the assessment of the chamber angle structures and for accurate classification of glaucoma. Anterior segment optical coherence tomography (AS-OCT) has also established itself as a completely noninvasive procedure that allows accurate measurement and documentation of the anterior chamber (normal values in Table 1).

S. J. Lang
Department of Ophthalmology, University Hospital of Freiburg, Kilianstrasse 5, 79106 Freiburg, Germany
e-mail: stefan.lang@uniklinik-freiburg.de

R. S. Grajewski (✉)
Department of Ophthalmology, University Hospital of Cologne, Kerpener Strasse 62, 50937 Köln, Germany
e-mail: rafael.grajewski@uk-koeln.de

© The Author(s), under exclusive license to Springer Nature Switzerland AG 2022
L. M. Heindl and S. Siebelmann (eds.), *Optical Coherence Tomography of the Anterior Segment*, https://doi.org/10.1007/978-3-031-07730-2_11

Table 1 Normal dimensions of anterior chamber

Corneal thickness central	520 μm
Anterior chamber depth (VKT)	3.0–3.6 mm
Anterior chamber diameter (VKD)	12.33 ± 0.57 mm
Chamber angle width	0–45°
Iris diameter	12 mm
Iris thickness (iris root)	3.0 mm
Iris thickness (iris ruff)	0.5 mm
Pupil diameter (miosis-mydriasis)	0.5–9.0 mm

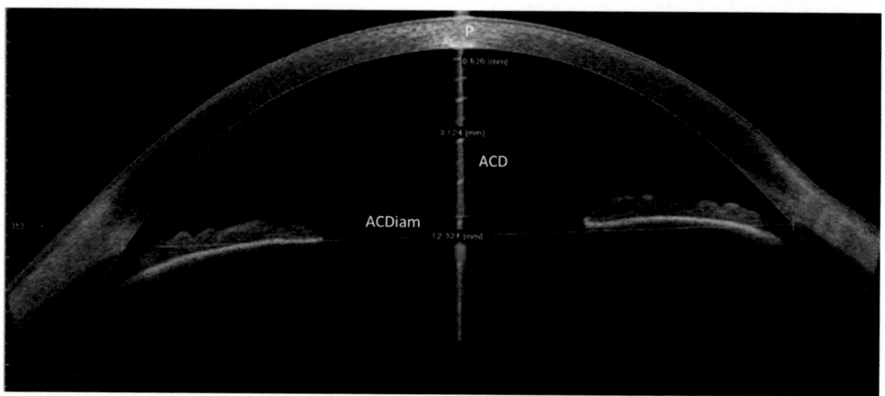

Fig. 1 Measurement of the anterior segment of the eye: diameter and depth of the anterior chamber

For example, accurate measurement of the anterior chamber angle, anterior chamber depth (ACD), and anterior chamber diameter (ACDiam) is possible (Fig. 1). The anterior chamber depth and consequently the chamber angle (Fig. 2) can change due to variations of the limiting structures. Thus, an increase in size of the lens with age also leads to a flattening of the anterior chamber (Fig. 3). If there is a structural predisposition, this leads to an increased risk of angle closure. In the case of nanophthalmos, an anterior chamber is often found to be very shallow with a severely narrowed chamber angle (Figs. 4, 5 and 6).

In clinical routine, the chamber angle classification according to Spaeth has proven to be useful. It includes documentation of relevant aspects, such as.

- Insertion of the iris root (in front of or behind the Schwalbe′s line, on or behind the scleral spur),
- angular width (10–20°: narrow, 30–40° wide), and the
- configuration of the peripheral iris (steep, anterior convex, regular, planar, and anterior concave).

A finer subdivision of the chamber angle width is found in Shaffer′s classification:

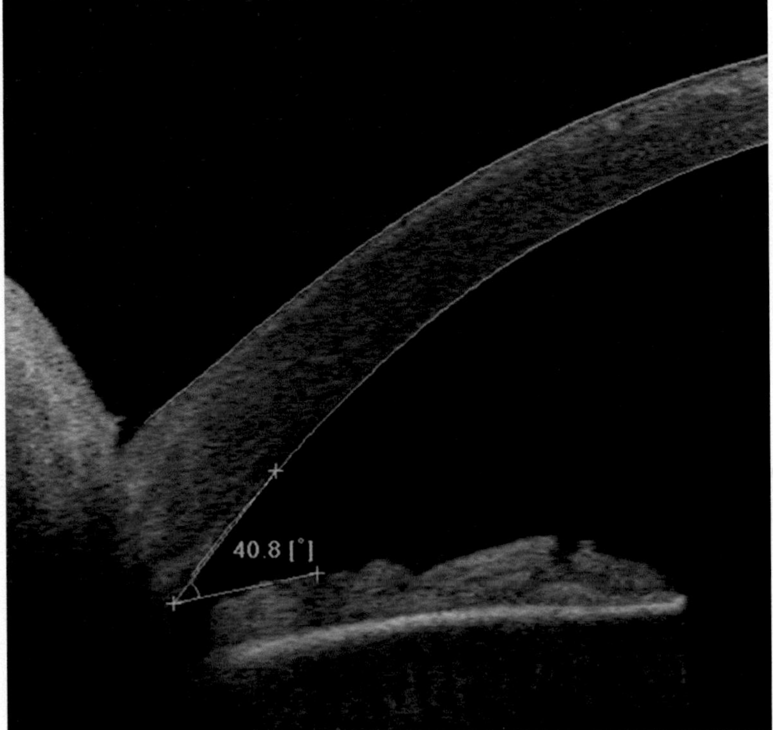

Fig. 2 Measurement of the anterior segment of the eye: chamber angle

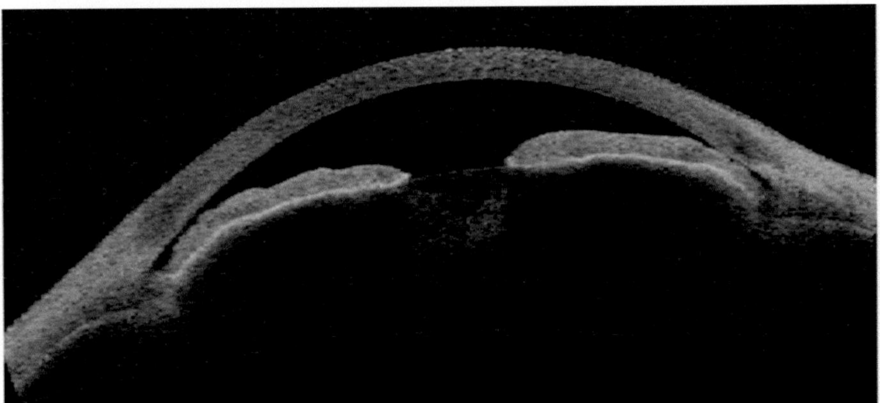

Fig. 3 Flat anterior chamber

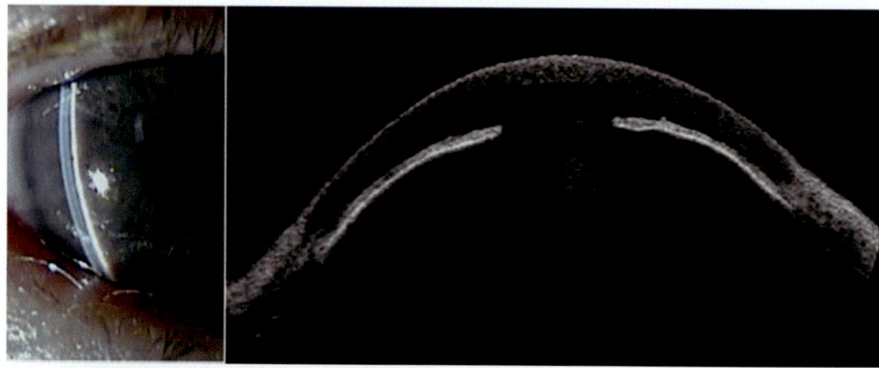

Fig. 4 Nanophthalmos

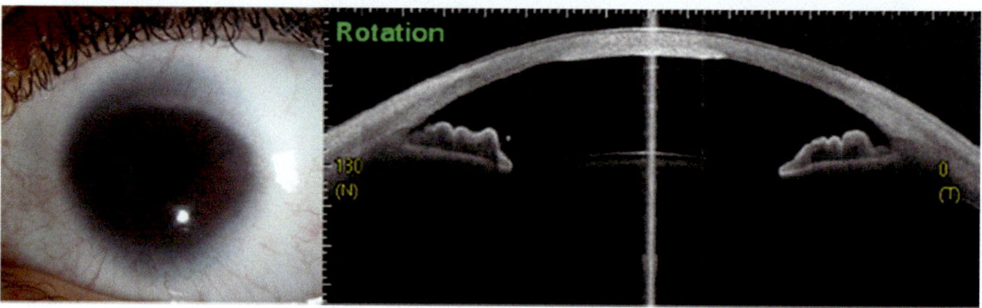

Fig. 5 Flat anterior chamber configuration in cornea plana

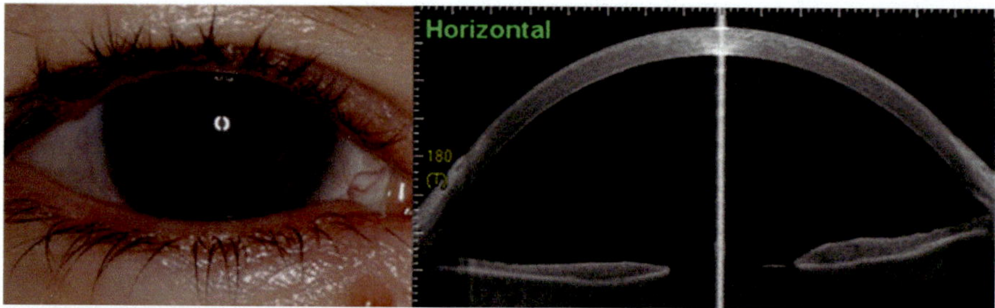

Fig. 6 Deep anterior chamber configuration in megalocornea

- Grade 0 (0°): closed chamber angle with iridocorneal contact.
- Grade I (10°): very narrow chamber angle, only Schwalbe´s line visible (high risk of occlusion)
- Grade II (20°): moderately narrow chamber angle (trabecular meshwork visible, occlusion possible)

- Grade III (20–35°): open chamber angle (visible up to scleral spur, occlusion unlikely)
- Grade IV (35–45°): very wide chamber angle (ciliary body ligament visible, occlusion not possible).

Using AS-OCT, these aspects can all be accurately measured and documented.

Pathologies in the area of the chamber angle are of great clinical relevance, since they have an influence on the outflow of aqueous humor and can thus contribute to the development of glaucoma.

Congenital diseases in the area of the chamber angle include various malformations, which are classified as mesodermal dysgenesias. A prominent Schwalbe line (embryotoxon posterius) occurs both in isolation and without disease value in about 15% of the population, and in combination with other clinically relevant changes, such as congenital glaucoma (then referred to as Axenfeld syndrome) (Fig. 7). In Axenfeld-Rieger syndrome, the Schwalbe line shifts anteriorly into the clear cornea, making it visible (Fig. 8). In addition, peripheral iris fibers span the chamber angle, resulting in the development of early glaucoma in approximately 50% of cases.

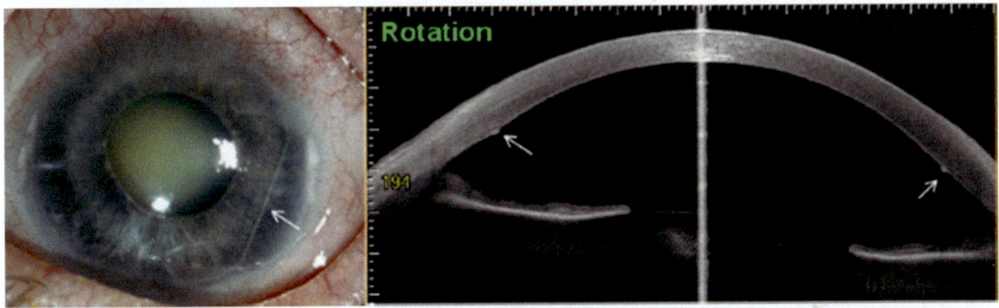

Fig. 7 Embryonotoxon posterius with congenital glaucoma

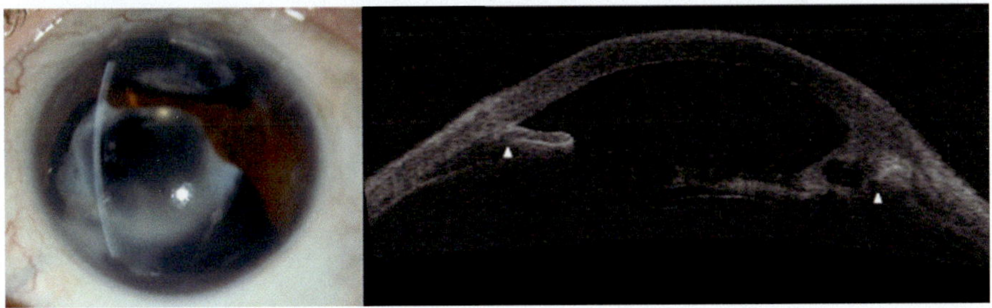

Fig. 8 Axenfeld-Rieger syndrome

In Rieger syndrome, these changes consist of pupillary malformations (corectopy, dystonia) and iris stromal hypoplasia.

Peter's anomaly is a sporadic malformation of the cornea with leukoma of the cornea and iris fibers extending to its edges. Despite the central corneal opacities, the iris fibers can often be well visualized on AS-OCT (Figs. 9, 10 and 11).

In addition to congenital malformations, inflammatory processes, e.g., after surgery or after anterior uveitis, can also lead to changes in the anterior chamber structure. Here, adhesions of the iris with the cornea and the chamber angle (anterior synechiae) or the anterior surface of the lens (posterior synechiae) are predominant and are promoted by inflammatory exudates such as fibrin and hypopyon (Figs. 12, 13, 14 and 15).

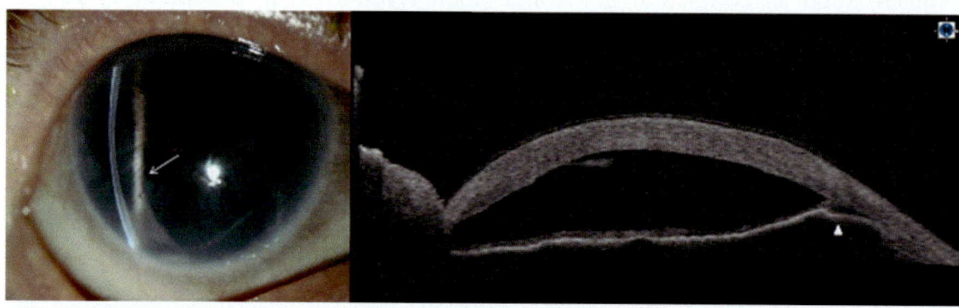

Fig. 9 Peters anomaly

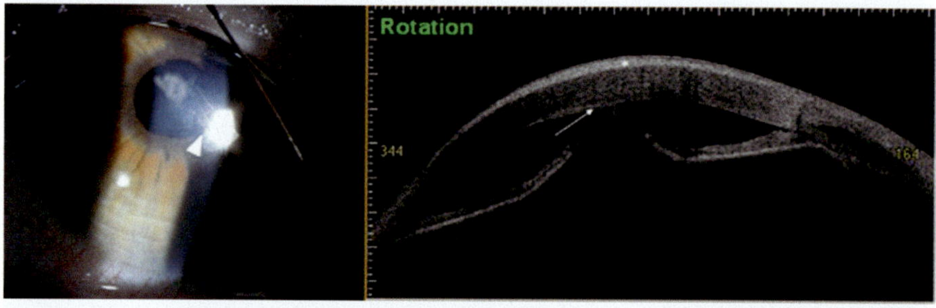

Fig. 10 Peters anomaly

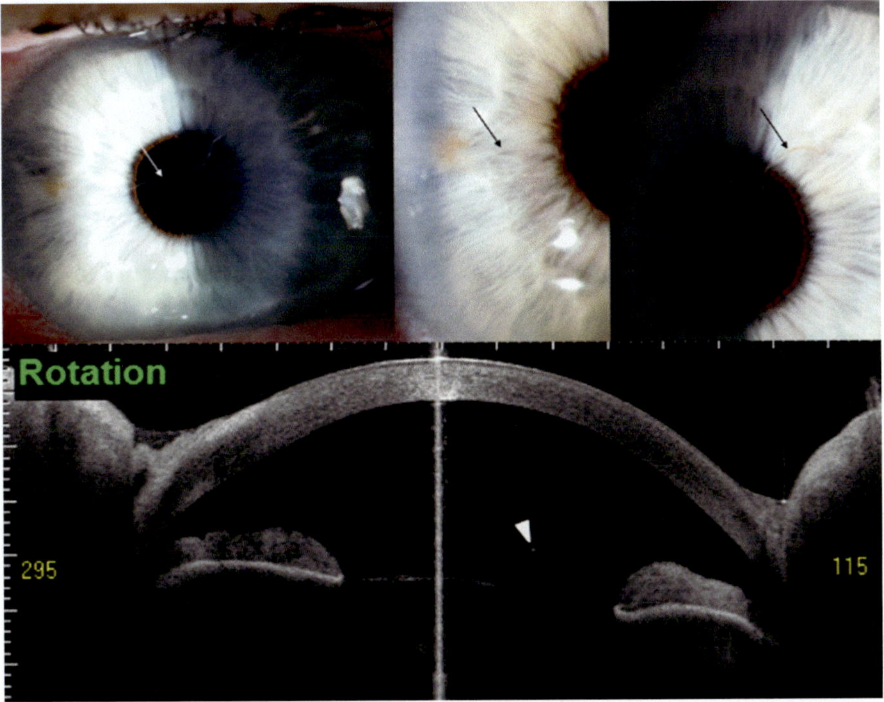

Fig. 11 Persistent iris vessel in the anterior chamber

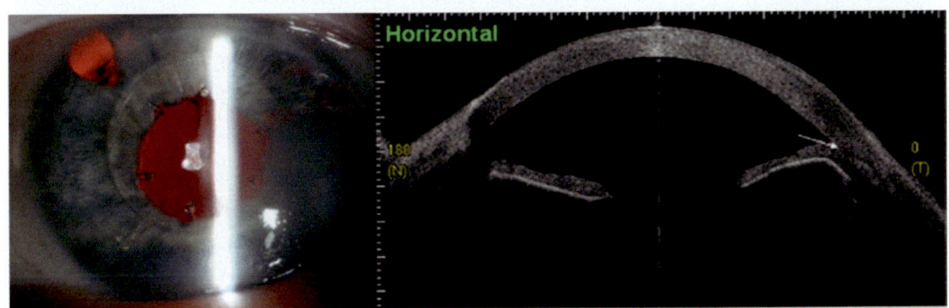

Fig. 12 Anterior synechiae in iris-fixed anterior chamber lens (Sputnik)

Postoperative assessment of precise positioning of intraocular implants, such as intraocular lenses and glaucoma implants, is also possible with AS-OCT. Here, even changes that are hardly visible in the slit lamp image, such as a vitreous traction to the tunnel incision after cataract surgery (Fig. 16), can be visualized.

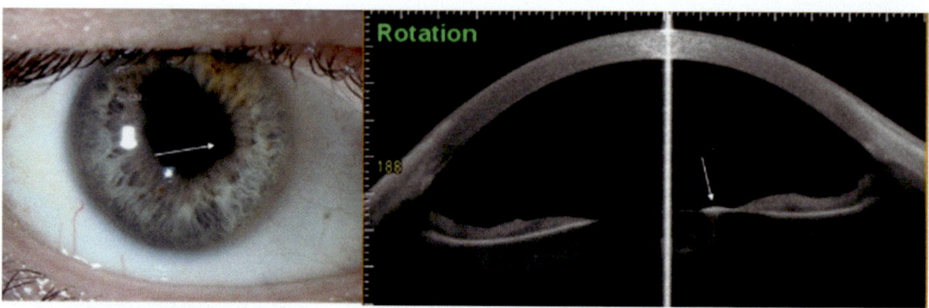

Fig. 13 Posterior synechiae

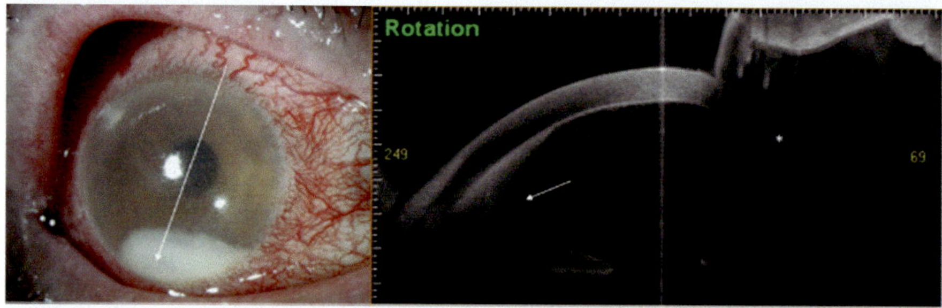

Fig. 14 Hypopyon in endophthalmitis

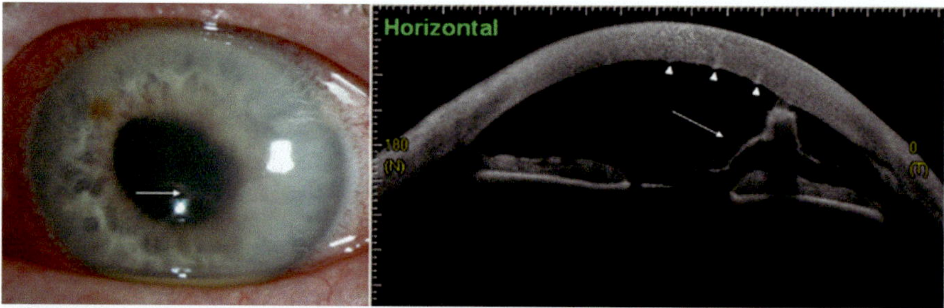

Fig. 15 Fibrin in anterior chamber

Regarding the position of a Baerveldt implant, the distance to the corneal endothelium can be measured exactly (Fig. 17).

Measurements using AS-OCT can also be used to assess deeper changes, such as the location of a phakic intraocular lens in the sulcus ciliaris (Fig. 18).

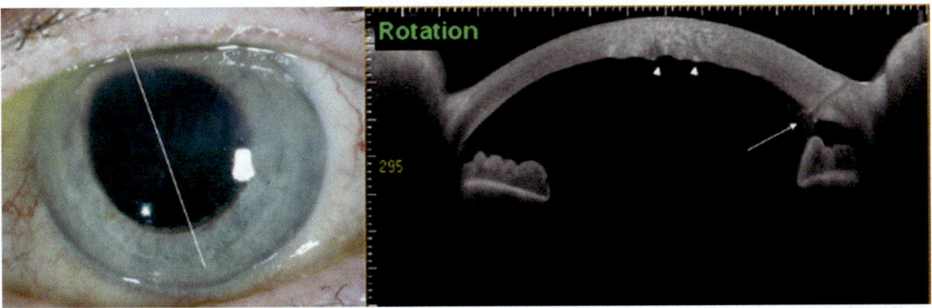

Fig. 16 Vitreous traction to the tunnel after cataract surgery

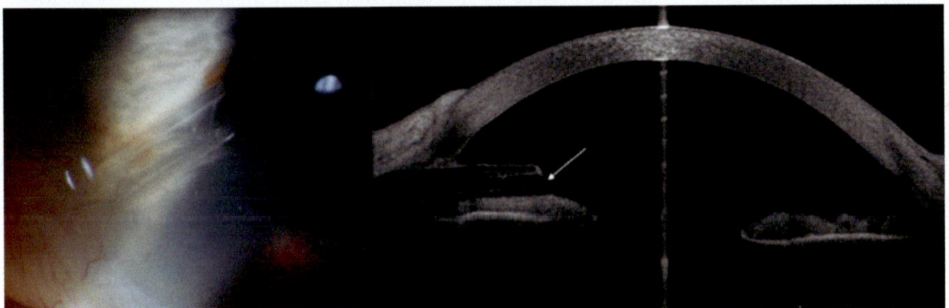

Fig. 17 Baerveldt implant in anterior chamber of eye

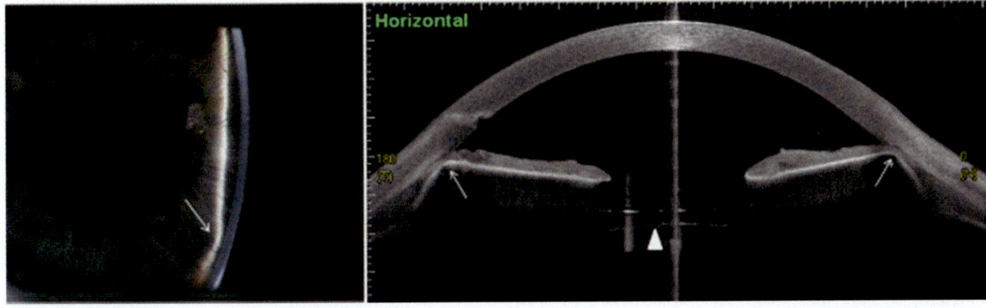

Fig. 18 Phakic IOL (ICL) "upside-down"

2 Possible Applications of Optical Coherence Tomography for the Analysis of the Anterior Chamber and the Chamber Angle

OCT of the anterior segment of the eye allows the collection of numerous measurement parameters, which are of interest for various questions.

P: Pachymetry of the cornea.

ACD: anterior chamber depth.

ACDiam: anterior chamber diameter.

The determination of the chamber angle is also possible with OCT. Shown is a very wide chamber angle, corresponding to grade IV (35–45°) according to Shaffer's classification. Thus, a closure of the chamber angle in the sense of an angle block is not possible.

Flat anterior chamber with very narrow chamber angle and anterior position of the lens, corresponding to grade I (10°) according to Shaffer, where gonioscopically only the Schwalbe line is visible (high risk of closure) and partly grade 0 (0°) with partially closed chamber angle and iridocorneal contact. The finding would be an indication for an iridotomy by YAG-laser or a basal surgical iridectomy. Prior to this, diagnostic mydriasis should be avoided with such a finding.

Very shallow anterior chamber with severely narrowed chamber angle in nanophthalmos. Already in the slit image (figure on the left), only a very narrow gap between the light slit of the cornea and the light slit of the iris can be seen in the Van Herrick test, which corresponds to a very narrow chamber angle with a high probability for an angle block.

A flat anterior chamber configuration is seen in cornea plana with sclerocornea. The refractive power of the cornea is 30 dpt with a radius of 11.2 mm. It is a rare bilateral disease, inherited autosomal-dominantly in milder forms and autosomal-recessively in severe forms (the opacity may affect the entire cornea). Sporadic variants are also relatively common. There are also two variants of cornea plana without associated sclerosis and opacification. Variant 1 (CNA1) is less severe (than CNA2).

A deep anterior chamber configuration in megalocornea is seen. Megalocornea is present when the corneal diameter exceeds 13 mm (normal is 10–13 mm in adults, below 10 mm is microcornea). It usually occurs bilaterally and is inherited x-linked recessively (rarely autosomal dominant or recessive). Association with various syndromes, such as Marfan or Apert syndrome is common.

The prominent anteriorly displaced Schwalbe line (arrows) can be seen on both the clinical image and OCT. Further details in the text (introduction).

Clinically, there is iris hypoplasia with corectopy. OCT shows the chamber angle displaced by the present iris parts (arrowheads). Further details in the text (introduction).

Clinically, there is iris stromal hypoplasia (arrow) and anterior synechiae at the chamber angle. This is visible on OCT (arrowhead). More details in the text (introduction).

In the clinical image, this shows a corneal opacity (arrowhead). OCT shows iridocorneal synechiae (arrow) with surrounding higher reflectivity at the level of Descemet's membrane, as well as in the anterior region of the cornea (*). More details on Peters anomaly can be found in the text (Introduction).

Clinically, there is a bright structure extending from the iris stroma into the anterior chamber, which runs in front of the pupil (white arrow). At higher magnification, a vessel is visible (black arrows). OCT shows a reflective structure (arrowhead). Basically, different residual structures of the hyaloidea artery, which originates from the optic disc during the embryonic period and supplies vitreous and lens during this time (tunica vasculosa), are possible. Depending on the localization a distinction is made between: Mittendorf spot: opacity in the area of the posterior lens capsule. Bergmeister papilla on the nasal side of the optic disc and pupillary membrane and vascular loops (95% of which are arterial) that attach as filaments to the anterior surface of the lens. It is important not to confuse pigmented remnants of the pupillary membrane on the anterior surface of the lens with pigment after anterior uveitis!

Anterior synechiae (arrow) with iris-fixed lens in place.

After anterior uveitis, posterior synechiae exist almost circularly. The corresponding posterior synechiae were marked with an arrow in the OCT and clinical image. These "adhesions" between the iris and the anterior surface of the lens are caused by proteins and especially fibrin released during uveitis. In circular synechiae, aqueous humor formed in the ciliary epithelium can no longer drain through the pupil into the anterior chamber. The resulting pressure buildup in the posterior chamber pushes the iris anteriorly with subsequent formation of a bombata ("cupcake") configuration (see "Epithelial Mapping", Fig. 11) and secondary angle block. In the long term, posterior synechiae also favor accelerated cataract formation.

Postoperative endophthalmitis with hypopyon. This can be well visualized on OCT (arrow). The arrow in the clinical image corresponds to the position of the OCT cross-sectional image. The OCT does not show the entire anterior chamber. The upper lid obscures the upper third of the cornea and anterior chamber (*).

Fibrin formation in the anterior chamber (arrows). OCT also shows corneal edema with Descemet's folds (arrowheads). The most common cause of acute fibrinous iridocyclitis is HLA-B27-associated anterior uveitis. Hypopyon formation may also occur in Behcet's disease, but typically with much less fibrin than in the HLA-B27-associated form.

There is incarceration of the vitreous into the tunnel (arrow). In addition, there is corneal edema with Descemet's folds (arrowheads). The line in the clinical image corresponds to the axis of the OCT section. The sectorial dilation is also visible here. An IOL is not visible in the clinical image nor in the OCT, this was dislocated into the vitreous cavity.

The tube of the Baerveldt implant comes to rest on the iris in this case. The lumen of the tube is visible (arrow). In this image, the distance of the tube to the corneal endothelium can be assessed. Other glaucoma implants, such as the Ahmed implant, can also be assessed in this way using OCT.

Status after implantation of a phakic IOL into the sulcus ciliaris. However, the posterior surface of the IOL sits toward the anterior chamber, which is why the iris is pushed anteriorly (arrows). The optics of the IOL are also visible on OCT (arrowhead) (Figs. 19, 20 and 21).

At the time of imaging, a bandage lens was on the ocular surface (*). The ulcer perforation is tamponaded by iris tissue (arrow). This is already visible in the clinical slit image.

Epithelial implantation cyst in the anterior chamber (arrow). This had developed after implantation of an ICL. The depth extension is visible in OCT (arrowhead). If such secondary cysts are progressive, which is usually the case, excision should usually be attempted to avoid further complications to the corneal endothelium and by development of secondary glaucoma.

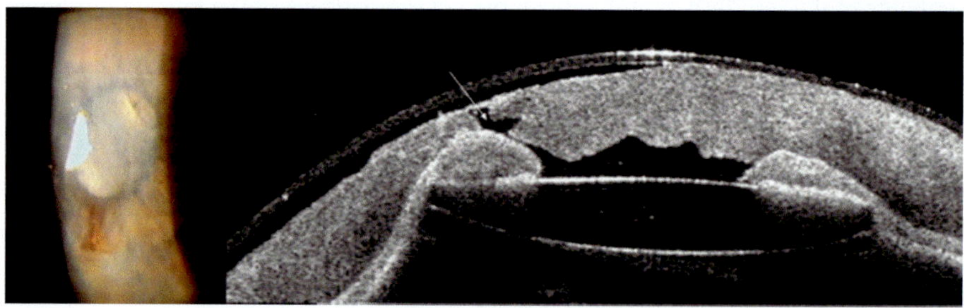

Fig. 19 Iris tamponade in perforated corneal ulcer

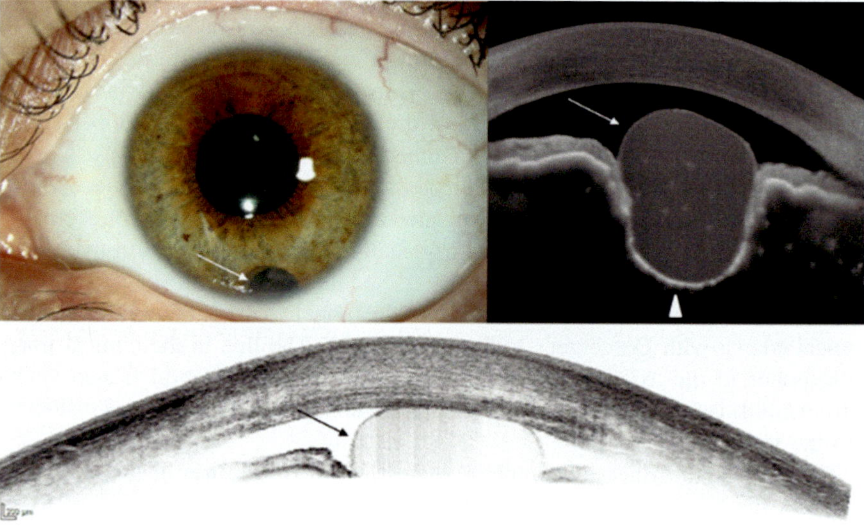

Fig. 20 Epithelial implantation cyst

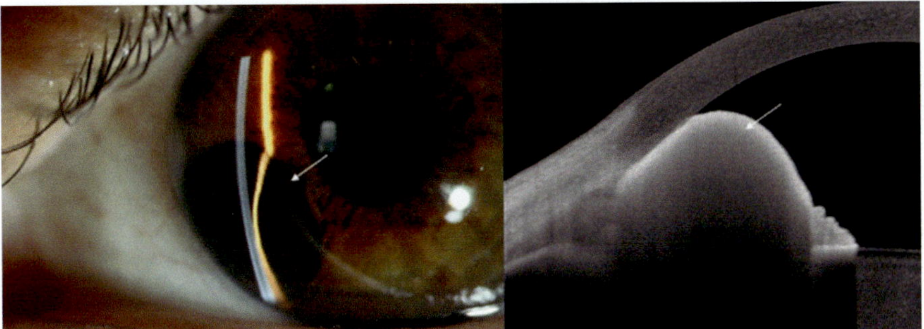

Fig. 21 Ciliary body melanoma

Ciliary body melanoma with invasion of the anterior chamber (arrow). The insidious thing about ciliary body melanoma is that it is often discovered very late, after it has broken through into the anterior chamber. Due to its location outside the optical axis, it also leads to symptoms only very late. In this case it is always advisable for the ophthalmologist to take a careful look at the "immediate surroundings", where often characteristic so-called "sentinel vessels" can be seen as circumscribed episcleral vascular dilatations in the area of the tumor base (indicated in the clinical figure). Naumann coined the term "Bonamour sign" for this. The therapeutic gold standard is still the complete block excision of the tumor (cornea, sclera, ciliary body and iris en bloc) with tectonic corneoscleral plasty.

3 Conclusion and Summary

Optical coherence tomography of the anterior chamber and chamber angle provides a noninvasive method for accurate measurement and follow-up of the configuration of the anterior chamber and chamber angle, including associated pathologies. In contrast to contact-required examination methods such as gonioscopy and ultrasound biomicroscopy, there is no interference with the structures under examination. It is important to examine under standardized conditions (miosis) and in different sectional planes and in each quadrant (upper, lower, nasal and temporal).

OCT allows accurate measurement of the chamber angle, anterior chamber depth (ACD), and anterior chamber diameter (ACD) to detect, for example, flattening of the anterior chamber with age or in the context of congenital changes, such as nanophthalmos, which lead to an increased risk of angle closure if there is a structural predisposition. Both the chamber angle width and the morphological classification of the chamber angle (e.g., according to Spaeth and according to Shaffer) can be precisely determined with OCT and reliably monitored in the course.

Pathologies in the area of the anterior chamber angle, which include various malformations that are classified as mesodermal dysgenesias (embryotoxon posterius, Axenfeld syndrome, Axenfeld-Rieger syndrome, Rieger syndrome, and Peter anomaly) can also be documented excellently using OCT.

Postoperative assessment of accurate positioning of intraocular implants, such as intraocular lenses and glaucoma implants, is now routinely performed by AS-OCT.

Conflict of Interest The authors have no financial, political, or economic conflicts of interest related to the content of this article.

References

Ang M, Baskaran M, Werkmeister RM, Chua J, Schmidl D, Aranha Dos Santos V, Garhofer G, Mehta JS, Schmetterer L. Anterior segment optical coherence tomography. Prog Retin Eye Res. 2018;66:132–56.

Chan PP, Lai G, Chiu V, Chong A, Yu M, Leung CK. Anterior chamber angle imaging with swept-source optical coherence tomography: comparison between CASIAII and ANTERION. Sci Rep. 2020;10:18771.

Chang TC, Summers CG, Schimmenti LA, Grajewski AL. Axenfeld-Rieger syndrome: new perspectives. Br J Ophthalmol. 2012;96:318–22.

Duru Z, Altunel O. Using anterior segment optical coherence tomography to assess angle anatomy in patients with Neurofibromatosis Type 1. Optom vis Sci. 2020;97:68–72.

Hashida N, Asao K, Maruyama K, Nishida K. Cornea findings of spectral domain anterior segment optical coherence tomography in Uveitic eyes of various etiologies. Cornea. 2019;38:1299–304.

Lang SJ, Cucera A, Lang GK. Applications of optical coherence tomography in the anterior segment. Klin Monbl Augenheilkd. 2011;228:1086–91.

Lang SJ, Heinzelmann S, Bohringer D, Reinhard T, Maier P. Indications for intraoperative anterior segment optical coherence tomography in corneal surgery. Int Ophthalmol. 2020;40:2617–25.

Lucisano A, Ferrise M, Balestrieri M, Busin M, Scorcia V. Evaluation of postoperative toric intraocular lens alignment with anterior segment optical coherence tomography. J Cataract Refract Surg. 2017;43:1007–9.

Mularoni A, Imburgia A, Forlini M, Rania L, Possati GL. In vivo evaluation of a one-piece foldable sutureless intrascleral fixation lens using ultrasound biomicroscopy and anterior segment optical coherence tomography. J Cataract Refract Surg. 2020.

Nongpiur ME, Tun TA, Aung T. Anterior segment optical coherence tomography: is there a clinical role in the management of primary angle closure disease? J Glaucoma. 2020;29:60–6.

Porporato N, Baskaran M, Aung T. Role of anterior segment optical coherence tomography in angle-closure disease: a review. Clin Exp Ophthalmol. 2018;46:147–57.

Porporato N, Baskaran M, Tun TA, Sultana R, Tan M, Quah JH, Allen JC, Perera S, Friedman DS, Cheng CY, Aung T. Understanding diagnostic disagreement in angle closure assessment between anterior segment optical coherence tomography and gonioscopy. Br J Ophthalmol. 2020;104:795–9.

Wang D, Lin S. New developments in anterior segment optical coherence tomography for glaucoma. Curr Opin Ophthalmol. 2016;27:111–7.

Wang SB, Cornish EE, Grigg JR, McCluskey PJ. Anterior segment optical coherence tomography and its clinical applications. Clin Exp Optom. 2019;102:195–207.

Optical Coherence Tomography of the Iris

Rafael S. Grajewski and Stefan J. Lang

1 Introduction

The anterior surface of the iris is readily assessable by slit lamp examination (with the exception of the transition to the chamber angle and assuming clear refractive media). However, changes in the stroma and on the posterior surface cannot be assessed in this way or only indirectly. This has been the domain of ultrasound biomicroscopy (UBM), which, however, requires the placement of a water- or gel-filled funnel on the cornea as a contact medium, since ultrasound conducts extremely poorly in air. Here, anterior segment optical coherence tomography (AS-OCT) has become very well established as a completely non-contact examination method. Since the iris also varies in shape and thickness due to changes in pupil width, standardized examination conditions should be established by pilocarpine eye drop administration prior to OCT examination. Under these conditions, iris lesions can then be accurately measured in height, width, and depth.

A prerequisite for accurate assessment of OCT images of the iris is detailed knowledge of its macroscopic and microscopic anatomy:

The posterior surface of the iris is formed by a double epithelial layer, which is a continuation of the bilaminar ciliary body epithelium. Here, it is important to note that the anterior epithelium of the iris is the anterior of the two layers, but lies posterior to the iris stroma. Thus, the anterior epithelium of the iris does not lie on the anterior surface of the iris, as its name suggests. The anterior surface of the iris is formed by the stroma, whose collagenous structures are present in a condensed

R. S. Grajewski (✉)
Department of Ophthalmology, University Hospital of Cologne, Kerpener Strasse 62, 50937 Köln, Germany
e-mail: rafael.grajewski@uk-koeln.de

S. J. Lang
Department of Ophthalmology, University Hospital of Freiburg, Kilianstrasse 5, 79106 Freiburg, Germany

L. M. Heindl and S. Siebelmann (eds.), *Optical Coherence Tomography of the Anterior Segment*, https://doi.org/10.1007/978-3-031-07730-2_12

form in this area. This modified iris stroma also contains increased fibroblasts and melanocytes located in a layer posterior to it. The surface of a brown iris is much smoother than that of a blue iris due to increased intercalation of stromal melanocytes, in which numerous crypts and delineable stromal trabeculae are evident. The posterior epithelium is heavily pigmented and forms the pigment sheet of the iris. The pigment sheet is well demarcated from anterior epithelium and stroma (both with intermediate reflectivity) on AS-OCT due to its hyperreflectivity.

Both epithelial layers of the iris (as well as the epithelium of ciliary body and retina) originate from the neuroectodermal eye cup, whereas the iris (and ciliary body) stroma originate from the head mesenchyme.

This also results in the different iris pathologies, whereby essentially neoplastic, inflammatory and degenerative changes can be distinguished.

OCT plays a particularly important role in the follow-up and assessment of the dignity of benign and malignant neoplastic lesions (Figs. 1, 2, 3, 4 and 5). The benign iris tumors can be divided into cystic (about 20%) and solid tumors (about 80%) originating either from the iris stroma or the iris pigment epithelium (Figs. 1 and 2).

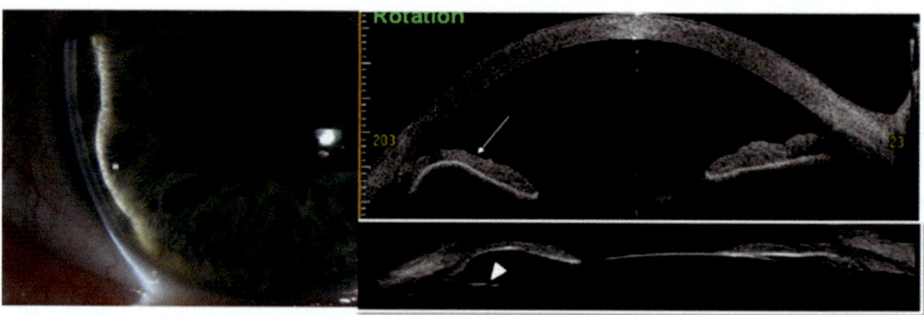

Fig. 1 Iris cyst

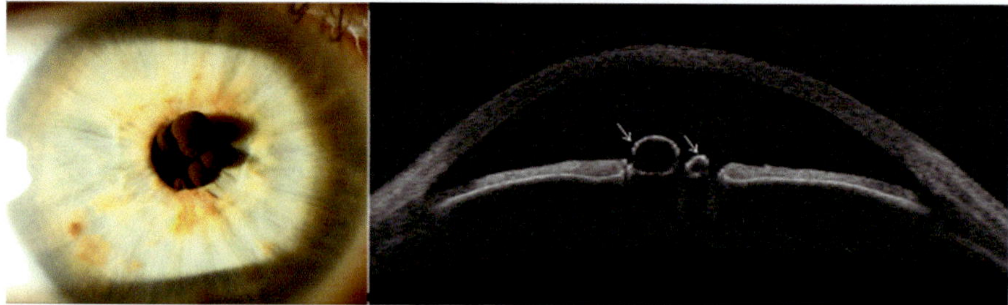

Fig. 2 Iris cysts in the pupillary region

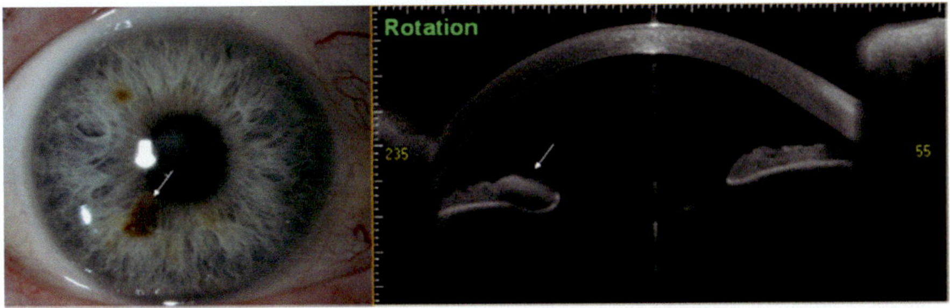

Fig. 3 Iris nevus

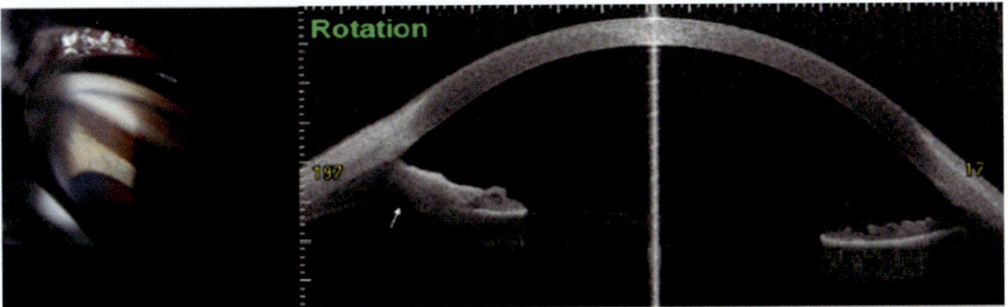

Fig. 4 Melanocytic iris lesion

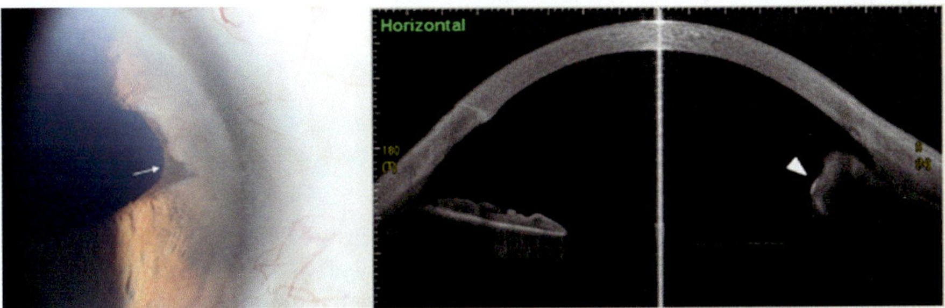

Fig. 5 Iris melanoma

Accordingly, cystic lesions include iris stromal and iris pigment epithelial cysts, with anatomic distinctions made among the latter between central, midzonal, peripheral, and other cysts (see Table 1).

Solid benign lesions include iris nevus (Fig. 3) and iris melanocytoma. AS-OCT allows differentiation of cystic and solid space lesions of the iris and ciliary body. The exact measurement in all three spatial axes also enables a very precise follow-up. Iris nevi belong to the very frequent iris lesions (to be distinguished from the harmless "freckles"), while iris melanomas (Fig. 5) are very rare. The

Table 1 Classification of iris cysts according to Shields

Primary cysts	
Iris pigment epithelial cyst	Iris stromal cyst
1. Pupillary	1. Congenital
2. Midzonal	2. Accuired
3. Peripheral	
4. Dislocated	
5. Free floating	
Anterior chamber or vitreous	
Secondary cysts	
Epithelial	Secondary to intraocular tumors
	(or parasitic)
1. Postoperative	1. Medulloepithelioma
2. Posttraumatisc	2. Uveal melanoma
	3. Uveal nevus

differentiation from nevi is often very difficult, especially since numerous variations of iris melanomas are possible. Specifically, circumscribed, diffuse, and iris melanomas of the tapioca or trabecular meshwork type are distinguished (Fig. 4).

It is important to always keep in mind that imaging techniques can only be a partial aspect of making a diagnosis. The overall assessment starts with the identification of possible risk factors for malignant transformation, which are often summarized in the so-called ABCDEF rule:

A: Age young.
B: Blood (hyphema).
C: Clock hour inferior.
D: Diffuse.
E: Ectropion.
F: Feathery margin.

Important clinical parameters that can also be measured by AS-OCT include an increase in size and depth of malignant lesions, as well as secondary changes, such as an ectropium uveae (also possible in nevus) or chamber angle invasion, which can often lead to secondary glaucoma.

This also allows OCT to contribute to the accurate TNM classification of iris melanomas (see Table 2).

The vasculature of the iris is supplied by the long posterior and anterior ciliary arteries, which anastomose in the iris to form a circulosus arteriosus major at the iris base, which is connected to the circulosus arteriosus minor at the collarette by radial vessels. Vascular anomalies with marked increase in lumen size also show correlates on OCT but can be better visualized via the newer technique of OCT angiography and fluorescence angiography. These vascular tumors include racemose (Fig. 19), cavernous, and capillary hemangiomas, as well as iris varix and microhemangiomatosis.

Table 2 TNM classification of iris melanoma

T1: tumor limited to iris
T1a: <3 o'clock affected
T1b: >3 o'clock affected
T2: ciliary body involved
T2a: with secondary glaucoma
T3: T2 with extrascleral extension
T3a: with secondary glaucoma
T4: with extraocular growth
T4a: <5 mm
T4a: >5 mm

Other tissue neoplasms of the iris may develop reactively after previous inflammation (granulomatous nodules) or in the context of genetic diseases. The latter include, for example, neurofibromatosis type 1, which may be associated with brownish nodules of the iris (Figs. 6 and 7). As a result of developmental disorders, both rudimentary remnants of tissue may remain, such as the pupillary membrane with portions of pigment, and tissue may be absent, as in iris coloboma (Fig. 8), which is usually localized nasally inferiorly. In congenital aniridia, the iris is completely absent except for a stump, which can be well visualized on AS-OCT

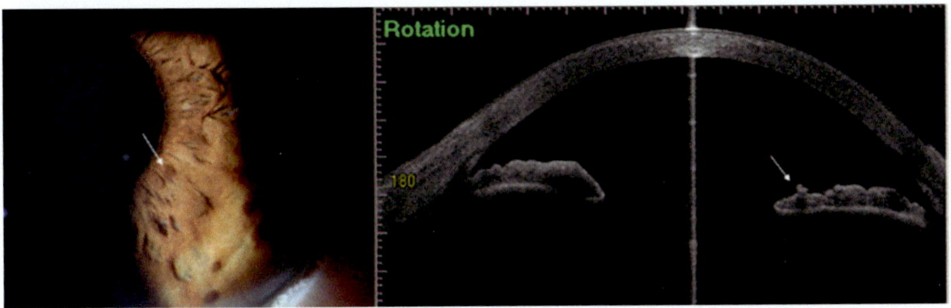

Fig. 6 Lisch nodule

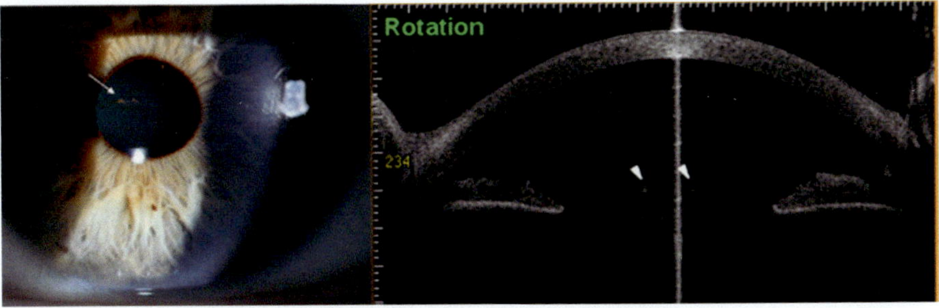

Fig. 7 Persistent pupillary membrane

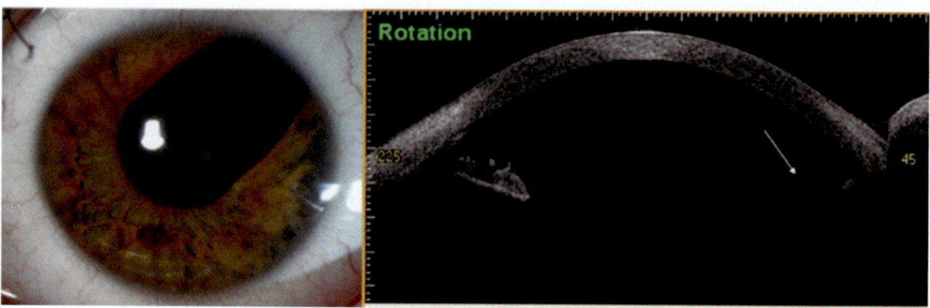

Fig. 8 Coloboma of the iris

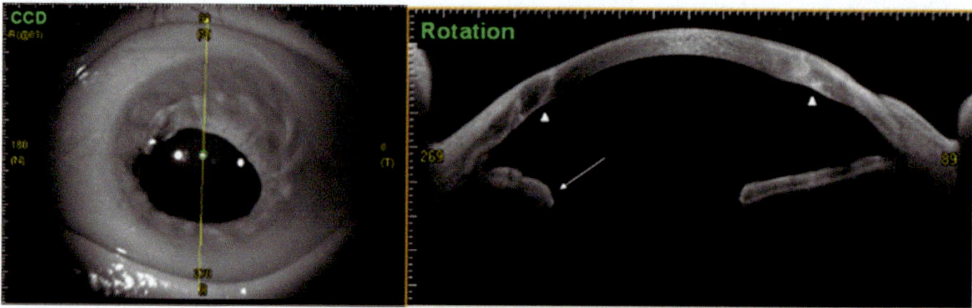

Fig. 9 Traumatic iris defect

(Fig. 10). Missing tissue may also result from trauma (Fig. 9). A desirable iatrogenic substance defect of the iris, can be created by surgical iridectomy or by YAG iridectomy, e.g., in case of impending angle closure and displacement of the chamber angle by an iris bombata ("cupcake iris") after anterior uveitis (Fig. 11a–c). Undesirable iatrogenic iris defects include, e.g., pigment loss due to friction of an intraocular lens on the iris posterior surface. The positioning of intraocular lenses, especially haptics, can be verified by AS-OCT. Finally, a completely missing iris can be replaced by an artificial iris.

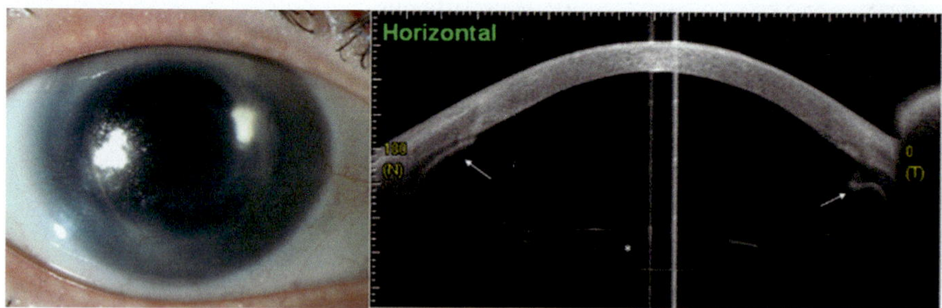

Fig. 10 Aniridia

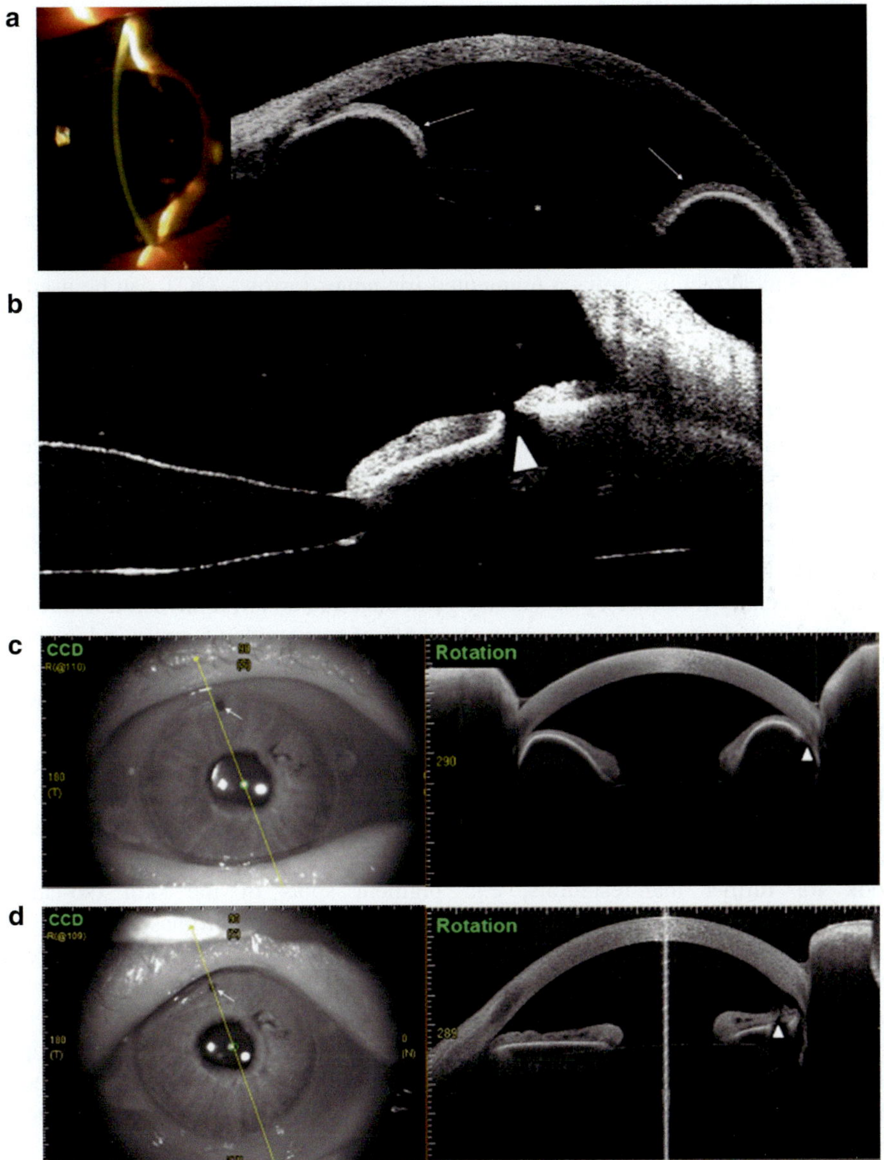

Fig. 11 **a** Iris bombata, **b** YAG Iridotomy, **c** Iris bombata, **d** YAG iridotomy

2 Possible Applications of Optical Coherence Tomography for the Analysis of the Iris

The clinical image shows the protrusion of the iris (*), which can also be visualized in OCT. However, the posterior surface of the cyst is shadowed in OCT and can only be visualized by UBM (arrowhead).

The clinical image shows pigmented structures in the pupillary region. OCT shows these as cysts without internal reflection (arrows).

The clinical picture shows a pigmented iris nevus (arrow). OCT can be used to document the progression. The iris nevus shows a higher reflectivity (arrow). Behind it, there is a slight acoustic extinction, although the pigment sheet is still recognizable.

Gonioscopy shows a pigmented change in the iris. OCT allows visualization, but the pigment sheet is already shadowed, so assessment of depth extent is not possible.

The clinical image shows a tumor of the iris with a consecutive ectropium uveae (arrow). OCT shows a tumor with high reflectivity and shadowing (arrowhead). Circumscribed iris melanomas up to 3–4 o'clock can be surgically excised, with iridectomy, iridocyclectomy, and iridocyclogoniectomy. Larger tumors involving more than half of the iris and trabecular meshwork (TMW) are treated by enucleation, especially if refractory secondary glaucoma due to TMW invasion is already present. Iris melanomas metastasize in about 5% of cases within 5 years and in about 10% within 20 years. The risk increases in advanced tumors with extraucular growth or extensive TMW invasion and secondary glaucoma (see above). Overall, however, prognosis is relatively good compared to other ocular melanomas.

Neurofibromatosis type 1 (Recklinghausen disease, NF type 1, NF1) with Lisch nodules. These are well recognizable in the clinical picture as well as in the OCT (arrows). Specific therapy is not required. However, Lisch nodules are by no means a sufficient criterion for a diagnosis of NF1. In this case, the ophthalmologist has to look for further manifestations, e.g. pigment spots of the skin (so-called "cafe-au-lait spots") and at the eyes for further small neurofibromas, especially at the eyelids and partly also in the area of the orbit and optic nerve. Furthermore, a plexiform neurofibroma of the upper eyelid is characterized by an S-shaped swelling of the eyelid (painless). Also at the fundus, so-called corkscrew vessels (without leakage in fluorescein angiography), choroidal hamartomas and multiple (hyperreflective in OCT) small pigmented nodules of the choroid are found in about one third of the patients. The presence of choroidal nevi in NF1 patients is associated with an increased risk of developing choroidal melanoma.

Rudimentary remnants of pupillary membrane with portions of pigment (arrow). These are visible as reflective structures on OCT (arrowheads). It is important not to confuse these pigmented remnants of the pupillary membrane on the anterior surface of the lens with pigment after anterior uveitis! See also "Degenerative Corneal Disorders", Fig. 11).

Congenital coloboma of the iris in the temporal upper quadrant. On OCT, only the missing iris tissue with a rudiment is noticeable at this location. This is unusual because colobomas of the iris are developmentally due to incomplete closure of the

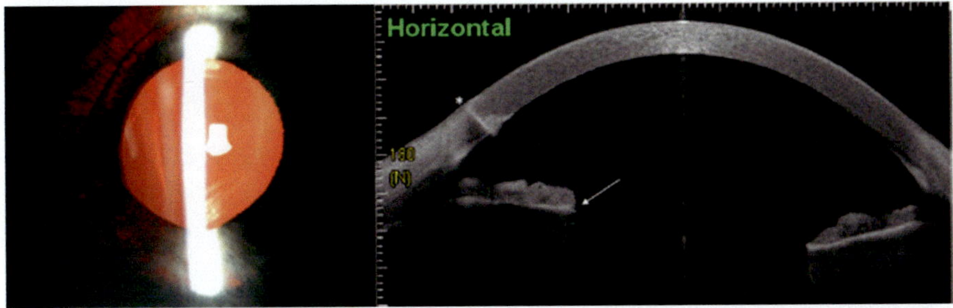

Fig. 12 Iris chafing

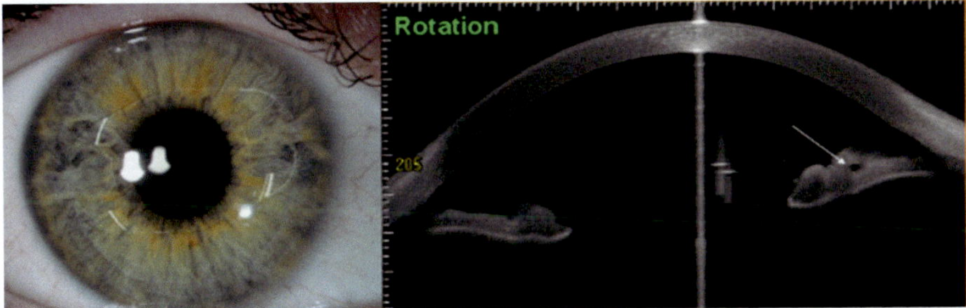

Fig. 13 Iris clip lens

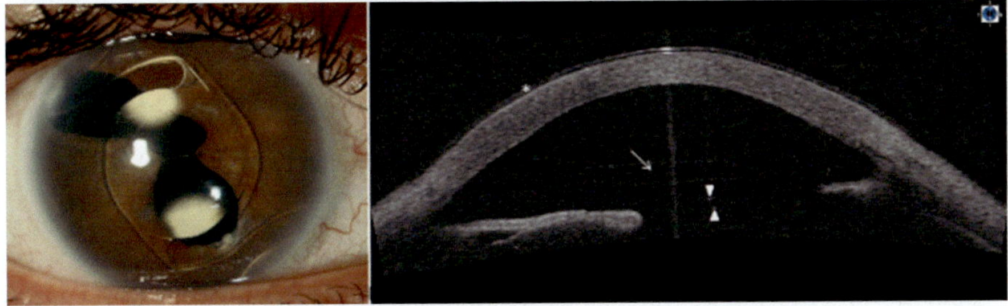

Fig. 14 Iris reconstruction and chamber angle supported intraocular lens (IOL)

orbital cleft, with the colobomas usually pointing nasally downward in accordance with the location of the orbital cleft (Figs. 12, 13, 14, 15 and 16).

The iris root is still preserved in the lower region after the injury (arrow). A keratoplasty scar is evident in the cornea (arrowheads). Injuries to the iris are also associated with deepening of the anterior chamber (recessus) and often lead to subsequent secondary glaucoma due to associated microtrauma in the trabecular meshwork, which can occasionally develop years later. Therefore, it is important to educate patients about this risk and document this.

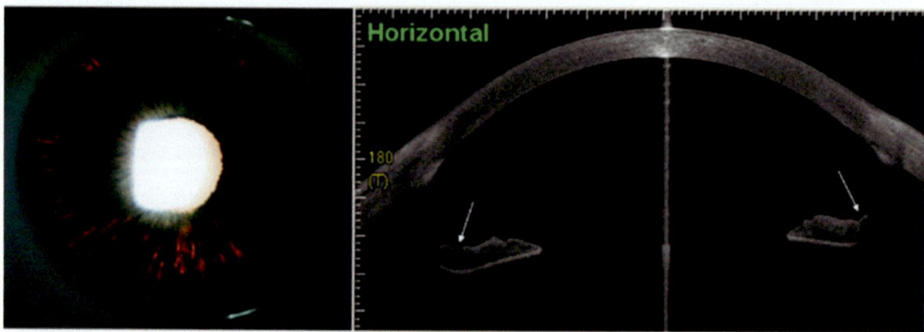

Fig. 15 Pigment dispersion

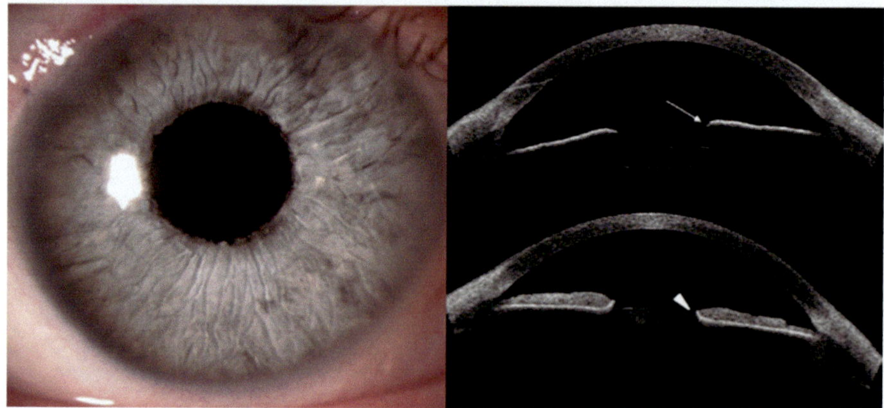

Fig. 16 Artificial Iris

Congenital aniridia. Remnants of the anteriorly displaced iris root are visible on OCT (arrows). In addition, there is a pseudophakia (*). The clinical picture also shows a circular limbal stem cell insufficiency. The autosomal-dominant inherited form of aniridia is without systemic associations, whereas the sporadic form carries a 30% risk for the development of a Wilms tumor of the kidneys. A very rare (about 1%) form of aniridia is inherited in an autosomal recessive manner and is associated with mental retardation and cerebellar ataxia. It is not associated with a mutation of the PAX6 gene, unlike the first forms mentioned.

Protrusion of the iris (arrows) with displacement of the angle of the anterior chamber in secclusio pupillae. The eye is pseudophakic (*). The aqueous humor formed in the ciliary epithelium of the ciliary body can no longer drain through the pupil into the anterior chamber, which can lead secondarily to the formation of the bombata ("cupcake") configuration (see "Epithelial Mapping", Fig. 11) with secondary angle block due to pressure increase in the posterior chamber of the eye (see also "Degenerative Corneal Disorders", Fig. 13). This example shows that therapeutic mydriasis (with residual pupil play during the day, e.g., by tropicamide) may be useful in anterior uveitis even in pseudophakic patients if the intraocular lens shows contact with the iris. This can be well demonstrated by AS-OCT.

After YAG iridotomy, the protrusion of the iris is no longer present. The iris shows a small defect anteriorly with a larger defect in the pigment sheet at the site of the iridotomy (arrowhead).

An iridectomy had been performed (arrow). OCT shows a defect in the pigment sheet at the corresponding site with the iris tissue still protruding (arrowhead).

After YAG iridotomy, the protrusion of the iris is also no longer present here. The iris shows a smaller defect anteriorly in this case, with a larger defect in the pigment sheet at the site of the iridotomy (arrowhead).

Transillumination of the iris due to loss of pigment. The cause is the position of the artificial lens being partly in the sulcus ciliaris. There is contact with the iris posterior surface (arrow). At this point a loss of the iris pigment occurs (iris chafing). A surgical approach site is also visible in the OCT (*).

In OCT, the fixation of the iris clip lens (arrow), as well as its position in the anterior chamber can be assessed.

The clinical image shows the iris defect, which was reduced with a suture. OCT shows the optics of the IOL (arrow), as well as a reflection of the suture (arrowheads). A bandage lens was in place at the time of imaging (*).

The clinical picture shows a clear iris transillumination in pigment dispersion syndrome. OCT shows a posterior bowing of the iris and a very deep anterior chamber. Young myopic males are particularly affected. In one third of the patients, secondary ocular hypertension develops within about 15 years, often with progression to pigmentary glaucoma.

Artificial iris tissue implanted after trauma. The clinical picture is hardly distinguishable from a real iris on cursory examination. There is a strong reflective band in the OCT (arrow) and shadowing of the tissue behind. The eye is pseudophakic. In comparison, the iris of the partner eye (arrowhead) shades only at the level of the pigment.

Status following procedure to change eye color (from brown to green). Green pigment (corneal tattoo) was introduced into the cornea into an annular cavity created by femtosecond laser (arrow) (Figs. 17, 18, 19 and 20).

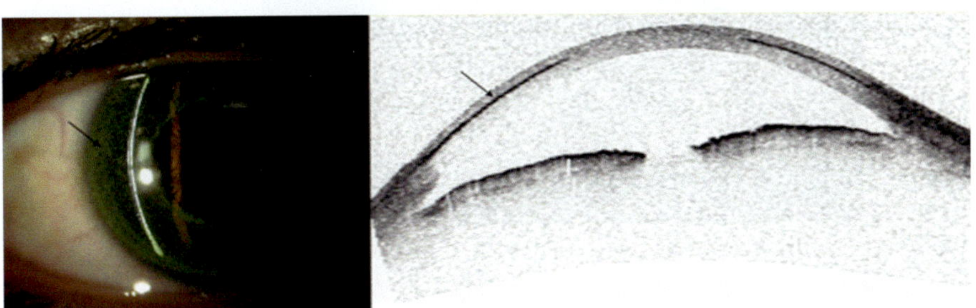

Fig. 17 Change of eye color by means of "corneal tattoo"

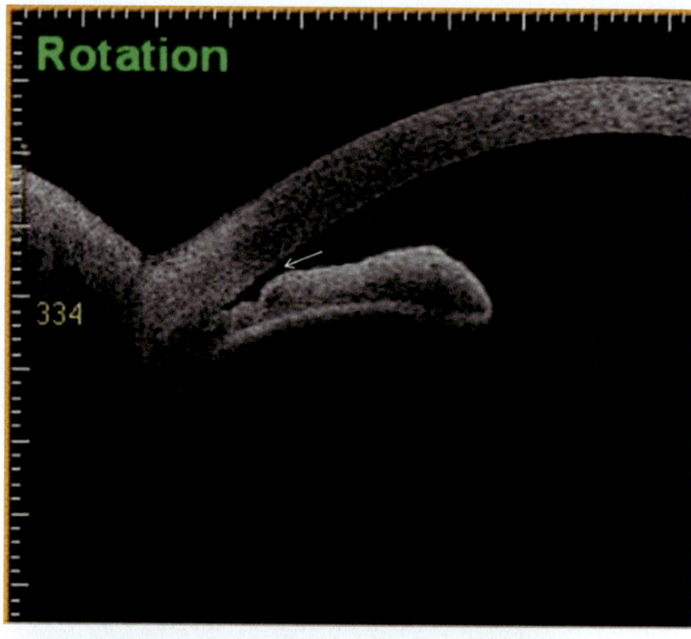

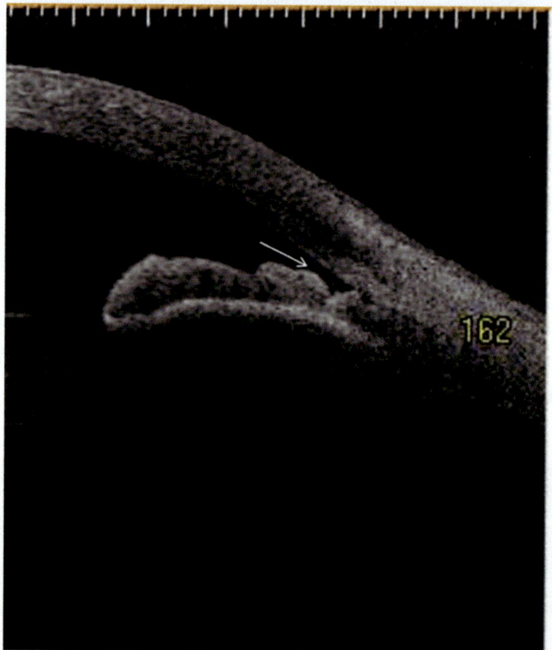

Fig. 18 Plateau iris

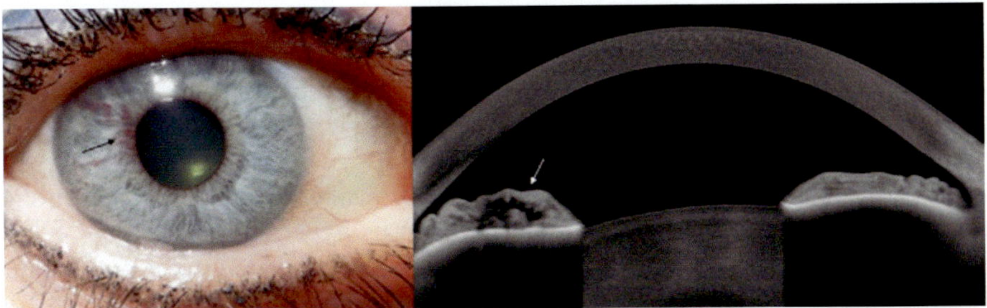

Fig. 19 Racemous hemangioma of the iris

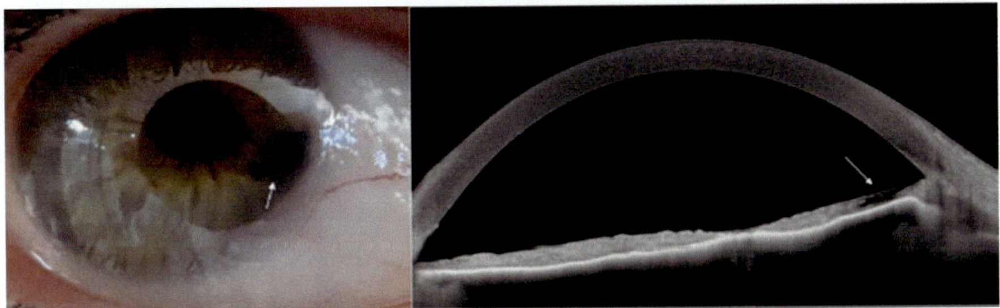

Fig. 20 Iris stromal atrophy

OCT shows a markedly constricted chamber angle (arrowheads) with a regular deep anterior chamber and flat iris configuration (plateau iris). The iris is thicker than average and, like the ciliary body processes, positioned anteriorly.

On clinical imaging, racemic hemangioma appears as a reddish change on the iris (arrow). In OCT, the hemangioma appears as a low-reflectance structure in the iris (arrow).

The clinical image shows atrophy of the iris stroma nasally (arrow). OCT shows thinning of the iris stroma at this location with areas of no reflection (arrow). The section of the OCT does not pass through the pupil but below it.

3 Conclusion and Summary

Optical coherence tomography of the iris provides a noninvasive method for accurate measurement and follow-up of the iris, including associated pathologies. Of particular note here is the differentiation of cystic from solid lesions and their accurate measurement that is readily comparable in progression.

Similar to ultrasound biomicroscopy (UBM), but without the invasiveness of direct corneal contact, anterior segment OCT, as a completely non-contact examination method, allows accurate assessment and measurement of changes in the iristroma that elude slit lamp examination due to localization. For standardized examination conditions, miosis should be achieved by pilocarpine eye drop administration prior to OCT examination to allow comparability of iris lesions in height, width, and depth over time.

The pigment sheet is readily distinguishable from anterior epithelium and stroma with intermediate reflectivity on AS-OCT due to its hyperreflectivity.

Iris pathologies that can be documented by OCT include neoplastic, inflammatory, and degenerative changes.

OCT plays a particularly important role in the follow-up and assessment of the dignity of neoplastic lesions. It is particularly helpful in clearly differentiating cystic and solid tumors.

It is important, despite the advantages of imaging techniques, to always consider the overall clinical picture, in which imaging techniques represent only one aspect of the diagnostic finding.

Conflict of Interest The authors have no financial, political, or economic conflicts of interest related to the content of this article.

References

Broaddus E, Lystad LD, Schonfield L, Singh AD. Iris varix: report of a case and review of iris vascular anomalies. Surv Ophthalmol. 2009;54:118–27.

Chien JL, Sioufi K, Ferenczy S, Say EAT, Shields CL. Optical coherence tomography angiography features of iris racemose hemangioma in 4 cases. JAMA Ophthalmol. 2017;135:1106–10.

Georgalas I, Petrou P, Papaconstantinou D, Brouzas D, Koutsandrea C, Kanakis M. Iris cysts: A comprehensive review on diagnosis and treatment. Surv Ophthalmol. 2018;63:347–64.

Kathil P, Milman T, Finger PT. Characteristics of anterior uveal melanocytomas in 17 cases. Ophthalmology. 2011;118:1874–80.

Lang SJ, Cucera A, Lang GK. Applications of optical coherence tomography in the anterior segment. Klin Monbl Augenheilkd. 2011;228:1086–91.

Marigo FA, Finger PT. Anterior segment tumors: current concepts and innovations. Surv Ophthalmol. 2003;48:569–93.

Shields JA, Bianciotto C, Kligman BE, Shields CL. Vascular tumors of the iris in 45 patients: the 2009 Helen Keller Lecture. Arch Ophthalmol. 2010;128:1107–13.

Williams BK Jr, Di Nicola M, Ferenczy S, Shields JA, Shields CL. Iris microhemangiomatosis: clinical, fluorescein angiography, and optical coherence tomography angiography features in 14 consecutive patients. Am J Ophthalmol. 2018;196:18–25.

Zheng ZK, Hu ZL, Li JJ. Iris cavernous hemangioma :a case report. Eye Sci. 2011;26:183–5.

Optical Cohenrece Tomography in Refractive Surgery

Toam Katz, Stephan Linke, Sebastian Siebelmann, and Fernando Gonzales-Lopez

1 Introduction

High-resolution and fast real-time imaging using spectral domain and swept source OCT is increasingly used in refractive surgery. In addition to Scheimpflug tomography as the gold standard in corneal imaging and the irreplaceable slit lamp microscope, OCT provides cross-sectional images of the cornea, anterior chamber, and its structures, as well as the anterior and partially posterior lens components, with an axial resolution in tissue of less than 10 μm.

In refractive surgery, OCT is useful both preoperatively and postoperatively, but also has the unique advantage of providing intraoperative imaging and measurement of tissues and implants. This can either be integrated into the surgical microscope as an intraoperative OCT or coupled directly to a surgical femtosecond laser.

In corneal laser refractive surgery, OCT imaging can be used to measure epithelial thickness, the depth and shape of a LASIK flap, a corneal scar to be ablated, the integrity of the Bowman, Descemet or endothelial layer. In addition, this technology can also be used intraoperatively to monitor primarily intrastromal

T. Katz (✉) · S. Linke
Care-Vision GmbH, Hamburg, Germany
e-mail: tkatz@care-vision.com

T. Katz · S. Linke
UKE, Augenklinik, Hamburg, Germany

S. Linke
Zentrum Sehstärke, Hamburg, Germany

S. Siebelmann
Department of Opthalmology, University Hospital of Cologne, Cologne, Germany

F. Gonzales-Lopez
Clinica Baviera, Instituto Oftalmologico Europeo, Madrid, Spain

L. M. Heindl and S. Siebelmann (eds.), *Optical Coherence Tomography of the Anterior Segment*, https://doi.org/10.1007/978-3-031-07730-2_13

operations when performing small incision lenticle extraction (SMILE), to visualize manually created or femtosecond laser-generated corneal tunnels, intracorneal pockets for corneal inlays and intra-stromal corneal rings, and corneal arcuate astigmatic incisions (Lai et al. 2006; Monteiro et al. 2018; Titiyal et al. 2017; Urkude et al. 2017; Sharma et al. 2017).

This allows non-contact measurement of, for example, stromal and flap thickness in both SMILE and LASIK (Fig. 1) (Lai et al. 2006). In addition, OCT technology allows the individual scans of the cornea to be reconstructed to map the anterior and posterior corneal elevations and curvatures, producing a corneal tomography map similar to Scheimpflug imaging. New-generation OCT devices such as the Casia2 (Tomey, Japan) produce 3-dimensional tomography of the cornea, anterior chamber, and even the anterior lens. With the help of special software (Casia2, Tomey, Japan), lower and higher order aberrations of the corneal surfaces can be calculated. The advantage of OCT over Scheimpflug imaging of the cornea is the simultaneous visualization of corneal densitometry in scars as well as pathologies of the endothelium in direct correlation to the anterior and posterior radii of the cornea as well as corneal thickness. Additional advantage of OCT compared to Scheimpflug tomography is the better imaging of the cornea around the limbus, especially the superior limbus without the known artifacts caused by the upper eyelid including reflections through the eyelashes and a better imaging of the chamber angle and its structures at the iris base (See comparison OCT versus Scheimpflug tomography, Table 1). In corneal scarring the Scheimpflug imaging is prone to artefact in corneal thickness calculation, but the OCT visualise the accurate pachymetry.

In phakic lens implantation, OCT is very helpful to image the size and relationship of the iris, corneal base and chamber angle and in 360° the anterior chamber preoperatively. This is important to avoid intraoperative or postoperative contact between the implanted lens and the chamber angle or posterior cornea with adjacent endothelium. Postoperatively, OCT also allows accurate measurement of the static and dynamic relationships between the implant and the anterior lens capsule (vault), as well as the implant periphery, iris, and cornea.

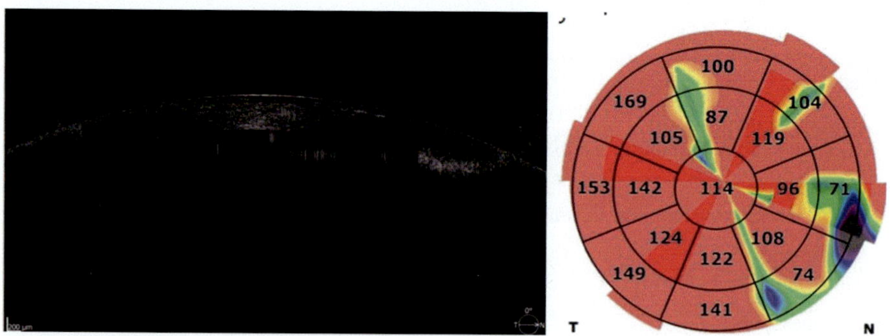

Fig. 1 Left: Freshly cut LASIK flap in OCT. Right: Correlated flap thickness in OCT

Table 1 Comparison between anterior segment OCT and Scheimflug tomography

Target tissue/implant	Anterior segment OCT	Scheimpflug tomography
Anterior and posterior corneal surfaces, corneal thickness	++	++
Pathological keratometries statistically analized	+	+++
Corneal high order aberrations	+	++
Corneal anatomy (layers, Flap, opacities)	+++	–
Corneal densitometry	+++	+
Corneo-iris angle, iris configuration	+++	+
Position of phakic IOLs	+++	–
Lens densitometry	++	++
Anterior segment morphology in scarred cornea	+++	+

Phacoemulsification for refractive lens exchange is increasingly performed femtosecond laser-assisted (FLACS). In this context, FLACS platforms usually include OCT for visualization and in vivo planning of the laser-guided cuts through the cornea, capsulorhexis, and dissection of the lens nucleus without damaging the posterior capsule. The accuracy and progression of FLACS would not be possible without constant OCT input.

2　OCT in the Implantation of Phakic Intraocular Lenses

Over the past 30 years, refractive surgery has emerged as a new specialty in ophthalmology. There have also been significant developments in the field of phakic lens implantation, leading to significant improvements in achieving optimal refractive outcomes. Various lens models have been tested over the years, their use abandoned or their design and materials improved. In general, a distinction can be made between posterior chamber and anterior chamber lenses. Anterior chamber lenses are further divided into phakic and aphakic anterior chamber lenses. Previously used anterior chamber lenses are e.g. the i-care or Cachet which are no longer used. Commonly used iris-fixed anterior chamber lenses are for example the Artisan (Verysize) or the Artiflex (Ophtec, Groningen, Netherlands). The phakic posterior chamber lenses are divided into PRL (Zeiss Meditec) and ICL (Staar, Lake Forest, California, USA) and recently also the "Implantable Phakic Contact Lens" (IPCL) (care Group, Gujrat, India). These are all sulcus-supported implants designed to be placed between the back of the iris and the front of the lens (Figs. 2 and 3). Most commonly used today are the ICL and IPCL models to correct myopia, hyperopia, and astigmatism that are outside the scope of excimer lasers (myopia higher than 8 D, hyperopia higher than 4 D) or are within the excimer range but are contraindicated if keratoconus is suspected. Recently, they have also

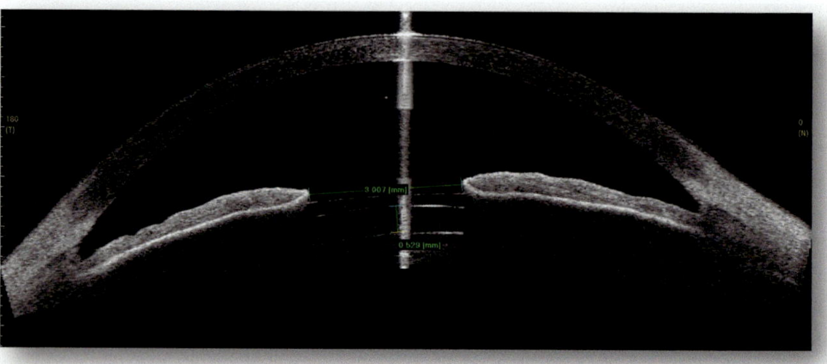

Fig. 2 Vault determination by OCT. The central vault is defined as the axial distance between the back of the phakic IOL and the front of the crystalline lens. The vault in this example is 529 μm

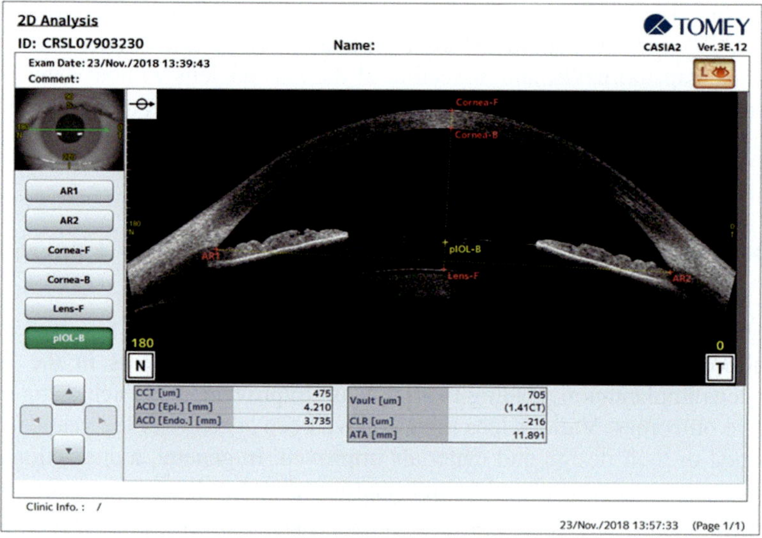

Fig. 3 Relationship of a myopic phakic ICL to anterior chamber structures in OCT. The dynamic vault is 274 μm (video made available online by publisher)

been used to correct presbyopia. The cases presented below focus on OCT imaging of the most commonly used today intraocular Collamer lenses. Of great importance for the safety of these lenses is the distance between the back of the ICL in relation to the lens capsule or front of the lens (vault). This should allow sufficient aqueous humor flow from the posterior to the anterior segment of the eye, thus maintaining the metabolism of the natural lens, avoiding the development of pupillary block glaucoma and angle block glaucoma, while ensuring the refractive effect of the ICL

(Lai et al. 2006). The generally soft haptics of the ICL should fit tightly to the sulcus without touching the iris pigment or dispersing it inside the eye due to resulting shear forces. In addition, the peripheral iris should also not be touched and thus pressed forward into the chamber angle. The size of the ICL is calculated preoperatively to estimate a correct position and location in the eye. An ICL that is too small may dislocate and provoke secondary glaucoma or a general inflammatory condition or uveitis with pigment dispersion. Furthermore, misalignment of e.g. a toric lens reduces the refractive outcome.

An ICL that is too small can be the cause of an insufficient vault and thus cause contact with the anterior lens capsule, resulting in a cataract (Fig. 4). On the other hand, an ICL that is too large pushes the haptics of the ICL forward causing a too high vault, which can lead to angle closure, in addition to pushing the optics forward, which leads to a shift of the refractive outcome into the myopic range (Fig. 5).

In addition to the standard preoperative white-to-white measurement by corneal tomography or biometry, Endothel photography and the postoperative slit lamp evaluation of the vault, OCT generates a variety of parameters with unsurpassed accuracy (Lai et al. 2006; Monteiro et al. 2018).

In general, the methodological approach to assessing ICLs distinguishes between static and dynamic OCT. Static OCT refers to an OCT acquisition at a specific time point under standardized conditions, whereas dynamic OCT examines, for example, the configuration of the anterior chamber as a function of accommodation. The relevant biometric parameters using static and dynamic OCT are anterior chamber

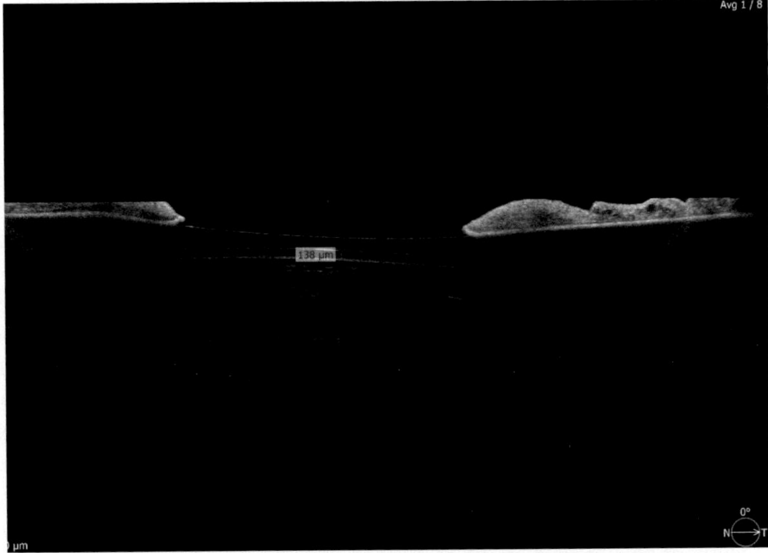

Fig. 4 Illustration of a too small vault in OCT imaging. Although the vault is 138 µm, the anterior lens capsule is not touched. The crystalline lens is still clear

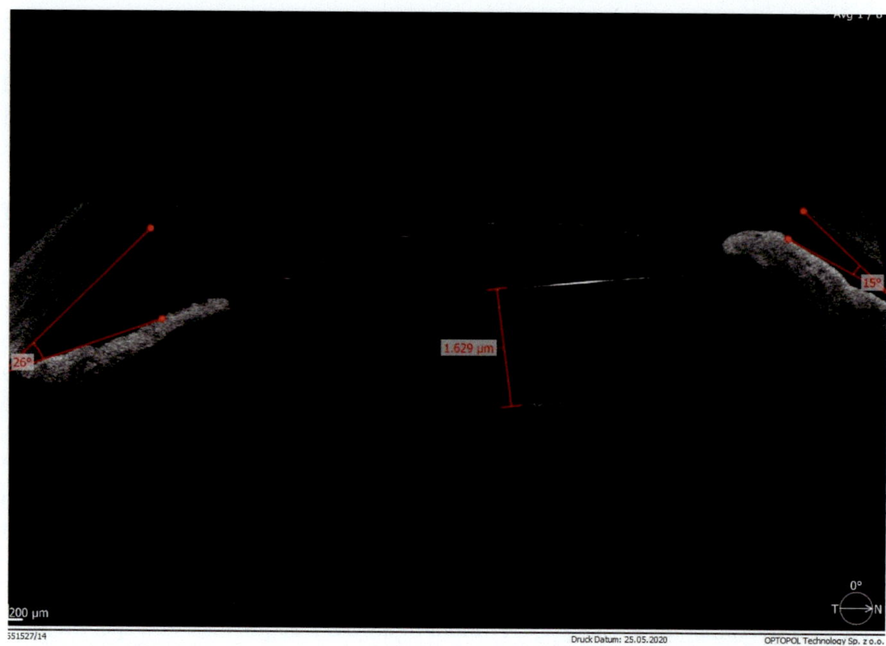

Fig. 5 Very large vault of 1629 µm after implantation of a hyperopic ICL. In addition, a very acute chamber angle is evident on OCT imaging. Urrets-Zavalia syndrome caused a permanently wide pupil, which allowed the ICL to tilt and move further forward

depth (ACD), crystalline lens rise (CLR), central vault, pupil size, angle-to-angle distance (AtA), anterior chamber width (ACW), and chamber angle (temporal and nasal). These OCT-based parameters are useful in extreme eyes and unexpected complications (Fig. 6a, b). Using the regression analysis of these multiple parameters, the NK formula and KS formula were developed to calculate the optimal ICL size with swept-source OCT of the anterior chamber (Fig. 7) (Monteiro et al. 2018). The ICL is placed behind the iris in the sulcus. All measurements from the other measurable anatomical features mentioned above as well as the prediction formulas try to estimate the correct level of the ICL on the sulcus. Nevertheless, direct measurement of the sulcus diameter (Sulcus-to-Sulcus, StS) is only possible with high frequency ultrasound (UBM). The most important single parameter for ICL safety after implantation is the Vault calculated preoperatively and measured postoperatively. A normal vault ranges from a minimum of 250 to a maximum of 800 µm. An extreme vault may cause short- or long-term complications and should be treated surgically by rotation or exchange of the ICL. Another safety feature to prevent pupillary block is the hole (aquaport) in the center of the myopic ICL, which allows the flow of aqueous humor through the ICL iris diaphragm (Fig. 8).

Prediction of the correct vault is further complicated by several unavoidable factors: The sulcus diameter is not homogeneous and is usually larger in the vertical

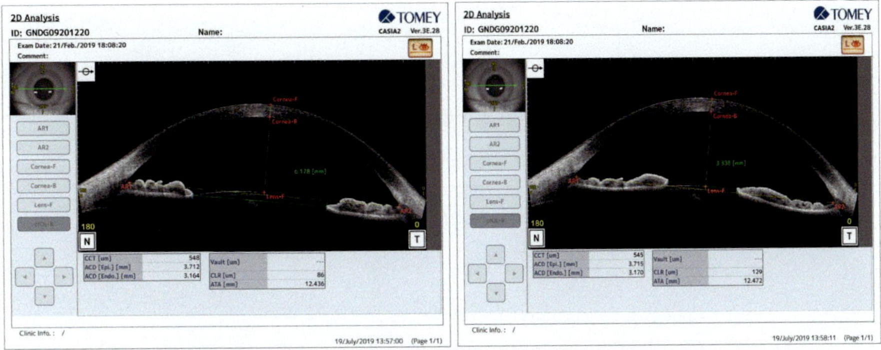

Fig. 6 Preoperative dynamic anterior segment measurements in the 0–180° axis under scotopic (left) and photopic (right) extraneous light environments: Measurable are corneal thickness, anterior chamber depth and width, crystalline lens rise (CLR), and pupil size

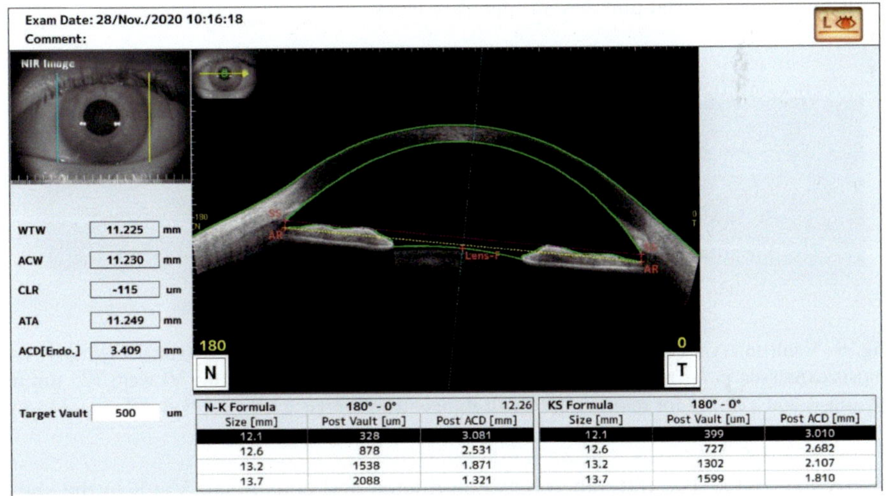

Fig. 7 Display "ICL-Size" with NK formula and KS formula for calculating the ICL size in the Casia2 from Tomey. The calculation is performed directly from the anterior segment OCT

meridian, the horizontal sulcus diameter (StS) is not measured directly but extrapolated from the measurement of the horizontal corneal diameter (white-to-white, WtW) or the angular diameter, and the ICL diameter is only available in 4 sizes (12.1, 12.6, 13.2, and 13.7 mm). In addition, natural pupil constriction due to light and accommodation and water flow cause dynamic changes in anterior chamber volume and depth preoperatively and in the vault of the ICL postoperatively (Figs. 9, 10 and 11), (Lai et al. 2006). In a study light-induced pupil constriction and dilation, which cause a difference in the vault due to thickness increase of the iris and displacement of the iris-lens diaphragm, were tested in

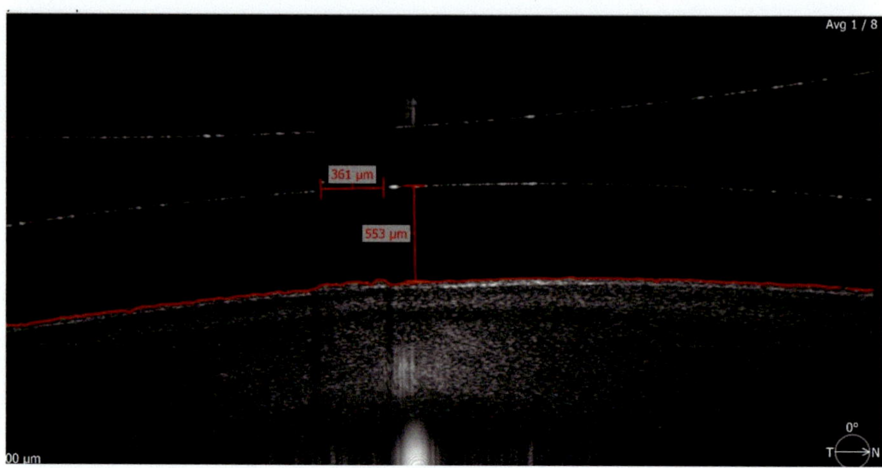

Fig. 8 Example of a normal vault of an ICL implanted in a myopic patient. The central opening of the ICL (aquaport) of 360 µm, prevents pupillary block

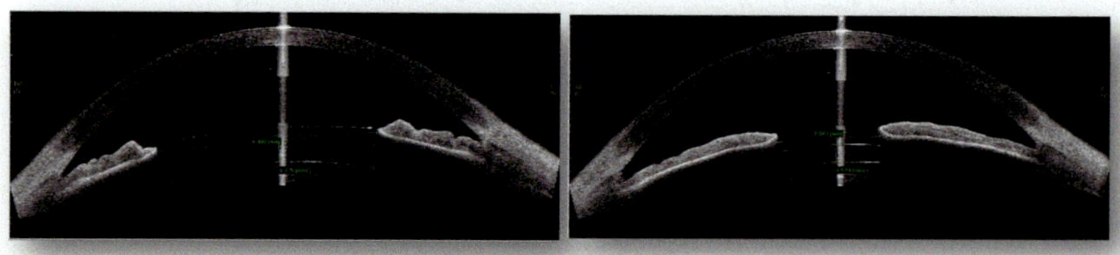

Fig. 9 Vault interval (VI) refers to values of central vault measured in maximal mydriasis and miosis expressed in micrometers after light-induced pupil changes. Here, the VI were 775 µm for mydriasis and 529 µm for miosis. The Vault Range, the difference between both VI, was 246 µm

39 myopic ICLs. The difference between dilated and constricted Vault in the same eye was defined as Vault-Interval (VI). Vault-range (VR) is the difference between maximal and minimal VIs in the same eye (Ref. 1). A photopic pupil pushes the ICL posteriorly and reduces the Vault by an average of 167 ± 70 µm compared to a scotopically dilated pupil. In eyes with low vault, the VI changed less with illumination than in eyes with high vault. The width of the ventricular angle can be measured dynamically and shows constriction due to mesopic dilation of the pupil. It may also become narrower if an ICL pushes the iris diaphragm forward.

Correction of high hyperopia with an ICL in the rare cases where the anterior chamber is deeper than 3 mm is more prone to pupillary block in the absence of an aquaport and with narrow preoperative chamber angles. Such surgery should include one or more iridotomies. OCT is an excellent noninvasive tool to assess dynamic patency and thus functionality of iridotomies (Fig. 12a, b).

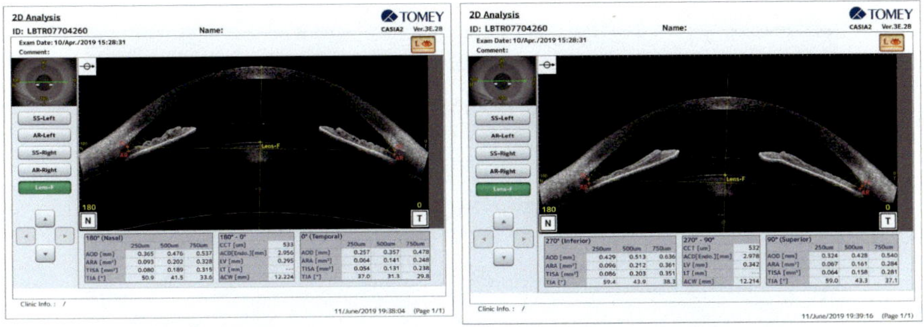

Fig. 10 Anterior chamber angle measured in ambient light after drug-induced maximal mydriasis (**a**) and in miosis (**b**). Using software integrated in the OCT device, the anterior chamber angle can be measured under different illumination conditions and pharmacological influences. (TIA 500 measurements -temp/nasal- (mydriasis): 31.3°/41.5° TIA 500 measurements -temp/nasal- (miosis): 43.3°/43.9°)

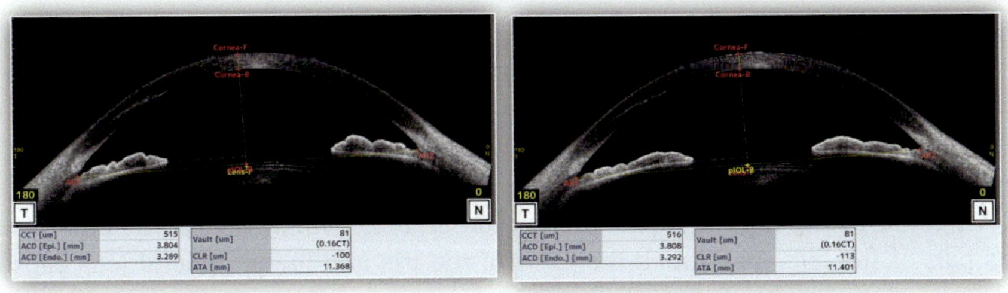

Fig. 11 Dynamic example of an ICL with low Vault and no variation in Vault Range. VI = 81 to 81 μm (VR 0 μm). (Insert video by publisher)

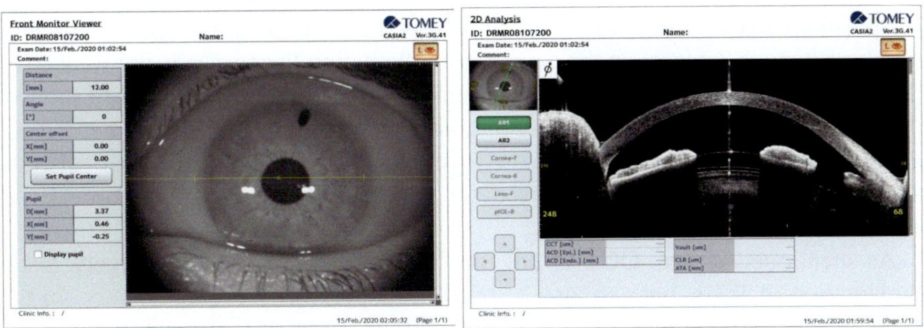

Fig. 12 Left: Surgical iridectomy in an ICL to correct hyperopia. Right: OCT shows well in the vertical section that the basal iridectomy is open at 12 o'clock

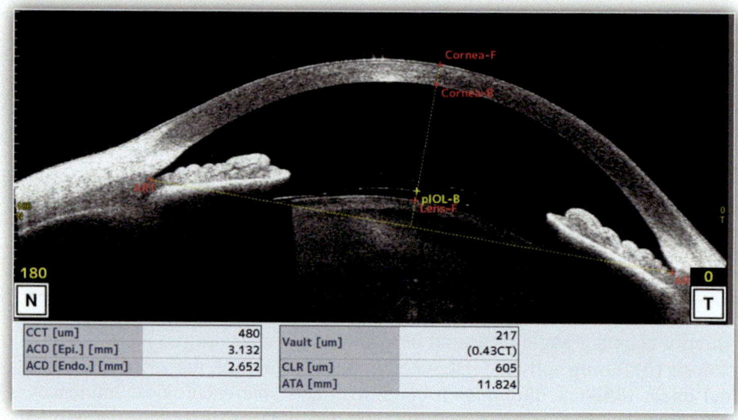

Fig. 13 Dynamic example of a good central vault of a −17 D 12.6 mm ICL (VI = 217 a 183 μ (VR 34 μ)) but a peripheral contact between ICL and anterior crystalline lens. The ICL was subsequently replaced with a wider ICL (13.2 mm)

All these parameters reduce the predictability of the ICL vault. The intraoperatively measured Vault is also different from the postoperative Vault measured on the first postoperative day. Only after at least one week postoperatively can the Vault be expected to remain constant.

When correcting high myopia, we implant an ICL with thicker peripheral optics. This part of the lens may touch the back of the iris and the peripheral lens capsule and cause pupillary block or anterior subcapsular cataract, even if the central vault is high enough and the angles are open. Such a relationship between the ICL and iris indicates that an ICL may need to be replaced (Fig. 13).

Other postoperative complications that can be identified by OCT include deposition of pigment on the ICL anterior surface or even in the aquaport, unnoticed damage or misplacement of the ICL haptics, and misplacement of the ICL due to a posterior iris anomaly (Fig. 14a, b). A toric ICL can be used especially in eyes with keratoconus, because in the course of implantation the cornea is not weakened, in contrast to a phototrefractive keratectomy (PRK). In this case, sizing of the lens to be implanted is particularly important, as rotation of the ICL should be avoided and a "touch-up" excimer treatment is contraindicated. The ICL can also be combined with other procedures used for keratoconus, such as intracorneal ring segments (Fig. 15a–d).

As mentioned above, OCT is not only useful pre- and postoperatively in the implantation of ICLs, but can also be used intraoperatively during surgery. In this context, the integration of OCT technology into a surgical microscope (microscope-integrated intraoperative OCT, MI-OCT) allows visualization of the surgical area in real time and in near histological resolution. By means of MI-OCT, the position of the implant can be controlled and adjusted in vivo in this context (Fig. 16a, b). The intraoperative OCT measured vault correlates well with the

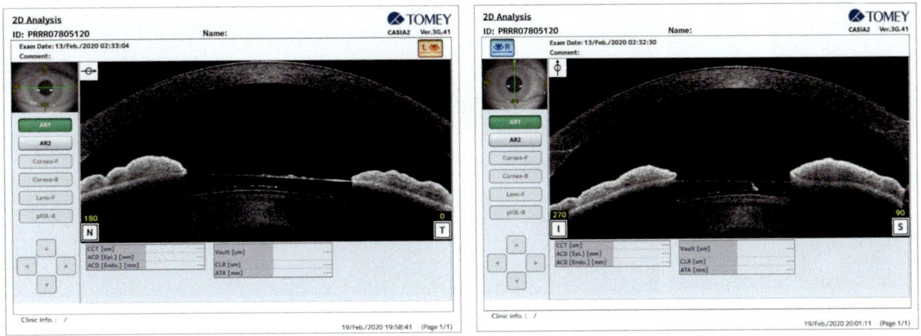

Fig. 14 Left: OCT imaging shows iris pigment deposited on the anterior surface of the pIOL in cross-section (ICL V4c −12/12.1); Right: This can also be found in the aquaport of the ICL after 6 years

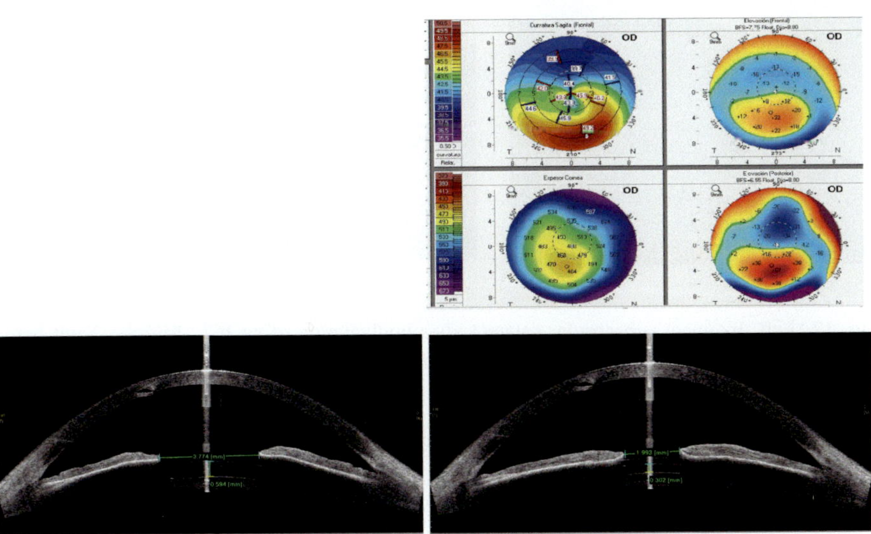

Fig. 15 Top right: Topography of the right eye of a patient with keratoconus after keraring implantation. There is a clear residual refraction. Bottom right: Illustration of the ICL under scotopic conditions and Bottom right: under photopic conditions. In addition, the cross-section shows the keraring in the cornea. (Keraring 5 mm/160° & ICL EVO + −7/ + 4.50 13.2. VI = 594 to 302μ (VR 292μ))

postoperative vault and can be used in the detection of a critical vault configuration. It also enhances the safety of the surgical procedure by providing a real-time representation of the maneuvers performed intraoperatively (Ref. 2). Rotating an ICL with too high a vault from the horizontal to the vertical axis allows more vertical space for the lens, reducing the vault to a safer value. Measuring and adjusting the vault in vivo using MI-OCT could save future explantation and additional corrective surgery.

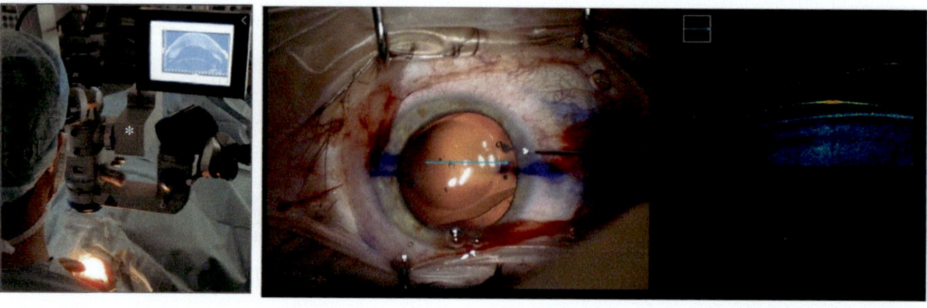

Fig. 16 Left: Intraoperative setup of the Haag Streit iOCT (Haag Streit Surgical, Wetzlar, Germany) during implantation of an ICL. Right: Intraoperative imaging of the ICL during rotation using the Rescan 700 mI-OCT from Zeiss (Zeiss Meditec, Jena, Germany)

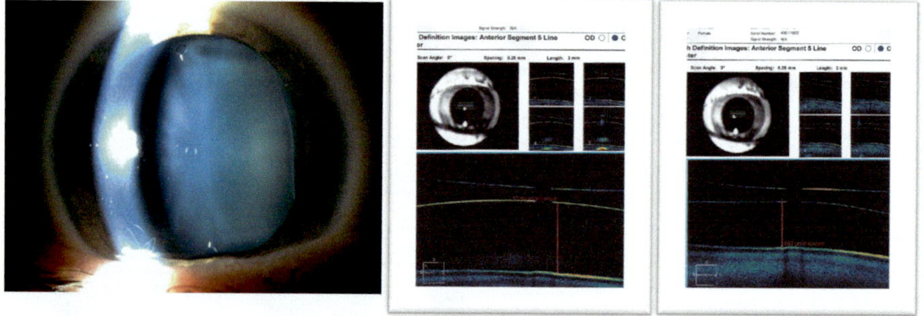

Fig. 17 Left: Incipient subcapsular cataract after implantation of an ICL. Middle: Vault before vertical rotation: 1028 μm. Vault after lens rotation is 692 μm after vertical rotation

In summary, OCT provides a wealth of information in refractive lens implantation, and can be used preoperatively during planning, intraoperatively during the surgery itself, and postoperatively to assess lens fit (Fig. 17).

Infobox:

High-resolution and fast real-time imaging OCT is increasingly used in refractive surgery. OCT provides cross-sectional images of the cornea, anterior chamber, and its structures, as well as the anterior and partially posterior lens components, with an axial resolution in tissue of less than 10 μm.

This can either be integrated into the surgical microscope as an intraoperative OCT or coupled directly to a surgical femtosecond laser.

In corneal laser refractive surgery, OCT imaging can be used to measure epithelial thickness, the depth and shape of a LASIK flap, Intrastomal Implants and their tunnels, a corneal scar to be ablated, the integrity of the Bowman, Descemet or endothelial layer and SMILE lenticle. This chapter dexcribes the clinical uses of OCT in refractive surgery today.

References

Gonzalez-Lopez F, Mompean B, Bilbao-Calabuig R, Vila-Arteaga J, Beltran J, Baviera J. Dynamic assessment of light-induced vaulting changes of implantable collamer lens with central port by swept-source OCT: pilot study. Translational Vision Science & Technology. 2018;7(3):4–4.

Igarashi A, Shimizu K, Kato S, Kamiya K. Predictability of the vault after posterior chamber phakic intraocular lens implantation using anterior segment optical coherence tomography. J Cataract Refract Surg. 2019;45(8):1099–104.

Lai MM, Tang M, Andrade EM, et al. Optical coherence tomography to assess intrastromal corneal ring segment depth in keratoconic eyes. J Cataract Refract Surg. 2006;32(11):1860–5.

Monteiro T, Alfonso JF, Franqueira N, Faria-Correia F, Ambrósio R, Madrid-Costa D. Predictability of tunnel depth for intrastromal corneal ring segments implantation between manual and femtosecond laser techniques. J Refract Surg. 2018;34(3):188–94.

Sharma N, Urkude J, Chaniyara M, Titiyal JS. Microscope-integrated intraoperative optical coherence tomography-guided small-incision lenticule extraction: New surgical technique. J Cataract Refract Surg. 2017;43(10):1245–50.

Takagi Y, Kojima T, Nishida T, Nakamura T, Ichikawa K. Prediction of anterior chamber volume after implantation of posterior chamber phakic intraocular lens. PLoS ONE. 2020;15(11): e0242434.

Titiyal JS, Rathi A, Kaur M, Falera R. AS-OCT as a rescue tool during difficult lenticule extraction in SMILE. J Refract Surg. 2017;33(5):352–4.

Urkude J, Titiyal JS, Sharma N. Intraoperative optical coherence tomography–guided management of cap–lenticule adhesion during SMILE. J Refract Surg. 2017;33(11):783–6.

Zhang X-F, Li M, Shi Y, Wan X-H, Wang H-Z. Repeatability and agreement of two anterior segment OCT in myopic patients before implantable collamer lenses implantation. Int J Ophthalmol. 2020;13(4):625.

Correction to: Physical Principles of Anterior Segment OCT

Correction to:
Chapter "Physical Principles of Anterior Segment OCT"
in: L. M. Heindl and S. Siebelmann (eds.),
Optical Coherence Tomography of the Anterior Segment,
https://doi.org/10.1007/978-3-031-07730-2_2

The original version of chapter 2 was inadvertently published prematurely, before incorporating the final corrections as regards to Figures and Section, which have now been updated.

1. Chapter authors affiliations are updated.
2. The following figure labels are translated from German to English language: Figures: 1, 3, 4, 5, 6, 8, 9, 10, 11, 12, 13, 14, 15, 16.
3. Figures citations are replaced accordingly.
4. Section 6.2 and figure 16 are removed from content.

The correction chapter and the book have been updated with the changes.

The updated version of this chapter can be found at
https://doi.org/10.1007/978-3-031-07730-2_2

  C1
L. M. Heindl and S. Siebelmann (eds.), *Optical Coherence Tomography of the Anterior Segment*, https://doi.org/10.1007/978-3-031-07730-2_14

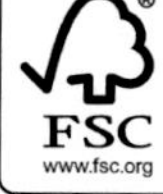